THE SCIENCE OF REAL-TIME DATA CAPTURE

THE SCIENCE OF REAL-TIME DATA CAPTURE

Self-Reports in Health Research

Edited by
Arthur A. Stone
Saul Shiffman
Audie A. Atienza
Linda Nebeling

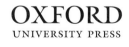

UNIVERSITY PRESS

2007

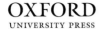

OXFORD
UNIVERSITY PRESS

Oxford University Press, Inc., publishes works that further
Oxford University's objective of excellence
in research, scholarship, and education.

Oxford New York
Auckland Cape Town Dar es Salaam Hong Kong Karachi
Kuala Lumpur Madrid Melbourne Mexico City Nairobi
New Delhi Shanghai Taipei Toronto

With offices in
Argentina Austria Brazil Chile Czech Republic France Greece
Guatemala Hungary Italy Japan Poland Portugal Singapore
South Korea Switzerland Thailand Turkey Ukraine Vietnam

Copyright © 2007 by Oxford University Press, Inc.

Published by Oxford University Press, Inc.
198 Madison Avenue, New York, New York 10016

www.oup.com

Oxford is a registered trademark of Oxford University Press

Library of Congress Cataloging-in-Publication Data
The science of real-time data capture : self-reports in health research / edited by
Arthur A. Stone . . . [et al.]. p. ; cm.
Includes bibliographical references and index.
ISBN: 978-0-19-517871-5
1. Human experimentation in medicine–Congresses. 2. Self-evaluation.
I. Stone, Arthur A. [DNLM: 1. Data Collection—methods. 2. Computer Systems.
3. Research—methods. 4. Self Disclosure. 5. Technology. 6. Time. WA 950 S4159 2007]
R853.H8S35 2007
610.72'4—dc22   2006027397

9 8 7 6 5 4 3 2 1

Printed in the United States of America
on acid-free paper

Foreword

Self-reported data are essential to social and behavioral sciences research. Although less obvious, it is also clear that self-reports are heavily relied upon in biomedical research. Within that domain, the clinical and population sciences, which include medicine, nursing, epidemiology, demography, and health services research, depend on self-reported states, characteristics, and behaviors to understand disease etiology, prevention, and treatment outcomes. For that reason, I believe that the science of self-report is a critical but frequently overlooked domain of research that deserves greater attention and support.

The importance of self-reported health information for biomedical research was previously recognized by the National Institutes of Health through a conference and subsequent publication examining "The Science of Self-Report: Implications for Research and Practice" (Stone, Turkkan, Bachrach, et al., 2000). Since the publication of that volume, the ever-growing sophistication and power of computer technology has facilitated the ability of researchers to gather self-reported health information in real time in the real world. Ecological Momentary Assessment (EMA) (Stone & Shiffman, 1994), a methodology derived from Experience Sampling Methodology (Csikszentmihalyi & Larsen, 1987), represents one framework to guide researchers who plan to conduct studies that capture self-reported health information in real time. In recent years, however, the number of investigators, techniques, and applications of real-time data capture methods has grown and diversified.

In September 2003, the National Cancer Institute convened scientists engaged in methodological and applied studies utilizing EMA and related approaches to discuss the opportunities for and challenges of conducting this type of research. Drs. Arthur Stone and Saul Shiffman, who have been instrumental in conceptualizing and operationalizing EMA, served as co-chairs. This conference, "The Science of Real-Time Data Capture: Self-Reports in Health Research," served as a catalyst for subsequent efforts by NCI to stimulate work in this area. After considering the demand for additional workshops and training, we decided it made more sense to pull together the body of work discussed at the conference into a single reference volume in order to reach the broadest audience possible.

Our enthusiastic support was based in part on the fact that, despite their potential, real-time data capture methods had yet to be applied in a substantial way to many domains of cancer prevention and control behavioral research. Given the importance of tobacco use, diet, physical activity, decision-making, and coping to cancer prevention and control, we believed that many investigators supported by NCI could strengthen the rigor of their research by either utilizing real-time methods or considering the sobering implications of the evidence generated by these methods for their own work. In facilitating the publication of this text, based in part on the 2003 conference, we hope to broaden the awareness and utilization of this important body of work in behavioral medicine and public health research. In addition, many of the methodological and statistical challenges encountered by the authors forecast issues that are likely to emerge from the entire range of real-time data capture methods emerging from new fields such as molecular imaging, nanotechnology, biosensing, and social neuroscience.

This publication would not have been possible without the dedicated and diligent work of numerous individuals both at the NCI and in the extramural scientific community. The scientists who have contributed to this volume are pioneers in this burgeoning research area and their efforts are greatly appreciated. For the reader, this book will provide a clearer understanding of self-reported health and more effective strategies for collecting valid information to address important scientific questions. It is my hope that this publication will encourage more investigators to incorporate these insights and accelerate progress in reducing the heavy burden of illness and disability.

Robert Croyle, PhD
Director
Division of Cancer Control and Population Sciences
National Cancer Institute

References

Csikszentmihalyi, M., & Larsen, R. E. (1987). Validity and reliability of the experience sampling method. *Journal of Nervous and Mental Diseases, 175,* 526–536.

Stone, A. A., & Shiffman, S. (1994). Ecological Momentary Assessment (EMA) in behavioral medicine. *Annals of Behavioral Medicine, 16,* 199–202.

Stone, A. A., Turkkan, J. S., Bachrach, C. S., Jobe, J. B., Kurtzman, H. S., & Cain, V. S. (2000). *The science of self-report: Implications for research and practice.* Mahwah, NJ: Lawrence Erlbaum Associates.

Contents

Part III: Future Developments in Real-Time Data Capture

Contributors

ELVA M. ARREDONDO, PhD
San Diego State University–Graduate
    School of Public Health
San Diego, CA

AUDIE A. ATIENZA, PhD
National Cancer Institute, Division of
    Cancer Control and Population Sciences
Bethesda, MD

BARBARA BAQUERO, MPH
San Diego State University–Graduate
    School of Public Health
San Diego, CA

KAREN BASEN-ENGQUIST, PhD, MPH
University of Texas, M.D. Anderson
    Cancer Center
Houston, TX

TASHA BURWINKLE, PhD, PsyD
University of Washington School of
    Medicine
Seattle, WA

BRIAN L. CARTER, PhD
University of Texas, M.D. Anderson
    Cancer Center
Houston, TX

PAUL M. CINCIRIPINI, PhD
University of Texas, M.D. Anderson
    Cancer Center
Houston, TX

R. LORRAINE COLLINS, PhD
Research Institute on Addictions
    State University of New York–Buffalo
Buffalo, NY

ROBERT CROYLE, PhD
National Cancer Institute, Division of
    Cancer Control and Population Sciences
Bethesda, MD

SUSAN X DAY, PhD
University of Houston
Houston, TX

JOHN P. ELDER, PhD, MPH
San Diego State University–Graduate
    School of Public Health
San Diego, CA

BRIAN FLAY, DPhil
University of Illinois at Chicago
Chicago, IL

KAREN GLANZ, PhD, MPH
Rollins School of Public Health
Emory University
Atlanta, GA

MATTHEW S. GOODWIN, MA
University of Rhode Island
Department of Psychology
Providence, RI

CHAD J. GWALTNEY, PhD
Brown University
Providence, RI

DONALD HEDEKER, PhD
University of Illinois at Chicago
Chicago, IL

BETTINA B. HÖPPNER, MA
University of Rhode Island
Cancer Prevention Research Center
Providence, RI

MICHAEL R. HUFFORD, PhD
invivodata®, inc., Pittsburgh, PA

STEPHEN S. INTILLE, PhD
Massachusetts Institute of Technology
Cambridge, MA

DENISE L. JANICKI, MS
University of Pittsburgh
Pittsburgh, PA

THOMAS W. KAMARCK, PhD
University of Pittsburgh
Pittsburgh, PA

RANDY J. LARSEN, PhD
Washington University in St. Louis
St. Louis, MO

SIMON MARSHALL, PhD
San Diego State University–Graduate
    School of Public Health
San Diego, CA

ROBIN MERMELSTEIN, PhD
University of Illinois at Chicago
Chicago, IL

CARL DE MOOR, PhD
University of Texas–Houston Health
Science Center, School of Public Health
Houston, TX

MATTHEW F. MULDOON, MD, MPH
University of Pittsburgh
Pittsburgh, PA

MARK MURAVEN, PhD
State University of New York–Albany
Albany, NY

SUZANNE MURPHY, PhD, RD
Cancer Research Center of Hawaii
University of Hawaii
Honolulu, HI

LINDA NEBELING, PhD, MPH, RD FADA
National Cancer Institute
Division of Cancer Control and
    Population Sciences
Bethesda, MD

PAMELA E. PAULSON, PhD
University of Michigan
Ann Arbor, MI

JOSEPH E. SCHWARTZ, PhD
Stony Brook University
Stony Brook, NY

NORBERT SCHWARZ, PhD
University of Michigan
Ann Arbor, MI

SAUL SHIFFMAN, PhD
University of Pittsburgh
Pittsburgh, PA

MELONIE SHOWLUND, BA
University of Washington
    School of Medicine
Seattle, WA

KAREN FARCHAUS STEIN, PhD
University of Michigan
Ann Arbor, MI

ARTHUR A. STONE, PhD
Stony Brook University
Stony Brook, NY

KIM SUTTON-TYRRELL, DrPH
University of Pittsburgh
Pittsburgh, PA

DENNIS C. TURK, PhD
University of Washington
    School of Medicine
Seattle, WA

THEODORE A. WALLS, PhD
University of Rhode Island
Providence, RI

DAVID W. WETTER, PhD
University of Texas
M.D. Anderson Cancer Center
Houston, TX

Introduction

Audie A. Atienza, Arthur A. Stone, Saul Shiffman,
Linda Nebeling

Health researchers often rely on self-reports as the main source of information (Stone, Turkkan, Bachrach, et al., 2000), particularly within the social and behavioral sciences (as noted by Schwarz in chapter 2). The proliferation of ubiquitous, ever more powerful electronic devices and computer technology has created opportunities for researchers to capture time-intensive data about health as experienced in real time and in the real world (Collins, Kashdan, & Gollnisch, 2003; Patrick, Intille, & Zabinski, 2005). Yet, methodological challenges have also arisen with the plethora of self-reported information that can be gathered with these technologies. These methodological opportunities and challenges become even more pronounced as researchers begin to integrate self-reported information with physiological states, environmental conditions, and other sources of information that do not rely on self-reports (e.g., motion detection, geographic position, electronic medicine bottle caps), and implement real-time data capture within an intervention context.

This book represents a primer, illustrating not only the promise and opportunities of conducting research using Ecological Momentary Assessment (EMA), but also the challenges and difficulties of such research. As such, it is not meant to offer a comprehensive discussion of real-time data capture research. Still, major conceptual and methodological issues are discussed in depth. The book is organized into three general sections.

The first section discusses the historical, methodological, statistical, and conceptual aspects of EMA. Stone and colleagues link EMA to preexisting real-time data capture methodological traditions and briefly discuss the rationale behind EMA. In chapter 2, Schwarz provides a thought-provoking discussion of the various dimensions of self-reported data and biases that can occur with retrospective reports. He also offers an engaging discussion of the rationale, challenges, and limitations of capturing concurrent (i.e., real-time) self-reported information. Shiffman and colleagues then focus on the intricacies of EMA protocols and research designs, emphasizing the crucial roles that theoretical issues and study hypotheses play in sampling designs and the study protocol. In chapter 4, by Hufford, the fundamental methodological issues of subject compliance, reactivity, subject burden, usability, and psychometric properties are addressed.

At the conclusion of this first section, Schwartz and Stone provide readers with a practical guide to the analysis of the complex, multilevel data that are typically obtained with EMA, illustrating seven separate questions that can be addressed with EMA and providing the reader with examples of SAS syntax for each question. While chapter 5 is written to provide statistically minded researchers with a sense of the analytic decisions that need to be made in conducting real-time research, others may find the chapter's general concepts helpful in understanding the analytic strategies used in the research exemplars presented in the second section of this book. Taken together, these chapters provide the foundation to understand the chapters in the next sections.

The second section provides exemplars of EMA research in various content areas, with a particular emphasis on lessons learned from the different studies. Health behaviors are first illustrated. Mermelstein and colleagues (chapter 6) discuss a longitudinal study using EMA that examines the natural history of adolescent smoking, highlighting the relationship between subjective moods and decisions to smoke or not smoke. In chapter 7, EMA research examining the health-promotion behavior of physical activity using pagers and pedometers among Hispanic/Latino women is illustrated by Arredondo and colleagues, while Glanz and Murphy discuss diet research using a personal digital assistant (PDA) system in chapter 8. A notable aspect of these health-promotion studies is the incorporation of behavioral feedback to participants into the study design in an effort to encourage behavior change. In chapter 9, Stein and Paulson also focus on eating behavior using EMA, but from an eating disorders (i.e., anorexia nervosa and bulimia nervosa) perspective within a clinical intervention context. In their study, PDAs were used as a tool to assess specific eating disorder behaviors. Next, Collins and Muraven (chapter 10) demonstrate how EMA can be used to test a particular conceptual model of alcohol consumption in a series of studies with community and college student samples and provide a brief but thoughtful discussion of how some newer technology (e.g., interactive voice recognition, cellular phones) can enhance the richness and quality of the EMA data that are collected.

EMA studies examining symptom-related behaviors in patient populations are discussed by Turk and colleagues (chapter 11), who used EMA to study the experiences of fibromyalgia syndrome patients, and by Basen-Engquist and de Moor (chapter 12), who applied EMA to investigate fatigue and physical activity among ovarian cancer patients. EMA studies focused on psychological states are then discussed in two chapters. Larsen (chapter 13) presents a persuasive argument that EMA can be useful in understanding the temporal nature of personality, mood, and health. Finally, in chapter 14, Kamarck and colleagues present innovative research integrating the study of psychological experiences (i.e., subjective demand and control) with physiological states (i.e., ambulatory blood pressure) in real time to test a particular conceptual model (i.e., job-strain model). As can be seen from these chapters, EMA represents a cross-cutting methodology that can be useful in the study of phenomena in various content areas. However, unique challenges and difficulties are also present depending on the content area and discipline of interest.

The third section of the book moves the discussion of real-time data capture beyond the assessment of self-reported experiences. While some of prior chapters briefly mention momentary interventions, Carter and colleagues, in chapter 15, provide a more detailed discussion of the complexities of ecological momentary health interventions and new technologies that may better enable real-time interventions to be effective. Intille (chapter 16) goes even further in the discussion of emerging technology and offers a unique, forward-thinking perspective in which sensors and other digital information are seamlessly integrated with the assessment of self-reported information (via smart cellular phones) in a context-sensitive manner. He also discusses possible intervention applications of these emerging technologies and addresses key ethical and practical issues. Given the enormous amount of time-intensive longitudinal data that can be collected now using EMA (with even large multimodal databases possible in one device, based on 7/24/365 data capture possibilities in the future), traditional statistical methods are inadequate to analyze the richness of the real-time information being collected. To address this issue, Walls and colleagues, in chapter 17, offer a cogent discussion of the nature of intensive longitudinal data and describe current and emerging statistical approaches that may adequately analyze the information gathered.

The goal of this book is to help the reader understand the opportunities and complexities of Ecological Momentary Assessment (EMA)/Ecological Momentary Intervention (EMI) research. As noted by Schwarz, real-time data capture may not be warranted in all situations; thus, this publication also provides a general framework for scientists to discern the appropriateness and relevance of EMA/EMI to their research. Some of the chapters begin to raise intriguing conceptual issues that need to be addressed in future research. For example, Turk and colleagues note that real-time reports are empirically distinct from retrospective reports. This raises questions as to which reports are most predictive of health outcomes (e.g., morbidity, mortality, disease states, psychopathology), or which aspects of health are most determined by which types of reports (and why). As another example, Mermelstein and colleagues stated that cooperation and permission from schools was obtained to allow students to use the technology. As such, the specific elements of the broader organizational and environmental context, where EMA research can effectively occur, remain important to delineate. These examples underscore that fact that much work remains to be done.

In the concluding chapter, Stone offers his reflection on a number of these conceptual and provocative issues. The acceptability of and willingness to use sophisticated electronic devices to capture real-time experiences will likely increase, especially with the proliferation and ubiquitous nature of newer technology (e.g., cell phones, instant messaging devices) in the general population. With most of the general population reporting that they own a cell phone, and groups of concern increasing their adoption of technology (e.g., 50% to 60% of older adults now own cell phones) (Pew, 2005), the ability to use ubiquitous technology to understand and change health is now more than ever a distinct possibility. It is our hope that the conceptual and methodological issues discussed in this book, as well as the lessons learned from the illustrative research studies, will advance and direct future research in this promising area.

References

Collins, R. L., Kashdan, T. B, & Gollnisch, G. (2003). The feasibility of using cellular phones to collect ecological momentary assessment data: Applications to alcohol consumption. *Experimental and Clinical Psychopharmacology, 11*(1), 73–78.

Patrick, K., Intille, S. S., & Zabinski, M. F. (2005). An ecological framework for cancer communication: Implications for research. *Journal of Medical Internet Research, 7*(3), 1–7.

Pew Research Center (2005). Pew Research Center Biennial News Consumption Survey. http://people-press.org/reports/pdf/215.pdf

Stone, A. A., Turkkan, J. S., Bachrach, C. A., Jobe, J. B., Kurtzman, H. S., & Cain, V. S. (2000). *The science of self-report: Implications for research and practice.* Mahwah, NJ: Lawrence Erlbaum Associates.

PART I

THE SCIENCE AND THEORY OF REAL-TIME
DATA CAPTURE: A FOCUS ON ECOLOGICAL
MOMENTARY ASSESSMENT (EMA)

1

Historical Roots and Rationale of Ecological Momentary Assessment (EMA)

Arthur A. Stone, Saul Shiffman, Audie A. Atienza, and Linda Nebeling

This chapter provides a brief introduction to the capture of real-time data referred to as Ecological Momentary Assessment (EMA) (Stone & Shiffman, 1994), which we hope sets the stage for the remainder of the book. We briefly define EMA, trace some of its historical antecedents, and discuss the core rationale for EMA methodology. Subsequent chapters deal in greater detail with specific aspects of EMA methods and present a wide array of studies using EMA to address substantive problems.

EMA methods are characterized or defined by the repeated collection of real-time data on participants' momentary states in the natural environment. Examples include studies in which participants: report their mood several times daily when they are "beeped" by a computer; make notes on an index card each time they interact with a friend; have their blood pressure periodically taken by an automated device; record everything they eat at the end of each meal; report on symptoms related to cancer treatments; or complete a diary about the day's stresses at the end of the day. While the methods, technologies, and content of these examples differ, they all focus on assessing real-world experience or behavior more or less "live" in participants' typical environments and do so repeatedly over time. Thus, the key elements of EMA are real-time collection of data about momentary states, collected in the natural environment, with multiple repeated assessments over time.

Historical Roots of EMA

The EMA framework encompasses a range of preexisting methods that also are based on real-time, real-world data collection. These approaches arose within particular disciplines to meet specific research needs but share the common features of EMA methods. Several traditions have been historically prominent.

Diaries

Diaries have long been used for collection of research data about participants' daily experience and behavior (Favill & Rennick, 1924). They have varied from open-ended narratives to structured daily assessments and have been used to gather self-reports on a diverse array of content, ranging from humorous experiences (Kambouropoulou, 1926) to coping styles (Affleck, Tennen, Keefe, et al., 1999; Stone, Porter, & Neale, 1993), to sexual behavior (Althof, Rosen, DeRogatis, et al., 2005). At times, diaries are combined with monitoring of physiological functions such as blood pressure, heart rate, cortisol, and glucose.

Behavioral Observation

Direct observation and coding of participants' behavior was used by sociologists and psychologists who were interested in the effect of situational contexts on behavior (Barker, 1978). Observational methods were also often used by researchers who focused on behavior (vs. subjective states) as the only legitimate target of observation and intervention, and who were suspicious of self-report. In these methods, a trained observer tracked and coded particular behaviors, usually for short periods and in particular contexts. These methods tended to be burdensome and limited the range of contexts and behaviors that could be observed and the duration of observation.

Self-Monitoring

These methods have long been used in behavioral research to gather data about target events, ranging from smoking a cigarette to marital conflict (Coxon, Coxon, Weatherburn, et al., 1993). Participants typically were asked to record each event, along with some information about the event, such as its antecedents and the participants' responses. Self-monitoring was particularly associated with behaviorist psychology and behavior therapy and was often used to assess behaviors targeted for change in behavior therapy (Best & Best, 1975; Romanczyk, Tracey Wilson, & Thorpe, 1973; Sieck & McFall, 1976). In this context, it was recognized that monitoring alone could sometimes stimulate behavior change (Sieck & McFall, 1976).

Time Budget Studies

Dating back to the beginning of the 20th century, these studies were concerned with describing how people spent their time (Robinson & Godbey, 1997). In this research, participants were asked to make a written note each time they changed activities, or to record their activities every 15 minutes at the end of a day, or they were asked to recall their time use at the end of the day for the whole day. Often sponsored by government or international agencies, time budget studies have been used to contrast the activity profiles of people in different countries or cultures (Szalai, 1966). Time use surveys have also been used to provide national estimates of time spent in labor force and nonmarket-related activities to address a range of economic and sociological issues.

Experience Sampling Method (ESM)

The idea of gathering data about people's ordinary lives by periodically "beeping" them at random or prearranged times was developed by pioneers of the Experience Sampling Method, or ESM (Csikszentmihalyi & Larson, 1987). Starting before technological advances such as palmtop computers, ESM researchers asked participants to carry pagers and arranged to beep them to prompt them to record their experience on paper for later collection and analysis. As the name implies, most ESM research time-sampled subjective experience, and these beeper studies advanced the development of models of subjective experience, such as Csikszentmihalyi's theory of "flow" (Csikszentmihalyi & Csikszentmihalyi, 1988).

Ambulatory Monitoring

Another tradition focused on collection of physiological or behavioral data over time in real-world environments. For example, as devices for assessing blood pressure became compact enough to travel and automated enough to operate independently, researchers studied variations in blood pressure by fitting participants with blood pressure monitors programmed to take and record readings at regular intervals as they went about their normal day. Participants were also often given diary cards to complete periodically so that activity and subjective states could be correlated with blood pressure readings (e.g., Schwartz, Warren, & Pickering, 1994).

Similar traditions evolved in other areas as devices for monitoring blood glucose, pulmonary function, heart rate, and other physiological parameters were developed. Physical monitors, such as motion detectors, have also been used to collect objective behavioral data in real time, often continuously and without requiring participants to provide self-reports (Bassett, 2000; Montoye, Kemper, Saris, & Washburn, 1996). Other studies have used prompting to periodically solicit biological samples (e.g., saliva samples for cortisol analysis) from participants in order to study variations over time, activity, and experience.

Each of these methodological traditions continues today, but with little systematic integration across the disciplines. Although the methods used in studies have increasingly converged (e.g., subjective self-report data being collected in ambulatory monitoring studies), each of these traditions has developed in isolation from the others. They are bounded by disciplinary traditions and appear in different scientific journals, impeding recognition of the common elements and potential synergies. The framework of EMA attempts to provide a unifying structure for these diverse methods, recognizing common aspects and systematizing the methodological issues, challenges, and opportunities inherent in these methodological traditions.

The Rationale for EMA

The core rationale for EMA methods rests on three core benefits of the EMA approach: (1) avoidance of recall and its attendant bias, by collecting data on momentary states; (2) realization of ecological validity by collecting data in the real world; and (3) achievement of temporal resolution, enabling analysis of dynamic processes over time. We discuss each one in turn.

Momentary Data and Avoidance of Recall Bias

Most self-reported data are collected by questionnaires or interviews that ask participants to summarize past experience over some period of time. For example, a pain questionnaire might ask about the intensity of last week's or last month's pain. Unfortunately, a growing mass of research data shows that human beings may not be able to accurately recall past experience, particularly experiences that are frequent, mundane, and irregular (see Schwarz, this volume; Bradburn, Rips, & Shevell, 1987; Hammersley, 1994). In contrast, people are able to report accurately on a wide range of their current here-and-now experiences and observations (Robinson & Clore, 2002a, 2002b; Ross, 1989). As noted by Schwarz (chapter 2, this volume), many of the experiences of interest to researchers (e.g., everyday, typical, routine behaviors) may be best captured with concurrent reports.

While it has long been recognized that retrospective data can be flawed, it was tacitly assumed that memory was generally accurate and that defects in recall would introduce only modest random error. However, research on autobiographical memory (memory from our own experiences) suggests that memory can be substantially inaccurate and can introduce systematic bias, not just random error, under certain circumstances. Memory is reconstructive and recall is heuristic (Gorin & Stone, 2001). In other words, we are not always able to retrieve a whole record of past experience on which to base self-reports; rather, we often reconstruct "what must have happened" based on mental shortcuts. Particularly when people are asked not only to recall but also to summarize their past experience—what is typically done in research settings (*"How intense was your average pain?"*)—biasing influences can creep in. These potential biases are summarized in the chapter by Schwarz (see also Bradburn et al., 1987). Importantly, these imperfect memory processes are fundamental to the operation of human memory. Thus, the biases they introduce can corrupt data even if the participant is being fully cooperative and has no motive to distort the data.

Concern about biases due to recall has led to a focus on reports of momentary experience: Robinson and Clore (Robinson & Clore, 2002a, 2002b) show that, in contrast to reports of past events and feelings, people can provide good reports of their experience in the here-and-now. Thus, EMA focuses on reports of momentary experience or very recent experience, aiming to minimize memory biases.

Ecological Validity and Real-World Experience

Researchers are typically interested in how participants behave and what they experience in real-world settings. As such, researchers have undertaken one of two strategies for projecting to real-world experience. One is to model the real world in the laboratory. For a long time, laboratory researchers assumed that the results of their experiments would generalize to the real world and, indeed, sometimes they did (e.g., basic learning and psychophysics). However, researchers also learned that an individual could be influenced by the context of the immediate environment (see Schwarz, chapter 2, this volume), altering the results of laboratory studies because the laboratory is not a typical environment. To take a single example, it is easy to imagine how one's reaction to a contrived stressor in a "safe" laboratory setting could be different from reaction to a real stressor. Another well-known example is the phenomenon known as "white coat hypertension," where blood pressure readings taken in a physician's office are higher than ambulatory readings taken in the real world (Pickering, James, Boddie, et al., 1988). Thus, results obtained with laboratory data may not necessarily generalize to the real world.

As we have discussed, the other strategy for assessing real-world experience is asking people to summarize it. Since such data can be subject to serious recall bias, particularly with frequent, mundane, and irregular experiences, EMA emphasizes real-time recording of momentary experience. But, since researchers are interested in real-world experience and not in the experience of the assessment setting, those moments must be assessed in real-world settings. Data are said to have "ecological validity" when they apply or generalize to the real world (Brunswik, 1943).[1] EMA research ensures ecological validity by collecting data in the real world, ensuring that the data represent the full range of real-life experience.

When researchers solicit global, retrospective reports of experience, they implicitly assume that the respondent will provide full and representative coverage of his or her experience. (Of course, respondents don't: for example, recent and salient events are overrepresented.) The EMA researcher, in contrast, relies on momentary "snapshots" of real-world experience. This requires thinking about the EMA data points as samples of experience that are then used to represent the whole. Considering the EMA data set as a sample has profound implications for EMA design. One obvious and compelling implication is that sufficient data points need to be collected: a single point will seldom be reliable. Thus, considering EMA assessment as a sampling strategy brings in considerations such as sample size (how many assessments are enough to adequately characterize an individual or time period?) and sampling design (is the sample representative and unbiased?). These issues are addressed in Shiffman's chapter on design (chapter 3).

Studying Process Over Time

Our discussion, thus far, has implicitly emphasized the use of data to characterize participants' experience in a summary way (e.g., their average pain in the past week). However, such static data do not address how processes unfold over time.

Researchers increasingly seek data with enough temporal resolution to test dynamic associations among variables that unfold over time (e.g., Affleck, Urrows, Tennen, & Higgins, 1992; Bolger, DeLongis, Kessler, & Schilling, 1989; DeVries, 1987; Roghmann & Haggerty, 1972; Verbrugge, 1980; Zautra, Guarnaccia, & Dohrenwend, 1986). For example, to understand if and how certain thoughts (risk perception) precede other behaviors (e.g., engaging in healthful behaviors) or physiological outcomes (e.g., cardiovascular or endocrine changes), a high level of temporal resolution is needed. The repeated, dense sampling of experience, behavior, and events that characterizes many EMA designs provides such resolution and allows dynamic temporal associations to be observed. Thus, EMA data are particularly valuable for studying processes and relationships among processes over time.

Limitations of EMA

As noted by Schwarz (chapter 2, this volume), EMA may not be optimal for assessing all experiences. Experiences that are rare and important (e.g., graduations, weddings, birth of a child, divorce) may not require EMA. Some retrospective reports may also be more strongly predictive of health or behavioral outcomes than real-time assessments, if subsequent behavior is influenced by the recalled experience rather than by the momentary experience. Moreover, EMA may be most useful for those willing to use technology (e.g., hand-held computers) associated with EMA or those willing to enroll in studies requiring these intensive assessments. Individuals with visual or fine motor difficulties may also find the technology associated with self-reported EMA challenging to use. However, advances in technology, such as interactive voice recognition and smart cell phones, may make EMA more feasible or appealing for these individuals. Further research is needed to examine adherence and satisfaction issues among populations who have not considered enrolling in EMA-type studies.

Conclusion

EMA methods encompass a variety of approaches to collecting real-time data about momentary experiences in real-world settings. These approaches can provide uniquely rich insights into human behavior in real-world contexts. In this book, we aim to discuss the methodological issues that arise in EMA research and to illustrate the application of diverse EMA methods to a broad range of health-related behavior.

Note

1. We recognize that Brunswik's original definition of "ecological validity" is at variance with current usage and that his term for this concept was "representative design."

References

Affleck, G., Tennen, H., Keefe, F. J., Lefebvre, J. C., Kashikar-Zuck, S., Wright, K., Starr, K., & Caldwell, D. S. (1999). Everyday life with osteoarthritis or rheumatoid arthritis: Independent effects of disease and gender on daily pain, mood and coping. *Pain, 83,* 601–609.

Affleck, G., Urrows, S., Tennen, H., & Higgins, P. (1992). Daily coping with pain from rheumatoid arthritis: Patterns and correlates. *Pain, 51,* 221–229.

Althof, S. E., Rosen, R. C., DeRogatis, L., Corty, E., Quirk, F., & Symonds, T. (2005). Outcome measurement in female sexual dysfunction clinical trials: Review and recommendations. *Journal of Sex and Marital Therapy, 31,* 153–166.

Barker, R. G. (1978). *Habitats, environments and human behavior: Studies in the ecological psychology and ecobehavioral science of the Midwest Psychological Field Station: 1947–1972.* San Francisco: Jossey-Bass.

Bassett, D. (2000). Validity and reliability issues in objective monitoring of physical activity. *Research Quarterly for Exercise and Sport, 71,* 30–36.

Best, J. A., & Best, H. (1975). Client self-monitoring in clinical decision making. *Canada's Mental Health, 23,* 9–11.

Bolger, N., DeLongis, A., Kessler, R. C., & Schilling, E. A. (1989). Effects of daily stress on negative mood. *Journal of Personality and Social Psychology, 57*(5), 808–818.

Bradburn, N. M., Rips, L. J., & Shevell, S. K. (1987). Answering autobiographical questions: The impact of memory and inference on surveys. *Science, 236,* 157–161.

Brunswik, E. (1943). Organismic achievement and environmental probability. *Psychological Review, 50,* 255–272.

Coxon, A. P. M., Coxon, N. H., Weatherburn, P., Hunt, A. J., Hickson, F., Davies, P. M., & McManus, T. J. (1993). Sex role separation in sexual diaries of homosexual men. *AIDS, 7,* 887–882.

Csikszentmihalyi, M., & Csikszentmihalyi, I. S. (1988). Optimal experience: *Psychological studies of flow in consciousness.* New York: Cambridge University Press.

Csikszentmihalyi, M., & Larson, R. E. (1987). Validity and reliability of the experience sampling method. SKH. *Journal of Nervous and Mental Diseases, 175,* 526–536.

DeVries, M. (1987). Investigating mental disorders in their natural settings: Introduction to the special issue. Annals. *Journal of Nervous and Mental Disease, 175,* 509–513.

Favill, D., & Rennick, C. F. (1924). A case of family periodic paralysis. *Archives of Neurology and Psychiatry, 11,* 674–679.

Gorin, A. A., & Stone, A. A. (2001). Recall biases and cognitive errors in retrospective self-reports: A call for momentary assessments. In *Handbook of Health Psychology,* edited by A. Baum, T. Revenson, and J. Singer (pp. 405–413). Mahwah, NJ: Lawrence Erlbaum Associates.

Hammersley, R. (1994). A digest of memory phenomena for addiction research. *Addiction, 89,* 283–293.

Kambouropoulou, P. (1926). Individual differences in the sense of humor. *American Journal of Psychology, 37,* 268–278.

Montoye, H., Kemper, H., Saris, W., & Washburn, R. (1996). *Physical activity and energy expenditure.* Champaign, IL: Human Kinetics.

Pickering, T. G., James, G. D., Boddie, C., Harschfield, G. A., Blank, S., & Laragh, J. H. (1988). How common is white coat hypertension? *Journal of the American Medical Association, 259,* 225–228.

Robinson, J., & Godbey, G. (1997). *Time for life.* University Park, PA: Penn State Press.

Robinson, M. D., & Clore, G. L. (2002a). Belief and feeling: Evidence for an accessibility model of emotional self-report. *Psychological Bulletin, 128,* 934–960.

———. (2002b). Episodic and semantic knowledge in emotional self-report: Evidence for two judgment processes. *Journal of Personality and Social Psychology, 83,* 198–215.

Roghmann, K. J., & Haggerty, R. J. (1972). The diary as a research instrument in the study of health and illness behavior. *Medical Care, 10* (2), 143–163.

Romanczyk, R. G., Tracey, D. A., Wilson, G. T., & Thorpe, G. L. (1973). Behavioral techniques in the treatment of obesity: A comparative analysis. *Behaviour Research and Therapy, 11,* 629–640.

Ross, M. (1989). Relation of implicit theories to the construction of personal histories. *Psychological Review, 96,* 341–357.

Schwartz, J. E., Warren, K., & Pickering, T. G. (1994), Location and physical position as predictors of ambulatory blood pressure and heart rate: Application of a multi-level random effects model. *Annals of Behavioral Medicine, 16,* 210–220.

Sieck, W. A., & McFall, R. M. (1976). Some determinants of self-monitoring effects. *Journal of Consulting and Clinical Psychology, 44,* 958–965.

Stone, A. A., Porter, L. S., & Neale, J. M. (1993). Daily events and mood prior to the onset of respiratory illness episodes: A nonreplication of the 3–5 day "desirability dip." *British Journal of Psychology, 66,* 383–393.

Stone, A. A., & Shiffman, S. (1994). Ecological Momentary Assessment (EMA) in behavioral medicine. *Annals of Behavioral Medicine, 16,* 199–202.

Szalai, A. (1966). The multinational comparative time budget research project: A venture in international research cooperation. *American Behavioral Scientist, 10,* 30.

Verbrugge, L. M. (1980). Health diaries. *Medical Care, 18,* 73–95.

Zautra, A. J., Guarnaccia, C. A., & Dohrenwend, B. P. (1986). The measurement of small life events. *American Journal of Community Psychology, 14,* 629–655.

2

Retrospective and Concurrent Self-Reports: The Rationale for Real-Time Data Capture

Norbert Schwarz

Self-reports are the dominant method of data collection in the social and behavioral sciences, where they are used to assess respondents' behaviors, attitudes, and subjective experiences, like moods, emotions, or pain. Whereas overt behaviors can, in principle, be assessed with other methods, individuals' self-reports provide the only window on their inner states. Unfortunately, this window is often foggy, especially when respondents are expected to report on extended time periods. For example, the Health Interview Survey conducted by the National Center for Health Statistics asks respondents, *"Now, I'd like to read you a short list of different kinds of pain. Please say for each one, on roughly how many days—if any—in the last 12 months you have had that type of pain. How many days in the last year have you had headaches?"* (This question is repeated for backaches, stomach pains, joint pains, muscle pains, and dental pains.) I encourage readers to answer this question. Trying to do so quickly raises another question: Are we asking people for things that they can't tell us?

This chapter addresses what people can and cannot tell us and reviews what we know about the cognitive and communicative processes underlying retrospective self-reports. It draws on research at the interface of autobiographical memory, judgment, and research methodology and highlights the numerous sources of bias that threaten the validity of retrospective reports (for comprehensive reviews see Schwarz & Sudman, 1994; Sudman, Bradburn, & Schwarz, 1996; Tourangeau, Rips, & Rasinski, 2000). Some of these biases can be attenuated through the use of better interviewing techniques, like Event History Calendars (see Belli, 1998), but the room for improvement is limited by the limits of autobiographical memory. As an alternative, we can ask people to report on things they can tell us about, namely their current behavior and experiences. This is the promise of real-time data capture, which focuses on the collection of concurrent rather than retrospective self-reports. Real-time data capture, exemplified by Ecological Momentary Assessment (EMA) (see Stone, Shiffman, & DeVries, 1999),

Table 2-1. Types of information sought

Type	Real-time data capture	Retrospective reports
Historical Information *Ever? First?*	Not applicable	Feasible; reporting can be improved through the methodology of event history calendars
Frequency *How often?*		
a. Rare	Not applicable	Feasible when behaviors are distinct and important
b. Frequent and regular	Applicable but not needed	Extrapolation from rate information feasible
c. Frequent and irregular	Applicable and preferable	Estimation strategies dominate; bias likely
Intensity *How intense, pleasant, painful, etc.?*	Applicable and preferable	Likely to be biased, even after a short delay
Change over time *More or less...?*	Applicable and preferable, provided behavior is frequent	Theory-driven and biased
Covariation/causation *When and why?*	Applicable and preferable, provided behavior is frequent	Theory-driven and biased

attenuates or eliminates the memory-related biases inherent in retrospective reports. Unfortunately, it does not eliminate other potential sources of bias in self-reports, from problems of question comprehension to the influence of question order or response alternatives (for reviews see Schwarz, 1999a; Sudman et al., 1996).

Table 2-1 shows the main types of retrospective self-reports and summarizes key points discussed in the following sections. I first review the cognitive and communicative processes underlying these reports and identify what respondents can and cannot tell us. Throughout, I highlight how the underlying processes result in systematic bias. Following this review of retrospective self-reports, I turn to the cognitive and communicative processes involved in concurrent self-reports and identify open issues for future research.

Historical Information

Some retrospective questions pertain to historical information. Examples include: *Have you ever had an episode of back pain? In what year did you first have an episode of back pain?* Respondents' memories are usually the only available source of information on these issues and real-time data capture does not provide an alternative strategy. The best a researcher can do is to use interviewing techniques that take the structure of autobiographical memory into account to facilitate recall (for advice see Belli, 1998; Schwarz & Oyserman, 2001; Tourangeau et al., 2000).

The structure of autobiographical memory can be thought of as a hierarchical network that includes extended periods (like *"the years I lived in New York"*) at the highest level of the hierarchy. Nested within this high-order period are lower-level extended events pertaining to this time, like *"my first job"* or *"the time I was married to Lucy."* Further down the hierarchy are summarized events that correspond to the knowledge-like representations of repeated behaviors noted above (e.g., *"During that time, I was frequently ill"*). Specific events, like an illness, are represented at the lowest level of the hierarchy. To be represented at this level of specificity, however, the event has to be unusual. As these examples illustrate, autobiographical memory is organized primarily by time (the years in New York) and relatively global themes (first job, first marriage, illness) in a hierarchical network (see Belli, 1998, for a comprehensive review). This network "permits the retrieval of past events through multiple pathways that work top down in the hierarchy, sequentially within life themes that unify extended events, and in parallel across life themes that involve contemporaneous and sequential events" (Belli, 1998, p. 383). Such searches take considerable time and their outcome is somewhat haphazard, depending on the entry point into the network at which the search started. Hence, using multiple entry points and forming connections across different periods and themes improves recall.

These fortunate conditions are rarely met in research interviews. One promising method to instantiate them is offered by the Event History Calendar (see Belli, 1998, for a comprehensive review). It allows respondents to place their behavior in time and space and uses the hierarchically nested structure of autobiographical memory to facilitate recall. Moreover, it provides respondents with considerable time for the recall task and emphasizes the importance of accuracy. Finally, it explicitly encourages the correction of earlier answers as newly recalled information qualifies earlier responses. This correction opportunity is missed under regular interview formats, where respondents can rarely return to earlier questions.

To assess a respondent's health history, for example, respondents may begin by marking life periods such as being in school, living at home, getting a first job, and so on. Next, they may be asked to mark health-relevant events within these periods, changing the timing of already marked events as needed when newly recalled information requires corrections. Within the developing rich structure of associations, respondents are usually able to recall and date events with considerable accuracy (e.g., Freedman, Thornton, Camburn, et al., 1988; Caspi, Moffitt, Thornton, et al., 1996). Although costly in terms of interview time, this approach provides the most promising avenue for the assessment of historical information. Without such efforts, recall errors are highly likely, as illustrated by Cannell, Fisher, and Bakker's (1965) observation that 42 percent of a sample of patients failed to report an episode of overnight hospitalization when interviewed 1 year after the event.

Frequency Reports

Frequency questions ask respondents to report on how often a behavior or experience occurred during a specified reference period, often "last week" or "last month." Researchers typically hope that respondents will identify the behavior of interest, search the reference period, retrieve all instances that match the target behavior, and count these instances to determine the overall frequency of the behavior. However, respondents can follow such a recall-and-count strategy only under very limited circumstances. In most cases, they must rely on extensive inference and estimation strategies to arrive at an answer. Which strategy they use depends on the frequency, importance, and regularity of the behavior (e.g., Brown, 2002; Menon, 1993, 1994; Sudman et al., 1996).

Rare and Important Behaviors

Rare and important behaviors can be reported on the basis of autobiographical knowledge or a recall-and-count strategy. When asked, *"How often did you get divorced?"* most people can provide an accurate answer without extended memory search. On the other hand, when asked, *"How often did you relocate to another city?"* many respondents do not know immediately but can determine the appropriate answer by reviewing their educational and job history, following a recall-and-count strategy. Real-time data capture is not suited for such tasks because of the low frequency of the respective behavior and the extended time periods covered. Fortunately, respondents' answers will nevertheless be relatively accurate when the behavior is rare and important if they are encouraged to take the time necessary for extensive recall.

Frequent Behaviors

A respondent's task is considerably more demanding when the behavior is frequent. In this case, respondents are unlikely to have detailed representations of numerous individual episodes of a behavior stored in memory. Instead, the various instances of closely related behaviors blend into one global, knowledge-like representation that lacks specific time or location markers (see Linton, 1982; Strube, 1987). Frequent doctor visits, for example, result in a well-developed knowledge structure for the general event, allowing respondents to report in considerable detail on what usually goes on during their visits. But the highly similar individual episodes become indistinguishable and irretrievable, making it difficult to report on any specific one. This is most likely to occur for mundane behaviors of high frequency but has also been observed for more important events. Mathiowetz and Duncan (1988), for example, found that respondents were more accurate in recalling a single spell of unemployment than at recalling multiple spells of unemployment.

As a result of the knowledge-like representation of frequent behaviors and experiences, respondents cannot rely on a recall-and-count strategy. Instead, they need to resort to estimation strategies to arrive at a plausible frequency report. Which strategy they choose depends on the regularity of the behavior and the context in which the frequency question is presented.

RATE INFORMATION AND EXTRAPOLATION

When the behavior is highly regular, respondents can arrive at a frequency estimate on the basis of rate information (Menon, 1994; Menon, Raghubir, & Schwarz, 1995). Respondents who go to church every Sunday, or wash their hair daily, face little difficulty in computing a weekly or monthly estimate. Unfortunately, exceptions are likely to be missed and the obtained answers are accurate only when the behavior does conform to the assumed rate. A related estimation strategy relies on extrapolation from partial recall. When asked how often she took pain medication during the last week, for example, a respondent may reason, "I took painkillers three times today, but this was a bad day. So probably twice a day, times 7 days, makes 14 times a week." The accuracy of this estimate depends on the accuracy of the underlying assumptions, the regularity of the behavior, and the specifics of the day that served as input into the chain of inferences.

As these examples illustrate, respondents are unlikely to answer frequency questions on the basis of the recall-and-count strategy that most researchers hope for. Their answers are, at best, based on partial recall and extensive inferences, unless the behavior is rare and important, and hence highly memorable (for extended discussions see Brown, 2002; Schwarz & Oyserman, 2002). Other estimation strategies may even bypass any effort to recall specific episodes. One such strategy is respondents' reliance on information provided by the research instrument itself.

FREQUENCY SCALES

Respondents are often asked to report the frequency of their behavior by checking the appropriate alternative from a list of quantitative response alternatives of the type shown in Table 2-2. What is typically overlooked is that respondents believe that researchers construct meaningful scales that are relevant to the task at hand. Specifically, they assume that the scale reflects the researcher's knowledge about

Table 2-2. Frequency response alternatives for reporting physical symptoms

Low frequency scale	High frequency scale
( ) never	( ) twice a month or less
( ) about once a year	( ) once a week
( ) about twice a year	( ) twice a week
( ) twice a month	( ) daily
( ) more than twice a month	( ) several times a day

the distribution of the behavior, with values in the middle range of the scale corresponding to the "usual" or "average" behavior and values at the extremes of the scale corresponding to the extremes of the distribution. Given these assumptions, respondents can use the range of the response alternatives as a frame of reference in estimating their own behavioral frequency. This results in higher frequency estimates along scales that present high- rather than low-frequency response alternatives.

For example, Schwarz and Scheuring (1992) asked 60 patients of a German mental health clinic to report the frequency of 17 symptoms along one of the two scales shown in Table 2-2. Across 17 symptoms, 62 percent of the respondents reported average frequencies of more than twice a month when presented with the high-frequency scale, whereas only 39 percent did so when presented with the low-frequency scale, resulting in a mean difference of 23 percentage points. The impact of response alternatives was strongest for the ill-defined symptom of "responsiveness to changes in the weather," where 75 percent of the patients reported a frequency of more than twice a month along the high-frequency scale, whereas only 21 percent did so along the low-frequency scale. Conversely, the influence of response alternatives was least pronounced for the better-defined symptom "excessive perspiration," with 50 percent versus 42 percent of the respondents reporting a frequency of more than twice a month in the high- and low-frequency scale conditions, respectively. The differential size of the observed scale effects also illustrates that respondents are more likely to resort to estimation strategies, the less salient and memorable the respective behavior is (e.g., Schwarz, 1999b).

Higher frequency reports along high- rather than low-frequency scales have been observed across a wide range of behaviors, including health behaviors (e.g., Gaskell, O'Muircheartaigh, & Wright, 1994), television consumption (e.g., Schwarz, Hippler, Deutsch, & Strack, 1985), sexual behaviors (e.g., Tourangeau & Smith, 1996), and consumer behaviors (e.g., Menon et al., 1995). Several methodological implications deserve attention. First, these findings call the meaning of the absolute reports into question and show that reports provided along different scales are not comparable. Second, they illustrate that the impact of frequency scales is more pronounced the more poorly the behavior is represented in memory, as expected on theoretical grounds (Menon et al., 1995). When behaviors of differential memorability are assessed, this can either exaggerate or cloud actual differences in the relative frequency of the behaviors, undermining comparisons across behaviors. Third, respondents with poorer memory are more likely to be influenced than respondents with better memory (e.g., Knäuper, Schwarz, & Park, 2004; Schwarz, 1999b). This can undermine comparisons across groups that differ in memory performance (e.g., younger vs. older respondents; see Knäuper et al., 2004). Finally, for any given group, the use of frequency scales results in an underestimation of the variance in behavioral frequencies. Because all respondents draw on the same frame of reference in computing an estimate, the estimates they compute are more similar than warranted.

Summary

As this selective review illustrates, retrospective frequency reports are fraught with uncertainty. In particular when the behavior is frequent, mundane, and irregular, respondents can arrive at a frequency report only by relying on an estimation strategy. Unfortunately, many of the behaviors that health researchers are interested in fit these characteristics. Under these conditions, concurrent reports are highly preferable.

Intensity Reports

Other retrospective questions pertain to the intensity of an experience (*How pleasant, painful, etc. was it?*). Intensity reports show pronounced biases even after a very short delay, making real-time data capture the method of choice. In general, our subjective experiences, including the intensity of our feelings, are poorly represented in memory: once the experience ends, its characteristics can no longer be directly examined (see Robinson & Clore, 2002, for a review). Accordingly, respondents again need to rely on fragmentary recall and extensive inferences to arrive at an answer. I first address which moments of an extended experience are particularly likely to be remembered and how these moments influence the overall retrospective recall. Subsequently, I turn to respondents' inference strategies.

Memorable Moments: Peak and End Effects

Redelmeier and Kahneman (1996) asked patients undergoing a colonoscopy to provide concurrent ratings of their pain along a 10-point scale. Figure 2-1 shows the pain ratings of two patients, collected at 60-second intervals. Both patients experienced similar peak pain, but patient B's colonoscopy lasted more than twice as long as patient A's, resulting in an overall experience of more pain. A few minutes after the completion of the procedure, however, patient B evaluated the overall experience as **less** painful.

As numerous related studies demonstrated (for a review see Fredrickson, 2000), this surprising result reflects that retrospective assessments follow a peak-and-end heuristic. This heuristic draws on two pieces of information that are particularly relevant from a survival point of view, namely the peak (*"How bad does it get?"*) and end (*"How does it end?"*). Hence, patient B was left with a memory of "less pain" than patient A: although both experienced the same peak pain, the final moment of patient B's colonoscopy was more benign, resulting in a more favorable memory despite similar peak pain and longer pain duration.

Findings of this type have two important implications. First, they illustrate that the duration of experiences is not well represented in memory and hence largely neglected in retrospective reports, even after a very short delay. Second, they highlight that retrospective reports of the intensity of an experience are based on two distinct moments, the peak and the end, while neglecting the intensity at

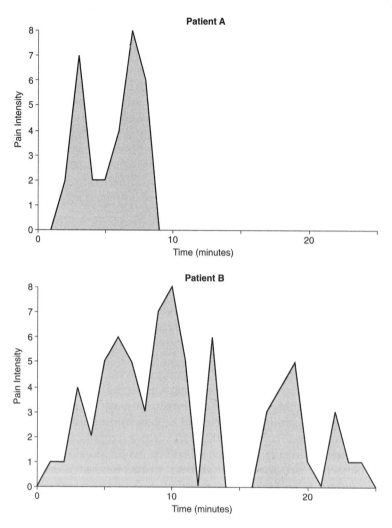

Figure 2-1. Concurrent reports of pain. Shown are real-time pain reports from two patients undergoing colonoscopy. The x axis represents time in minutes from the start of the procedure; the *y* axis represents the intensity of pain reported in real time on a visual analog scale (0 = no pain; 10 = extreme pain). (Adapted from Redelmeier and Kahneman, "Patients' memories of painful medical treatments," in PAIN, 1996. Reprinted by permission.)

other moments. Quite clearly, the concurrent measurement of pain, shown in Figure 2-1, provides a more accurate picture of these patients' experience than their retrospective reports. Reiterating this theme, Stone and colleagues observed peak-and-end effects in the retrospective pain reports of arthritis patients over a 1-week period (Stone, Broderick, Porter, & Kaell, 1997).

Despite their profound advantages in capturing people's actual experiences, concurrent measures may not always be the measure of choice. Suppose, for example, that the goal is to predict patients' compliance with the need for a subsequent follow-up colonoscopy. In light of his more benign memory of the procedure, patient B is more likely to comply than patient A, in contrast to what the concurrent measures of pain may suggest (for examples see Kahneman, Fredrickson, Schreiber, & Redelmeier, 1993; Redelmeier, Katz, & Kahneman, 2003). Given that people's decisions are based on their remembered experiences, retrospective reports may often be better predictors of their behavior, even though concurrent reports excel at capturing what was really going on. From a methodological perspective, this implies that a close link between retrospective reports and behavioral intentions does not validate the retrospective report; nor does a poor relationship between concurrent reports and behavioral intentions invalidate the concurrent reports. Instead, both observations merely reflect that we don't "learn from experience"—we learn from remembered experience.

Inference Strategies: The Role of Naïve Theories

In most cases, respondents have to rely on inference strategies to arrive at retrospective reports of intensity. Suppose a respondent is asked how bad her pain was last week. To answer this question, she may use her present pain as benchmark, asking herself if there is any reason to assume that last week was different. If she recalls such a reason, she will adjust her retrospective report accordingly; if not, she will report her current pain as a good approximation of last week's pain. As a result, her retrospective report of pain is a function of her current pain and her naïve theory about the stability of her pain over time.

In many domains, individuals assume an unrealistically high degree of stability, resulting in retrospective reports about past behaviors and experiences that are more similar to their present behaviors or experiences than is warranted. Accordingly, retrospective estimates of income (Withey, 1954) and of tobacco, marijuana, and alcohol consumption (Collins, Graham, Hansen, & Johnson, 1985) were found to be heavily influenced by respondents' income or consumption habits at the time of interview. The same holds for retrospective reports of pain. For example, Eich and colleagues (1985) asked chronic pain patients to report their current pain and the maximum, minimum, and usual pain they experienced during the previous week. When they compared these retrospective reports with patients' concurrent entries in daily pain diaries, they observed a familiar pattern: the retrospective reports were more similar to patients' pain at the time of recall than warranted. Thus, high current pain resulted in an overestimation of last week's pain, whereas low current pain resulted in an underestimation.

On the other hand, when respondents have reason to believe in change, they will detect change, even though none has occurred (see Ross, 1989). For example, Ross and Conway (1986) had students participate in a study skills training that did not improve their skills on any objective measure (and was not expected to do so). Following the training, researchers asked participants to recall how skilled they were before the training. Applying a plausible theory of change, namely that the training improved their skills, participants inferred that their prior skills must have been much worse than they were after training. Hence, they retrospectively reported having had poorer pretraining skills than they indicated before the training, apparently confirming the intervention's success. This result was obtained despite incentives to respondents to recall their earlier answers as accurately as possible. As Ross and Conway (1986) noted, you can always get what you want by revising what you had. The same logic, again, applies to retrospective reports of pain intensity. For example, Linton and Melin (1982) had back pain patients record their pain prior to a treatment program (baseline measurement). Following program completion, the patients were asked to recall their baseline pain. Reiterating Ross and Conway's (1986) finding, they now "recalled" more baseline pain than they had reported concurrently, apparently confirming the success of the treatment program. Again, concurrent measures of pain would provide a more accurate assessment.

Summary

The intensity of experiences is poorly represented in memory. Accordingly, respondents resort to inference strategies unless the episode is highly memorable. Even in the latter case, however, their retrospective reports are likely to be based on only a few moments of the episode, namely its peak and end. Accordingly, concurrent measures are preferable whenever their collection is feasible.

Reports of Change

The tasks posed to respondents sometimes go beyond mere retrospective reports. This is the case when researchers attempt to compensate for the lack of longitudinal data by asking respondents to report on change over time: *Do you have more or less pain now than you had at the beginning of the treatment?* As already seen in the preceding section, respondents' theory-driven inferences can make the past seem more or less similar to the present than warranted, resulting in systematic biases. Such theory-driven inferences are particularly likely, and problematic, when the context suggests an applicable theory, as is often the case in medical studies: believing that things get better with treatment (or why else would one undergo it?), patients are likely to infer that their past condition must have been worse than their present condition (e.g., Linton & Melin, 1982; for a review see Ross, 1989). This reliably results in overly optimistic assessments of change, which may explain the recent popularity of subjective change reports as "patient-reported outcomes." From a cognitive perspective, asking patients whether they feel better now than before their treatment is the most efficient way to "improve" the success rate of medical interventions.

As this discussion indicates, there is no substitute for appropriate study design, and respondents cannot compensate for the researchers' earlier oversights or lack of funds. If change over time is of crucial interest, concurrent measures at different points in time are the only reliable way to assess it.

Reports of Covariation and Causation

Similar problems arise when respondents are asked to report on covariation (*Under which circumstances?*) or causation (*Why?*). To arrive at an observation-based answer to these questions, respondents need an accurate representation of the frequency of their behaviors, the different contexts of these behaviors, and the intensity of related experiences. As already seen, respondents often cannot provide accurate reports on any of these components, making their joint consideration an unrealistically complex task. Once again, they are likely to draw on applicable naïve theories, resulting in systematic biases.

As an example, consider a study by McFarland and colleagues (1989), in which women kept daily diaries of their affect and physical symptoms. Following the diary period, the women were asked to recall their affect and physical symptoms for a particular day, either a day during their menstrual or their inter-menstrual phase. A comparison of their concurrent diary data and their retro-spective reports showed the pronounced impact of their beliefs about menstruation. Women who considered their menstruation a distressing event recalled feeling worse during the menstrual phase than they had reported con-currently, whereas these beliefs did not bias recall for a day during the intermen-strual phase.

Findings of this type illustrate that the reconstructed experience is itself a function of naïve theories of covariation (*"I feel bad during menstruation"*). This reconstruction, in turn, "confirms" the naïve theory, rendering its future appli-cation more likely. Note that this process is the opposite of what researchers hope for: instead of inferring covariation from accurately recalled behaviors and circumstances, respondents often draw on naïve theories of covariation to reconstruct the relevant behaviors in the first place. Accordingly, reports of covariation and causation are fraught with uncertainty unless they pertain to relatively simple and highly memorable events (*"I broke my leg because I fell off the ladder"*).

Again, there is no substitute for appropriate study design, and covariation and causation are best assessed with real-time data capture. EMA excels at this task by prompting respondents to report on their behavior, experiences, and circum-stances, allowing researchers to collect all the data needed for appropriate analyses, as the contributions to this volume illustrate. As already noted in the context of intensity reports, however, this does not render respondents' beliefs about covariation irrelevant. Respondents' behavioral decisions are likely to be driven by their own beliefs about covariation, inaccurate as those beliefs may be. Once again, assessing reality and capturing people's perceptions of reality are different enterprises, with different purposes and payoffs.

Real-Time Data Capture: Promises and Challenges

As this selective review indicates, retrospective questions often ask respondents for information that they cannot provide with any validity. The key promise of real-time data capture methods is that they pose more realistic tasks by asking respondents for information they know: their current behavior, experiences, and circumstances. However, respondents' memory limitations are not the only source of biases in self-reports, and issues of question comprehension, response formatting, or social desirability arise in concurrent as well as retrospective reports (for reviews see Schwarz, 1999a; Sudman et al., 1996). To date, these complications have received little attention in methodological studies of real-time data capture. In this final section, I illustrate the needed research with three examples.

Question Comprehension

To provide a meaningful answer, respondents typically have to go beyond the literal meaning of a question to infer what the researcher is interested in. To do so, they make extensive use of contextual information, including features of the question that the researcher may consider tangential to the question's meaning (for reviews see Clark & Schober, 1992; Schwarz, 1996). Suppose, for example, that a respondent is asked how often he has been "angry" recently. To answer this question, the respondent needs to determine what kind of anger the researcher has in mind: minor irritations or major annoyances? One source of information that respondents draw on is the reference period specified in the question (Winkielman, Knäuper, & Schwarz, 1998). When the question pertains to "yesterday," respondents assume that the researcher has minor irritations in mind because "big anger" doesn't happen that often. Conversely, when the question pertains to the last 6 months, respondents assume that the researcher has major annoyances in mind because they can hardly be expected to recall all the minor irritations of life over such an extended period. As a result, respondents deliberately report on substantively different experiences, depending on the reference period specified in an otherwise identical question (Igou, Bless, & Schwarz, 2002; Winkielman et al., 1998).

This observation has potentially profound implications for real-time data capture, where the typical reference period is very short ("right now" or the last few hours). It suggests that EMA respondents may include relatively minor events in their reports, which would go unmentioned for any longer reference period. This renders differences between concurrent and retrospective frequency reports of "anger," for example, highly ambiguous. On the one hand, concurrent reports may indicate higher frequencies than retrospective reports because some episodes were simply forgotten. On the other hand, concurrent reports may do so because they include many minor episodes that respondents may consider irrelevant when asked a retrospective question, pertaining to a longer reference period. In the latter case, concurrent and retrospective reports would pertain to subjectively "different" questions, rendering the answers noncomparable.

Scale Use

A related issue arises with regard to scale use. When asked to indicate along a rating scale how angry they are, respondents need to determine the meaning of the scale numbers. They do so by anchoring the endpoints of the scale with low and high anger events. Accordingly, their current anger receives a lower rating, the more extreme the event is that serves as the high anchor (e.g., Daamen & de Bie, 1992; Parducci, 1965). Retrospective and concurrent assessments are likely to differ in terms of the comparison episodes that come to mind. When asked to rate a single past episode, the recalled episode is likely to be compared to other memorable instances—which are often memorable because they were extreme. But when asked to rate multiple episodes over the course of a single day, previously rated moderate episodes may still be highly accessible. Accordingly, retrospective and concurrent ratings may differ in the comparison points and scale anchors used, undermining the comparability of the obtained results.

Social Desirability

Not surprisingly, respondents sometimes hesitate to report behaviors or opinions that they consider undesirable (for a review see DeMaio, 1984). It seems likely, however, that such social desirability concerns are less pronounced for reports that pertain to very short reference periods. For example, a parent may report, "I couldn't stand my kids last night," a report that pertains to a specific, limited episode. Yet the same parent may hesitate to report, "I don't like being with my kids," given the more pervasive implications of this general statement. If so, it is conceivable that concurrent reports, pertaining to limited episodes, are less subject to social desirability bias and more likely to capture negative and undesirable thoughts and feelings. But how many episodic reports does it take until respondents become aware that reporting that they don't like being with their kids "right now" amounts to the same as reporting that they rarely like being with them? Does socially desirable responding increase over repeated measurements?

Research Needs

At present, we know nothing about the conjectures offered above. To date, methodological research on real-time data capture has largely focused on overcoming the limits of retrospective reports. While this focus is important, we also need systematic experimental research into the cognitive and communicative processes underlying **concurrent** reports. Without this work, we run the risk of merely replacing the known biases of retrospective reports with new, unknown biases of concurrent reports.

Conclusion

As this review illustrates, psychologists and survey methodologists have made considerable progress in understanding the cognitive and communicative processes underlying self-reports (for more comprehensive treatments see Schwarz, 1999a; Sudman et al., 1996; Tourangeau et al., 2000). Despite the progress made, however, human memory imposes limits on what people can validly report on. Under most of the conditions of interest to health researchers, respondents have to rely on partial recall and extensive inference strategies when asked to report on their past behavior and experiences. These strategies result in biases that are well understood and difficult to avoid. Methods of real-time data capture provide a promising alternative by asking people about things that they **can** report on: their current behavior and current experiences. Moreover, EMA as the prime example of real-time data capture methods offers unique opportunities to assess behaviors and experiences in their ecological context and to complement subjective reports with objective measures, as the contributions to the present volume illustrate. To fully develop the potential of real-time data capture, however, future research will need to attend to the cognitive and communicative processes underlying concurrent reports, thus complementing previous work on retrospective reports.

ACKNOWLEDGMENT

Preparation of this chapter was facilitated by grants AG024928 from the National Institute of Aging and AR052170 from the National Institute of Arthritis and Musculoskeletal and Skin Diseases.

References

Belli, R. (1998). The structure of autobiographical memory and the event history calendar: Potential improvements in the quality of retrospective reports in surveys, *Memory, 6,* 383–406.

Brown, N. R. (2002). Encoding, representing, and estimating event frequencies: Multiple strategy perspective. In P. Sedlmeier & T. Betsch (Eds.), *Frequency processing and cognition* (pp. 37–54). New York: Oxford University Press.

Cannell, C. F., Fisher, G., & Bakker, T. (1965). Reporting on hospitalization in the Health Interview Survey. *Vital and Health Statistics* (PHS Publication No. 1000, Series 2, No. 6). Washington, DC: U.S. Government Printing Office.

Caspi, A., Moffitt, T., Thornton, A., Freedman, D., Amell, J., Harrington, H., Smeijers, J., & Silva, P. (1996). The life history calendar: A research and clinical assessment method for collecting retrospective event-history data. *International Journal of Methods in Psychiatric Research, 6,* 101–114.

Clark, H. H., & Schober, M. F. (1992). Asking questions and influencing answers. In J. M. Tanur (Ed.), *Questions about questions* (pp. 15–48). New York: Russell Sage.

Collins, L. M., Graham, J. W., Hansen, W. B., & Johnson, C. A. (1985). Agreement between retrospective accounts of substance use and earlier reported substance use. *Applied Psychological Measurement, 9,* 301–309.

Daamen, D. D. L., & de Bie, S. E. (1992). Serial context effects in survey items. In N. Schwarz & S. Sudman (Eds.), *Context effects in social and psychological research* (pp. 97–114). New York: Springer Verlag.

DeMaio, T. J. (1984). Social desirability and survey measurement: A review. In C. F. Turner & E. Martin (Eds.), *Surveying subjective phenomena* (Vol. 2, pp. 257–281). New York: Russell Sage.

Eich, E., Reeves, J. L., Jaeger, B., & Graff-Radford, S. B. (1985). Memory for pain: Relation between past and present pain intensity. *Pain, 23,* 375–380.

Freedman, D., Thornton, A., Camburn, D., Alwin, D., & Young-DeMarco, L. (1988). The life history calendar: A technique for collecting retrospective data. In C. C. Clogg (Ed.), *Sociological Methodology,* Vol. 18 (pp. 37–68). Washington, DC: American Sociological Association.

Fredrickson, B. L. (2000). Extracting meaning from past affective experiences: The importance of peaks, ends, and specific emotions. *Cognition and Emotion, 14,* 577–606.

Gaskell, G. D., O'Muircheartaigh, C. A., & Wright, D. B. (1994). Survey questions about the frequency of vaguely defined events: The effects of response alternatives. *Public Opinion Quarterly, 58,* 241–254.

Igou, E. R., Bless, H., & Schwarz, N. (2002). Making sense of standardized survey questions: The influence of reference periods and their repetition. *Communication Monographs, 69,* 179–187.

Kahneman, D., Fredrickson, B. L., Schreiber, C. A., & Redelmeier, D. (1993). When more pain is preferred to less: Adding a better end. *Psychological Science, 4,* 401–405.

Knäuper, B., Schwarz, N., & Park, D. C. (2004). Frequency reports across age groups: Differential effects of frequency scales. *Journal of Official Statistics, 20,* 91–96.

Linton, M. (1982). Transformations of memory in everyday life. In U. Neisser (Ed.), *Memory observed: Remembering in natural contexts* (pp. 77–91). San Francisco: Freeman.

Linton, S. J., & Melin, L. (1982). The accuracy of remembering chronic pain. *Pain, 13,* 281–285.

Mathiowetz, N. A., & Duncan, G. J. (1988). Out of work, out of mind: Response errors in retrospective reports of unemployment. *Journal of Business and Economic Statistics, 6,* 221–229.

McFarland, C., Ross, M., & De Courville, N. (1989). Women's theories of menstruation and biases in recall of menstrual symptoms. *Journal of Personality and Social Psychology, 57,* 522–531.

Menon, G. (1993). The effects of accessibility of information in memory on judgments of behavioral frequencies. *Journal of Consumer Research, 20,* 431–440.

Menon, G. (1994). Judgments of behavioral frequencies: Memory search and retrieval strategies. In N. Schwarz & S. Sudman, S. (Eds.), *Autobiographical memory and the validity of retrospective reports* (pp. 161–172). New York: Springer Verlag.

Menon, G., Raghubir, P., & Schwarz, N. (1995). Behavioral frequency judgments: An accessibility-diagnosticity framework. *Journal of Consumer Research, 22,* 212–228.

Parducci, A. (1965). Category judgment: A range-frequency model. *Psychological Review, 72,* 407–418.

Redelmeier, D., & Kahneman, D. (1996). Patients' memories of painful medical treatments: Real-time and retrospective evaluations of two minimally invasive procedures. *Pain, 116,* 3–8.

Redelmeier, D. A., Katz, J., & Kahneman, D. (2003). Memories of colonoscopy: A randomized trial. *Pain, 104,* 187–194.

Robinson, M. D., & Clore, G. L. (2002). Belief and feeling: Evidence for an accessibility model of emotional self-report. *Psychological Bulletin, 128,* 934–960.

Ross, M. (1989). The relation of implicit theories to the construction of personal histories. *Psychological Review, 96,* 341–357.

Ross, M., & Conway, M. (1986). Remembering one's own past: The construction of personal histories. In R. M. Sorrentino & E. T. Higgins (Eds.), *Handbook of motivation and cognition* (pp. 122–144). New York: Guilford.

Schwarz, N. (1996). *Cognition and communication: Judgmental biases, research methods, and the logic of conversation*. Hillsdale, NJ: Erlbaum.

Schwarz, N. (1999a). Self-reports: How the questions shape the answers. *American Psychologist, 54,* 93–105.

Schwarz, N. (1999b). Frequency reports of physical symptoms and health behaviors: How the questionnaire determines the results. In Park, D. C., Morrell, R. W., & Shifren, K. (Eds.), *Processing medical information in aging patients: Cognitive and human factors perspectives.* Mahwah, NJ: Erlbaum.

Schwarz, N., Hippler, H. J., Deutsch, B., & Strack, F. (1985). Response categories: Effects on behavioral reports and comparative judgments. *Public Opinion Quarterly, 49,* 388–395.

Schwarz, N., & Oyserman, D. (2001). Asking questions about behavior: Cognition, communication and questionnaire construction. *American Journal of Evaluation, 22,* 127–160.

Schwarz, N., & Scheuring, B. (1992). Selbstberichtete Verhaltens- und Symptomhäufigkeiten: Was Befragte aus Antwortvorgaben des Fragebogens lernen. (Frequency-reports of psychosomatic symptoms: What respondents learn from response alternatives.) *Zeitschrift für Klinische Psychologie, 22,* 197–208.

Schwarz, N., & Sudman, S. (1994). *Autobiographical memory and the validity of retrospective reports.* New York: Springer Verlag.

Schwarz, N., & Sudman, S. (1996). *Answering questions: Methodology for determining cognitive and communicative processes in survey research.* San Francisco: Jossey-Bass.

Stone, A. A., Broderick, J. B., Porter, L., & Kaell, A. T. (1997). The experience of rheumatoid arthritis pain and fatigue: Examining momentary reports and correlates over one week. *Arthritis Care and Research, 10,* 185–193.

Stone, A. A., Shiffman, S. S., & DeVries, M. W. (1999). Ecological momentary assessment. In D. Kahneman, E. Diener, & N. Schwarz (Eds.), *Well-being: The foundations of hedonic psychology* (pp. 61–84). New York: Russell Sage.

Strube, G. (1987). Answering survey questions: The role of memory. In H. J. Hippler, N. Schwarz, & S. Sudman (Eds.), *Social information processing and survey methodology* (pp. 86–101). New York: Springer Verlag.

Sudman, S., Bradburn, N. M., & Schwarz, N. (1996). *Thinking about answers: The application of cognitive processes to survey methodology.* San Francisco: Jossey-Bass.

Tourangeau, R., Rips, L. J., & Rasinski, K. (2000). *The psychology of survey response.* New York: Cambridge University Press.

Tourangeau, R., & Smith, T. W. (1996). Asking sensitive questions. The impact of data collection, mode, question format, and question context. *Public Opinion Quarterly, 60,* 275–304.

Winkielman, P., Knäuper, B., & Schwarz, N. (1998). Looking back at anger: Reference periods change the interpretation of (emotion) frequency questions. *Journal of Personality and Social Psychology, 75,* 719–728.

Withey, S. B. (1954). Reliability of recall of income. *Public Opinion Quarterly, 18,* 31–34.

3

Designing Protocols for Ecological Momentary Assessment

Saul Shiffman

Ecological Momentary Assessment (EMA) methods emphasize capture of real-time data in real-world settings, using multiple assessments of momentary states collected over time to characterize human behavior and experience (Stone & Shiffman, 1994). Investigators apply EMA methods to many different research areas and with diverse objectives. The objectives of EMA methods may be the reliable assessment of the individual with minimal retrospective bias, documenting the flow of behavior and experience over time, or studying the impact of environmental events, among others. Most often, EMA studies focus on variation in behavior or experience over time and across contexts. To achieve their goals, investigators must think carefully about the arrangements for collecting EMA data: what moments will be sampled and how they will be sampled and assessed. This chapter deals with the design of EMA protocols for data collection.

EMA assessment protocols will necessarily be embedded in a larger study design that addresses how many subjects are recruited, how subjects are grouped in the design, how conditions are assigned and structured, and so on. It is a truism that investigators must thoughtfully plan the design of their research, taking into account their research questions and hypotheses, their knowledge of the phenomenon they are studying, practical and logistical considerations, and plans for analysis. The usual design considerations of an adequate and representative sample of subjects, unbiased assignment to experimental conditions, reliable and valid assessment instruments, etc., apply to studies using EMA assessment methods but are not the focus of this chapter; this chapter focuses on the EMA protocol itself. Just as investigators must thoughtfully plan the overall study, they must similarly consider and plan how many EMA assessments will be collected, on what schedule they will be collected, how they will relate to events people experience, and how they fit into the context of the overall study design and research questions. This chapter discusses the basic structure of EMA protocols and presents a number of design options useful in health-related EMA studies.

Since the core of EMA is repeated collection of assessments in the field, the key issue in EMA design is deciding how those assessments will be scheduled. Will they occur at regular intervals and, if so, how often? If they are to be scheduled at random, how will this be accomplished, and how will the schedule be communicated to the participants? Perhaps assessments are not going to be "scheduled" at all but dictated by the natural flow of relevant events. If so, how will participants know when to do them? These are concrete decisions that must be made in any EMA protocol. While these decisions involve practical considerations, they must, above all, be driven by the research question and the natural history of the behavior under study. The design of the EMA protocol will shape what questions the study can answer and how well it can answer them. Accordingly, investigators must think very hard about their research questions and hypotheses and ensure that the EMA protocol is designed to address them.

A key concept that must be considered is that EMA assessments represent a **sample** of the participant's experience. In traditional one-time, retrospective questionnaire assessment approaches, investigators assume they are capturing data about the person's full range of experiences in one fell swoop, directly characterizing the phenomenon they are interested in. EMA approaches are applied when the attribute being assessed varies over time, and the assessments are conceptualized as sampling the person's condition over time. This is most clear when EMA measures are used to assess the participant's immediate momentary state at random times throughout the day. In that instance, each assessment, each moment, is seen as a sample from the population of moments in that person's experience over time.

Perhaps less obviously, the sampling framework is also applicable when participants are asked to complete diaries once daily, as the assessments sample particular days from the flow of the participant's daily life. Moreover, the assessment may be influenced by his or her condition at the moment of assessment (e.g., mood congruence; Teasdale & Fogarty, 1979), making it useful to think of it as a momentary sample as well. Thus, designing an EMA protocol is essentially designing a sampling scheme for blocks of time in a person's life. A well-designed sampling scheme aims to efficiently produce reliable, representative data.

Sampling Discrete Events Versus Continuous Experience

A fundamental consideration in designing an EMA protocol is the assessment's target and whether the target phenomenon is best conceptualized as a continuous experience (e.g., mood) or as a discrete, episodic phenomenon (a panic attack, a meal). Discrete episodic phenomena lend themselves to event-based sampling approaches in which subjects are asked to make a recording each time a predefined "event" occurs (e.g., *"Make an entry each time you take a pill"*). The event itself essentially serves as the cue for initiating a recording.

Continuous experience (e.g., variations in mood) does not lend itself to this approach: there is no natural trigger and all moments are part of the population to be sampled. Sampling continuous experience lends itself to time-based sampling schemes, in which assessments are scheduled at intervals—at either regular or irregular (often random) intervals—to sample the participants' experience. Most of this chapter is taken up with a discussion of these two approaches and variations upon them. (This organization of EMA designs into event-based and time-based schema is based on prior conceptualizations by Wheeler & Reis [1991] and by Bolger, Davis, & Rafaeli [2003].) Table 3-1 summarizes the major approaches to EMA design.

Event-Based Sampling Strategies

Event-based approaches are suitable when the phenomenon under study is conceptualized as occurring in discrete episodes. Examples abound in health research: asthma attacks, headaches, sexual intercourse, meals, alcohol consumption, exercise episodes, taking medication, vomiting, missing work, smoking a cigarette, and so on. The approach of having participants record relevant events has a long tradition in behavioral science, notably in the literature on "self-monitoring" (McFall, 1977), which has long been considered a major mode of behavioral assessment. Event-based EMA recording is relatively straightforward: participants are asked to make a recording every time a predefined event occurs (e.g., *"Make an entry each time you eat a meal"*). The recordings themselves yield a count or frequency of events, which is often a useful parameter. More often, when subjects record the events, they are also asked about details, allowing the events to be characterized (e.g., *"What did you eat?"*).

DEFINING EVENTS

In event-based EMA, the investigator relies on the participant to identify and record target events, making it crucial that the investigator clearly define what constitutes an "event." This often turns out to be more complex and more difficult than it appears. A "migraine" may seem like a clear episodic event, but it is in fact complex. Does every headache meet the criteria to be recorded, or must certain other symptoms also be present to define a "migraine?" If the onset of a migraine is to be recorded, is the "aura" that often precedes head pain to be counted as part of the event? Or consider tracking of "meals." When does a "snack" become a "meal?" Is a meal defined by the quantity of food consumed, the organization of an eating occasion, or other criteria? Defining events such as "sexual intercourse" or "social interaction" obviously has its own challenges. It is crucial that the definitions be clearly set out by the investigator and not left to the participants' discretion.

Defining the target event is particularly challenging when the distinction between "events" and "nonevents" lies along a continuous dimension, as when an event represents an exacerbation of symptoms (namely, meeting some threshold to be considered an event). When does "discomfort" become "pain?" When does tightness in the chest become wheezing, and when does wheezing become an

Table 3-1. Summary of EMA designs

Approach	Definition	Targets	Example in this volume	Issues	Notes
Event-based	Recording triggered by event of interest	Defined "events" or episodes	Recording smoking (Chapter 6)	Events must be well defined; compliance hard to document	Multiple events may be tracked; no prompting device required
Time-based	Recording triggered based on a time schedule	Either continuous phenomena or summary of events over time			
Regular	Recordings scheduled at regular intervals				
Daily	Recording once daily, usually at end of day	Summary of day's experience or events	End of day stress assessment	Recall-based, may introduce bias Time of completion may introduce bias	Usually aims for coverage of whole day via recall and summary
Interval	Recording multiple times per day	Summary of experience or events	Symptom assessment morning, afternoon, night (Chapter 13)	Typically recall-based, but smaller recall intervals; Schedule may become entrained to events	Usually aims for coverage of whole day via recall and summary
Intensive	Recording very frequently (e.g., once/hr or more)	Fast-changing phenomena	Ambulatory blood pressure (Chapter 14)	Significant subject burden	Approaches randomly scheduled variable assessment in representativeness; usually automated or prompted

Variable, random	Recording scheduled at random, variable intervals	Continuous phenomena	Pain assessment at random within time blocks (Turk)	Requires device for scheduling and prompting	Aims to accrue representative sample of occasions; assessment usually focused on subjects' immediate state; allows sampling stratified and weighted sampling schemes

Combinations

Event or time + daily	Combining within-day event or time-based recording with end of day	Daily summary to supplement within-day momentary assessment	Noting plans for future drinking while tracking drinking events (Collins)	Daily and momentary can be independent; no coordination required	Daily assessment relies on recall and summary
Event + random	Combining event-based recording with randomly scheduled time-based recoring	Correlates, antecedents, and sequelae of events	Smoking + background (Mermelstein)	Must consider overlap of two schedules	Used for case-control designs and for retrospective and prospective analyses of event antecedents
Event + follow-up	Arranging time-based recordings following an index event	Sequelae of events	Track onset and offset of relief from medication (event) (not represented in this volume)	Requires on-line intelligence for responsive prompting schedule	Use either randomly or regularly scheduled prompts to assess sequelae of recorded events

asthma attack? While these definitional issues are challenging, phenomena like pain and drug craving demonstrate a course that mixes some continuously varying "background" level of intensity with punctuation by episodes of more intense symptoms that lend themselves to capture as events (Shiffman, 2000). For example, in a study of smoking cessation (Shiffman, Engberg, Paty, et al., 1997), subjects successfully monitored craving on a continuous scale, while also tracking episodic temptations, which were defined for them as occasions when craving suddenly "spiked" or when they were on the verge of smoking. Thus, it is possible to simultaneously monitor both continuous experience and episodic events, although both the programming and the interpretation are challenging.

In some instances, investigators may wish to allow for idiosyncratic subjective definitions of events, particularly when the participants' judgments are themselves of interest. For example, an investigator may wish to study occasions when subjects believe they have overeaten or drunk too much, regardless of the objective quantities (e.g., Stein, Chapter 9; Collins, Chapter 10, this volume). At the other extreme are special cases of event-based EMA where the event is not detected or defined by the participant at all but is detected automatically. For example, a heart-monitoring device could detect episodes of transient cardiac ischemia (short-lived blockage of blood flow to the heart) that can be detected from analysis of the EKG waveform but are not detectable subjectively (see Intille, Chapter 16, this volume). The device can then prompt the participant to complete an assessment of the circumstances surrounding the detected event. In this case, the algorithmic definition of the event is contained in the device.

Timing of Recording

Participants in event-oriented EMA studies must be given clear directions about **when** they are to record a target event: at its onset, at termination, or at another milestone (e.g., its peak). Considerations for selecting a target "trigger" include concern about reactivity (reactivity is maximized if recording is initiated at the onset of a target behavior, when there is still opportunity to redirect behavior) (McFall, 1977), ability to define the onset in advance (the subject may not know that an episode is going to end in binge drinking), and the focus of the research. Depending on the investigator's interests, it may be useful to record both onset and offset. This allows the duration of the event to be computed and also allows one to ask pre- and post-event questions separately (see, e.g., Collins, Chapter 10, this volume; cf. Mermelstein, Chapter 6, this volume). Of course, defining the onset or end of an event or episode is an extension of the challenge of defining the event itself. Some delay may occur between the onset or offset and subject recording; collecting data about any delays may help determine actual event times.

Kinds of Event Data

Event-based recording can be used for many purposes. Sometimes the main interest is simply in the count or frequency of events, as when one is testing a treatment for urinary incontinence and reducing event frequency is a goal. In these instances, it may not be necessary to collect any data about the event beyond the fact that it happened, requiring only a single key press or checkmark. With time-stamped records, this also provides a record of how events are distributed over time (e.g., whether they are more likely at certain times of day, whether they cluster together or tend to occur at regular intervals; see Rathbun, Shiffman, & Gwaltney, 2005). More often, we want to know something about the events (*How intense was the headache? How long did it last? Was medication taken?*) or their antecedents (*Where were you? How were you feeling?*), which requires collecting additional data.

Sometimes investigators are interested in the absence of target events: when the person failed to exercise or went without drinking. These can be approached by recording events, but noting when events have **not** been recorded. For example, in a study of smoking cessation (Shiffman, Paty, Gnys, et al., 1996), we were interested in detecting when participants quit smoking, which we defined as 24 hours without smoking. Participants were to record every instance of smoking on a palmtop computer. When the computer noted that no cigarettes had been reported in 24 hours, it declared that cessation had occurred and switched to a different protocol. However, the absence of event recordings might sometimes indicate poor compliance rather than behavior change. Accordingly, it is essential to validate the inference with the participant. Such protocols also place particular emphasis on good compliance with event recording.

Event-based protocols are not always limited to a single event: multiple events may be monitored simultaneously. For example, Stein (Chapter 9, this volume) monitored binge eating, vomiting, and laxative use; Mermelstein (Chapter 6, this volume) monitored occasions when participants smoked and when they decided not to smoke. When monitoring multiple events, it is essential that they be mutually exclusive and that they be especially clearly defined and distinguished. Participant burden, both the number of recordings and the cognitive decision making involved, obviously rises as the number of target events rises, so investigators must weigh the costs and benefits of monitoring multiple events and limit the number of event types.

Issues Related to Event Frequency

The direct capture of event data using event-based recording works well when the event frequency is moderate. However, when event frequency is high, recording every event may become unrealistically burdensome or intrusive (e.g., recording every sneeze during allergy season). In these instances, it may be possible to redefine the "event" as a larger unit, such as an episode of sneezing (or a bout of drinking; see Collins, Chapter 10, this volume). The investigator may also consider using time-based assessment to capture event frequency (e.g., by asking hourly for an estimate of the frequency of sneezing). However, such approaches reintroduce an element of retrospective recall that can potentially undo the benefits of real-time collection of momentary data. Indeed, evidence suggests that people are particularly poor at recalling the timing of events or placing them within a time frame (Huttenlocher, Hedges, & Bradburn, 1990). Thus, when asked an apparently simple question like, *"How many cigarettes did you smoke in the past 2 hours?"* participants may not be able to provide accurate responses. For this reason, real-time event entries are preferred. One should not underestimate a participant's ability to record many individual events if the task is made simple. In our studies of heavy smokers (Shiffman, Gwaltney, Balabanis, et al., 2002), it is not unusual for them to record 30 or more smoking occasions each day.

The other end of the event frequency spectrum—very infrequent events, such as migraines—poses a different challenge. For infrequent events, the challenge is that the burden of carrying a recording device at all times and remembering the recording protocol may seem disproportionate to the task of recording rare events. (A special class of infrequent events deals with cases where the research is trying to capture a unique instance of an event, such as the very first drink after a period of treatment and abstinence; even if lapses to drinking are common and drinking eventually becomes frequent, the probability of a first event is low on any given day.) In these cases, it may be adequate to implement time-based monitoring at some low level (e.g., asking daily whether a target event has occurred). However, this may not be adequate if real-time data are needed about the event itself. There are no hard-and-fast guidelines about which event frequencies lend themselves to direct event-based monitoring.

One issue that arises in event-based EMA is that the response burden is not under the investigator's direct control, it is potentially variable, and it is proportional to the event frequency. In other words, participants with more events (heavier smokers, those with more frequent migraines) will have a greater recording burden. Above, I described some strategies for cases where the burden of simply recording events is itself a concern. More often, the concern is magnified by the burden of completing assessments about the events. One solution is to limit and balance the number of event assessments by randomly sampling only a limited number, using algorithms programmed into palmtop computers running the EMA protocol. For example, one smoking study asked participants to record all cigarettes but randomly selected only a few each day for assessment (Shiffman, Gwaltney, Balabanis, et al., 2002). It is essential that the events sampled for assessment be selected at random (or in some other predetermined, systematic way); if the participant can decide which ones are assessed, a biased sample may result.

COMPLIANCE WITH EVENT MONITORING

It is often difficult to validate accurate and complete recording of events, because there is rarely a "gold standard" measure against which event reports can be validated. Some bias in event recording can arise from attempts by participants (deliberate or unconscious) to manage their image. Events might be deliberately underreported if they are considered embarrassing (e.g., unsafe sex) or overreported if they are considered positive (e.g., taking prescribed medication). A common concern is underreporting of events, either from the burden of recording or from inadvertent omission. This can be particularly problematic for frequent and unremarkable events that may be easily missed. While it is unlikely that a migraine sufferer would fail to take note of a migraine headache, a heavy cigarette smoker might easily smoke a cigarette "on automatic pilot" without noting it for recording (Tiffany, 1990).

The lack of a gold standard against which to compare EMA records makes validation difficult: we usually cannot know how many migraines were actually experienced or how many drinks were consumed. Comparing EMA event records with global self-reports (e.g., weekly recall of migraines or drinks) is unsatisfactory. The motivation for collecting real-time EMA data is often the suspicion or conviction that global reports are inaccurate and invalid, so departure from them may not indicate a problem with the EMA data; just the opposite, it may reflect the limitations of global self-report. In a few cases, it may be possible to validate event counts against objective measures, such as biochemical markers of smoking (Benowitz, 1983), motion sensors for tracking exercise (see Arredondo, Chapter 7, this volume), or instrumented pill bottles for tracking medication compliance (Cramer, Mattson, Prevey, et al., 1989).

Studies that have assessed compliance with event recording in electronic diaries using external criteria have suggested that subjects are adequately compliant with event recording (e.g., Shiffman & Paty, 2003), but more research of this sort is needed. In any case, it is unlikely that perfect compliance will be attained, so the researcher must think carefully about how noncompliance may affect the data. The effects of noncompliance can be more serious if failure to record events is biased in some way (e.g., failing to record asthma attacks when they are particularly severe) or if analyses focus on individual events, such as the very first occurrence of a symptom. Technological developments may improve instrumentation to detect some types of events without requiring subject initiative (see Intille, Chapter 16, this volume), but no fully satisfactory approach to achieving complete fidelity of event recording exists today.

SUMMARY

EMA methods are often used to collect data about events participants experience in day-to-day life. These protocols require clear definitions of what constitutes an event and careful consideration of event frequency. Participants' compliance with event recording is crucial to the validity of the data but often difficult to confirm.

Time-Based Sampling Strategies

In contrast to event-based strategies, which depend on a definable event to trigger recording, time-based strategies implement a time-based schedule for assessment and sampling, in which assessments are scheduled at regular or irregular intervals. Time-based sampling strategies are particularly well suited for studying phenomena that are present continuously but are expected to vary in intensity or character.

Examples relevant to health abound, including variations in pain, mood, fatigue, self-efficacy, motivation, activities, and location. They include an experience or behavior that varies continuously in intensity (pain) or categorically (kind of activity) and objective (blood pressure) and subjective (mood) targets.

COVERAGE STRATEGIES VERSUS SAMPLING STRATEGIES

When investigators arrange intermittent assessment of subjects, they may be following one of two strategies. A **coverage** strategy aims to have the participant's report cover every moment of the day. Thus, when assessed, participants are asked to recall and summarize their experience since the last assessment and, piecemeal, the assessments cover the entire day. As noted, this strategy requires some recall and retrospection and may pose an additional burden for the participant because of difficulty recalling what experience fell into the interval "since the last assessment." In contrast, a **sampling** strategy, best exemplified by randomly scheduled assessments, sees the moments selected for assessment as representative of the day and therefore usable as an unbiased estimate of the day's experience. It does not assume that we have "covered" every single moment of the day and, therefore, allows that specific moments may be missed, while relying on representative sampling to provide a representative picture of the day.

REGULAR AND VARIABLE ASSESSMENT INTERVALS

It is also useful to distinguish assessment-scheduling strategies that rely on regularly spaced assessment schedules and those with irregular, typically random, schedules. The choice of scheduling scheme is partially linked to selection of a coverage or sampling strategy, as described above. Random schedules are usually associated with sampling strategies, where the randomness of the assessments is seen as an essential element in a representative sampling strategy. (This is not a strict linkage, in that investigators sometimes include coverage questions in randomly scheduled assessments.) In a sampling strategy, the scheduling of assessment occasions is carefully planned to avoid bias, and regularly spaced assessments are seldom considered optimal for ensuring representative and unbiased sampling.

In contrast, regular assessment intervals are often associated with a coverage strategy. This approach always characterizes daily assessments and often characterizes more frequent regular assessments, where subjects might be asked to summarize their experience at the end of the morning, afternoon, and night (i.e., over a smaller recall interval). The scheduling of assessments is often based on convenience, or on the lack of a practical method for implementing a random schedule, rather than on representativeness, which is not relevant, because the assessments in aggregate are not considered to sample from the day, but to actually encompass the entire day.

REGULAR INTERVALS   Many diary studies have relied on a fixed-interval scheduling of assessment. The assessment interval has varied substantially, ranging from once daily, to several times daily, to intensive schedules of diary completion every 30 to 60 minutes (see Kamarck, Chapter 14, this volume). I discuss each in turn.

Daily Diaries   Daily diaries are one of the oldest forms of field-data collection and have often been used in health research. Participants complete an assessment once daily, usually near the end of the day or at bedtime (e.g., Duncan & Grazzani-Gavazzi, 2004; Freeman & Gil, 2004; McDonald & Almeida, 2004; Park, Armeli, & Tennen, 2004; Yip & Cross, 2004). Daily diaries have the advantage of being relatively undemanding (e.g., subjects need not carry their diary with them throughout the day or interrupt their activities to enter data). A day may also be seen as a natural unit for study (we talk about having "good days" and "bad days"). For these reasons, daily diaries are the most common implementation of EMA.

Investigators sometimes choose a daily diary approach on the assumption that the phenomenon under study does not vary meaningfully within the day, making the day a natural sampling unit. However, such assumptions are rarely tested and some phenomena thought to be relatively stable, when tested, have been found to have meaningful within-day variation (see, e.g., Gwaltney, Shiffman, & Sayette [2005]). Most often, the investigator recognizes within-day variation in the assessment target but relies on the participants' retrospection to summarize experience across time and variance. This erodes the "real-time" emphasis of EMA methods and reintroduces a degree of retrospection and possible recall bias. How significant this bias is has to be considered on a case-by-case basis.

Participants may be asked to sum up the day (e.g., average mood, severity of pain), to aggregate quantities (e.g., number of cigarettes smoked, calories consumed), or to recall and report on specific events (e.g., a migraine headache). Recalling whether one had a migraine today—an infrequent, highly salient event—is likely to be more accurate and less bias-prone than recalling how many cigarettes were smoked (frequent and "ordinary" events). Even with salient events like migraines, recall of intensity and other details may be subject to substantial distortion depending, for example, on how long ago it was and whether one is still in pain. When participants are asked not just about a specific episode but are also asked to summarize the day, characterizing its average qualities or giving counts of events, they must not only recall but also aggregate and summarize their experience. Research suggests that participants often use heuristic strategies to estimate their answers rather than explicitly recalling their experience and computing some algebraic average (Bradburn, Ripps, & Shevell, 1987).

A particular source of bias in daily diaries is the time at which they are completed, almost always near the end of the day. Recall of past experience is colored by one's state at the time of recall; for example, people who are in a sad mood are more likely to recall negative experiences and to interpret experiences negatively (Clark & Teasdale, 1982). Because the end of the day is an unrepresentative moment in daily life (e.g., one is more likely to be tired and sleepy, less likely to be under immediate stress) and because the condition being studied may be subject to diurnal rhythms, this has the potential to color end-of-day reports and to dampen true variation among days. (This is exacerbated when the timing of diary completion is left to participants' discretion or tied to a milestone event; see below.) Thus, daily summaries may be subject to considerable recall bias and may fail to adequately sample daily experience.

Interval Diaries   Many diary studies go beyond once-daily diary completion to collect assessments several times a day, corresponding to daily epochs (e.g., morning, afternoon, and evening) or at certain times of day (e.g., 10 a.m., 2 p.m., 6 p.m., 10 p.m.; see below on scheduling considerations). These approaches, like daily diaries, usually call for recall to capture experience but over shorter recall intervals. In addition to shrinking the recall interval, this strategy, by spreading assessments throughout the day, lessens the potentially biasing effect of a particular assessment occasion such as bedtime. When multiple assessments are scheduled at regular intervals throughout the day, a sampling strategy may be adopted, but careful consideration must be given to whether such regularly spaced occasions are representative of the subject's experience.

Intensive Diaries   At the extreme, the frequency of regularly spaced assessments can become so high that the dynamics of assessment change to more closely resemble those of randomly scheduled assessments. For example, in research on ambulatory monitoring of cardiovascular function (heart rate and blood pressure), it is not unusual to collect an assessment (often both self-report and physiological) every 25 or 45 minutes (see Kamarck, Chapter 14, this volume). These frequent assessments may implement either a coverage or sampling strategy, but the two are less differentiated when assessments become very frequent because (1) even if the assessments follow a coverage strategy based on recall, the recall interval is short; and (2) the frequency of assessment is so great that even a sampling strategy focused on momentary reports begins to approach full coverage of the day.

Considerations for Regular-Interval Schedules   Fixed-interval assessments have the advantage that they are evenly spaced. This can be a virtue or even a requirement for certain analyses, such as time series analysis, and lessens the challenge of modeling the autocorrelation structure of the data (the correlation among adjacent observations), because of the passage of equal amounts of time between observations. This advantage has become somewhat less important as newer statistical methods have become available for unevenly spaced data, however. Sometimes a device used to collect data (e.g., a blood pressure monitor) may support only regular intervals.

Regularity provides predictability for participants, but this can be a mixed blessing. On one hand, participants may find that predictability reduces the perceived intrusiveness of the data collection. On the other hand, they may come to anticipate the assessments in ways that change their experience (e.g., thinking about the target behavior as the scheduled assessment time approaches).

How the assessments are scheduled and prompted can be very important. Tying the assessment schedule to daily milestones (e.g., meals, bedtime) is appealing because it provides a natural prompt for the assessments. However, almost by definition, these milestone moments are unrepresentative and may introduce bias into the assessments. (There is a special case where these "milestones" are particularly apt occasions for a particular assessment, such as assessing ratings of sleep quality just after the person has awakened; see Collins, Chapter 10, this volume.) Scheduling by clock time (e.g., assessments at 10 a.m., 2 p.m., 6 p.m., 10 p.m.) can help avoid this problem. However, investigators must be aware that similar biases may creep in inadvertently. For instance, the "top of the hour" may be associated with particular activities or the assessment times may fall at work-break times for certain subjects (e.g., teachers switching classrooms).

When the instructions for scheduling are loose, participants implicitly have great discretion over when to complete assessments. For example, when assessments are to be completed "morning, evening, and night," different participants may interpret this differently, with one completing the "morning" assessment at noon and another at 7 a.m. Further, they may introduce systematic bias to their selection of moments for assessment. For example, participants in a pain study may systematically complete their assessments when they are in pain, because the pain reminds them that they are supposed to do an assessment during the evening. (Or, conversely, they may wait until pain-free moments to complete the assessment when they are not discomfited by pain. Or they may trade off among these practices and biases at different times.) Allowing participants to choose when they complete their assessments makes the task more convenient for them but opens the door to bias related to how these occasions are selected. These limitations of regular-interval assessments are a major motivation for implementing randomized assessments schedules supported by active prompting, as described below.

VARIABLE-INTERVAL ASSESSMENTS, RANDOM ASSESSMENTS   To avoid the potential for bias in regular-interval time-based assessment schedules, many studies have used variable intervals, usually random intervals. By arranging assessments at random times, the investigator can be assured of a representative sample of the person's experience. By providing a random sample of the person's experience, the assessments guarantee a representative, unbiased estimate of the whole, just as a randomly selected sample of individuals for participation in a study ensures population representativeness (though the representativeness of the sample may be undermined [e.g., by nonresponse] as described below). This innovation was developed by Csikszentmihalyi and colleagues (see Csikszentmihalyi & Larson, 1987), who conducted and inspired many studies using the Experience Sampling Method (ESM), typically by providing subjects with a "beeper" that was set off at random to prompt a diary entry. Since selecting moments at random cannot be left to the participant, random scheduling requires some device, under the investigator's control, that prompts the participant when it is time to complete an assessment. In addition to beepers, investigators have used wristwatches, cell phones, and palmtop computers (see section on devices).

Considering the scheduling of EMA assessments as a scheme for representative sampling of participants' experience puts at the EMA investigator's disposal a variety of sampling schemes that are used in population sampling. Simple random sampling is always a valid sampling scheme but can sometimes be improved upon. For example, stratified sampling is used in population studies when one needs to ensure adequate representation of participants with certain characteristics and the sample is not large enough to ensure balanced representation through simple random selection. Analogously, many EMA investigators have used stratified sampling schedules in which the day is divided into strata (e.g., 7–11 a.m., 11 a.m.–3 p.m., 3–7 p.m., 7–11 p.m.) and an assessment is scheduled at random within each of those blocks (e.g., Turk, Chapter 11, this volume), thus ensuring that assessments are spread evenly throughout the day.

Other sampling schemes may also be useful. In population sampling, investigators sometimes oversample a particular group of subjects of interest to ensure that the group is well represented (e.g., overrepresenting minority respondents in a survey comparing minority and majority attitudes), while using weighting to rebalance the sample for analysis. Similarly, investigators can oversample certain times that are of particular interest to ensure adequate data for analysis. In one example, we oversampled the first few waking hours of the day (by scheduling random prompts more frequently) because we were interested in how a particular medication might differentially affect morning symptoms (Shiffman, Elash, Paton, et al., 2000).

Summary

Particularly when the research focuses on continuous experience, EMA protocols often implement time-based assessment strategies. Regularly spaced assessments are often implemented when the investigator is prepared to rely on recall to achieve complete coverage of the day. More often, EMA studies rely on a random sampling strategy, characterizing subject experience through a series of randomly scheduled assessments to achieve representation of the subject's experience.

Combined Protocols

While some EMA designs use a single EMA schedule or strategy, it is often useful or essential to combine them, as illustrated below. Before discussing combinations of event-based and time-based recordings, which are among the most useful combination designs, I discuss the combination of daily fixed-time assessments with momentary assessments, whether event- or time-based.

Combining Daily and Momentary Assessments

Daily assessments are often used on their own to summarize a day's experience. In this sense, they are used in lieu of momentary assessments. However, daily summaries can be useful even when momentary assessments are also being completed, to capture information that does not lend itself to, or does not require, momentary assessment. For example, an investigator who is interested primarily in the association of nausea and mood might also wish to capture data about exercise, so that the analysis can factor in any differences between exercise and nonexercise days. In this instance, a daily assessment might inquire whether the subject had engaged in any exercise that day (or how much, subject to appropriate definitions, etc.). The end-of-day assessment of exercise may be less accurate and will lack exact information about the timing of the exercise but may be judged adequate for the intended purpose. In a sense, the investigator must weigh the convenience of collecting some data on a once-daily basis against the value to the particular study of having more refined momentary assessment. As always, the research questions, and the conceptualization of the variables being assessed, must provide the governing principles.

Daily diary assessments may also be particularly useful when the investigator specifically seeks the participants' retrospective judgment rather than their momentary response. While an end-of-day judgment about how stressful the day was may not always be a balanced representation of the participant's experience throughout the day, it may be a valuable piece of data and a subject of study in itself. For example, an investigator may wish to understand how end-of-day judgments relate to momentary experience, or may want to explore the possibility that this judgment, more than the momentary experience, affects subsequent behavior. In any case, end-of-day assessments have utility for collecting different kinds of data, even when momentary event- or time-based data are also being collected.

Combinations of Event- and Time-Based Assessments

CASE-CONTROL DESIGNS FOR EVENTS

Event-based EMA methods are often used to collect data about the circumstances or antecedents of the target events. How were subjects feeling before they drank? What had they eaten before the migraine started? What were they doing when the panic attack occurred? While these event data can be very useful in providing a description of the events' context, without additional data they cannot be used to establish an association between episodes and particular antecedents (much less causation; see Paty, Kassel, & Shiffman, 1992). Establishing that Joe was usually feeling depressed just before he drank does not tell us that depression is associated with drinking; he may have been just as depressed the rest of the time when he wasn't drinking. To understand the association between depression and drinking, we have to collect data on nondrinking occasions as well. Since "not drinking" cannot be tracked as an "event," such occasions can be sampled using time-based methods. Thus, an EMA protocol to study drinking antecedents might include random prompting and assessment in nondrinking situations, to serve as a control for the drinking situations (see Collins, Chapter 10, this volume; see Shiffman, Gwaltney, Balabanis, et al., 2002). This is essentially a within-person case-control design, also known as a case-crossover design

(Checkoway, 2004; Maclure, 1991): the "cases" are the drinking episodes and the "controls" are the nondrinking episodes, all within the same persons.

Comparing mood in drinking and nondrinking episodes tells us whether depression is in fact associated with drinking (just as comparison of fat intake in heart attack victims vs. healthy controls can establish an association between dietary fat and heart disease). As in other case-control designs, the logic of inference may seem reversed. We are interested in whether depression leads to drinking, but we actually sample both drinking and nondrinking episodes and "look back" to see how much depression was present in each. We can report how likely a person was to be depressed when drinking (vs. not drinking); we will not have data on how likely a person is to drink when he or she is depressed (though other designs and analyses can approximate this, analogous to a cohort design in epidemiology). As in case-control designs, statistics like the odds ratio can adequately express the association even without estimating these probabilities. This case-control design is a powerful EMA design combining event-based sampling with random time-based sampling (e.g., Collins, Chapter 10, this volume; Mermelstein, Chapter 6, this volume).

Unlike a between-person classical case-control design where differences among persons in the case and control samples can confound the inferences, the EMA-based case-crossover design makes comparisons between occasions within individuals, thus controlling for all person-level variables. Differences between occasions, however, still have the potential to confound the analysis. For example, differences in physical posture and activity, or reactions to the presence of others, might account for observed differences between blood pressure in calm and emotionally upsetting situations (see Kamarck, Chapter 14, this volume). Moreover, when the comparison involves both within- and between-person factors, careful controls are necessary to rule out confounding. For example, Shiffman and Paty (2006) found it necessary to control for time of day when comparing smoking (cases) and nonsmoking (control) occasions between groups of heavy and light smokers. Accordingly, it is essential to control for likely confounders in the analysis and to consider the potential influences of unmeasured third variables.

ANALYSIS OF EVENT ANTECEDENTS

The combination of event sampling and random time-based sampling can also be useful in exploring the antecedents of events, by examining whether the assessments in the period preceding an episode show a reliable pattern. For example, we observed that episodes in which smokers lapsed after quitting were preceded by escalating negative affect that was evident hours before the lapse event itself (Shiffman & Waters, 2004). In this instance, random time-based assessments that happened to fall in the hours preceding the event (whose timing was unpredictable) enabled the analysis to reconstruct the proximal history of the event.

Random time-based assessments can also be used to predict the likelihood of a succeeding event in an analogue of the prospective cohort study. For example, an investigator interested in whether negative affect leads to migraines could implement a protocol that combined tracking of migraines with frequent randomly scheduled time-based assessments. Each time-based assessment could be considered a prospective observation for assessing subsequent risk of migraine. For example, a logistic regression analysis could assess whether negative affect at each observation is related to the risk of a migraine event in the succeeding hour, or a survival analysis could look at the risk of subsequent migraine events over time, treating momentary affect as a time-varying covariate. This is similar to the preceding design but uses prospective logic to "predict" events rather than looking back from events toward their precursors.

FOLLOW-UP OF EVENT SEQUELAE

Combining event- and time-based assessments may also allow the investigator to analyze what happens after an event rather than what came before. For example, an investigator might be interested in the natural history of nausea following an episode of chemotherapy. With the chemotherapy episode entered as an event, subsequent time-based assessments could be analyzed to map out the time course of symptoms following the episode. Note that this requires an adequate density of time-based assessments in the period after the event; if randomly scheduled assessments are used, the uneven spacing of the observations may be inconvenient.

Rather than rely on the natural intersection of event- and time-based data collected in parallel, a more powerful approach is to arrange and schedule the time-based assessments to track the aftermath of the event. For example, a palmtop computer could be programmed so that the recording of the target event triggers a series of fixed-interval assessments at intervals that allow for systematic mapping of the time course of symptoms following the event. One important use of such designs is to assess time to onset for medication effects. For example, participants could be asked to record the onset of a migraine, at which time they are prompted to take a medication. A series of migraine assessments at regular intervals would then follow until symptoms had regressed to background levels. (Of course, the interval would be chosen to reflect the expected rate of change in symptoms, based on what is known about both the condition and the drug.) This would provide a complete account of the trajectory of symptoms following medication, from which time to effect can be computed. If patients are randomized to two drugs, or active and placebo drug, trajectories of relief can easily be compared.

GUARD PROMPTS FOR COMPLIANCE

A completely different reason to add interval assessments to an event-based protocol is to promote compliance with recording of events. The idea is to prompt the participant to monitor and record events on occasions when an unreasonable amount of time has passed since an event was last recorded. A recent study of overactive bladder (OAB) (McKenzie, Paty, Grogan, et al., 2004) illustrates the approach. Participants with OAB were asked to monitor episodes of urination (their primary symptom), recording them as events on a palmtop-based diary.

Based on knowledge of OAB symptoms and the patient population, it was determined that participants who had gone 8 hours without entering an event might be neglecting the protocol. Accordingly, after an interval of 8 hours without an event, they were prompted, reminded to monitor urination, and given an opportunity to report any urination events they had missed in the interim. The protocol was very successful in eliciting timely entry of urination events (McKenzie et al., 2004).

The use of reminder or guard prompts requires very careful consideration and design, however; prompting too often can have untoward effects. In a poorly designed protocol, the guard prompts may give participants the impression that they need not actively monitor events, but may simply wait for the guard prompt. Overly frequent guard prompts may also be highly reactive (e.g., prompting OAB patients to void voluntarily), thereby disturbing the phenomenon being measured. Used carefully, however, guard prompts can be useful for achieving good compliance in event-based monitoring.

EMA-Based within-Subject Experimental Studies

Of course, EMA methods data can be used as an assessment tool in the context of traditional between-person experimental studies. Beyond this, EMA methods can be extended to the experimental intervention itself, by randomizing treatment occasions (not people) to the experimental or control treatment. For example, when a participant in a headache study records a headache event, the EMA device can randomly direct him or her to take a nap (intervention #1) or take an aspirin (intervention #2) (or direct him or her to a particular pill from a dispenser that carries both test and control pills).

Randomization could also be stratified by headache severity or time of day, since these can be known at the time of randomization in the field. Follow-up observations, perhaps using the fixed-time follow-up approach described earlier, can assess the outcome of the intervention. Of course, such designs are useful only when the treatment is reactive to the target event, when the treatment has immediate effects and little carryover, and when such a crossover design is otherwise desirable. This design can be very powerful because it eliminates between-subject variation and provides for multiple assessments of the treatment effect.

Changes in EMA Protocol within a Single Study

Based on the objectives and design of a study, the investigator can often select an EMA approach that best fits the study. However, the study design and objectives may sometimes require shifting among multiple EMA protocols to accommodate different phases of the study or different patterns of subject behavior. For example, a clinical trial may include a transition from a baseline phase, in which no treatment is administered, to a treatment phase where the subject is instructed to take a pill at certain times or in response to emergent events. The EMA protocol may then need to shift to accommodate event-based recording of medication events, in addition to monitoring of symptoms.

Obviously, both protocols must be carefully designed to meet their respective objectives, and participants must be prepared for the transition and trained in both protocols. The trigger and process for transitioning must also be carefully thought through. The transition might be managed and activated by the investigative staff (as in the example above). But the transition can also be triggered "in the field," either by the passage of time (e.g., after n days of protocol #1) or by the content of the EMA data (e.g., after a certain number if events have been recorded, or when symptoms reach a predefined threshold). For example, in a recent study of smokers who were lapsing to smoking after a period of abstinence (Shiffman, Hickcox, Paty, et al., 1996), participants who had smoked at least five cigarettes on 3 consecutive days were considered to have fully relapsed. When this event was recognized, the computer-driven protocol changed so that participants were no longer asked to track lapse episodes.

Protocols with multiple EMA modalities place an extra burden on the investigator (for planning and programming) and on the participants (to learn both protocols), but they can often be optimal or even essential to collecting appropriate EMA data as transitions in experimental conditions or subject behavior occur. In sum, investigators must carefully consider the arrangement and scheduling of EMA assessments over the course of an EMA study.

Additional Considerations in EMA Protocols

Devices Used for EMA Data Collection

EMA data collection requires a device for collecting and recording data. It may be as simple as paper and pencil or as high-tech as a palmtop computer. The devices are used to support five functions:

1. Present assessment content (i.e., display questions and available response options), if self-report data are being collected;
2. Manage the logic of the assessment (e.g., enforce skip patterns, if applicable, test data for validity of the responses, etc.). In self-report data, formal validity tests may involve range checking and/or consistency with other responses; physiological data may be tested for range or conformity to other criteria;
3. Record the data in a secure form;
4. Time-stamp data to document time of completion; research has shown that subjects' reports of when data were entered are not reliable (Litt, Cooney, & Morse, 1998; Stone et al., 2002);
5. Manage the schedule of assessments (e.g., determine when an assessment is to be made). If the protocol calls for the scheduling to vary

with conditions, the device must be able to handle such responsive scheduling;

6. Prompt the subject, if the protocol involves active prompting.

Table 3-2 shows a range of devices and their support of various functions. For example, paper-and-pencil diaries present assessment content and record data, but they do not time-stamp the entries, and evidence indicates that some paper diaries are often hoarded and backfilled (Stone et al., 2002). Paper diaries also do not manage assessment schedules or enforce assessment logic and are notorious for generating out-of-range data, violations of skip patterns, etc. (Quinn, Goka, & Richardson, 2003).

In protocols requiring prompting, paper diaries may be combined with a separate prompting device such as a beeper or programmable watch to provide that function, but this does not necessarily ensure timely data recording (Broderick, Schwartz, Shiffman, et al., 2003). These auxiliary devices are not part of the diary itself (i.e., they have no data collection or recording capacity) but serve solely for prompting. Some studies have used automated telephone systems (interactive voice response [IVR]; Collins, Kashdan, & Gollnisch, 2003) to collect data. The IVR systems use normal phone calls to prompt subjects with prerecorded prompts and questions, and receive input via the telephone keypad and the tones it generates (*"If you had a migraine today, press 1...."*). The central system can manage assessment logic. The IVR systems have been used primarily to receive incoming calls, but they can in principle be extended to outbound calls, which would enable them to manage assessment schedules and support prompting (see Glanz, Shigaki, Farzanfar, et al., 2003). Portability would require the use of cellular phones. Palmtop computers are increasingly used in EMA studies; the on-board logic can manage intricate assessment protocols as well as complex and responsive scheduling, while built-in beeping or vibrating signals can support prompting, and the on-board clock makes time-stamping of entries or other events (e.g., missed assessments) possible. As seen in Table 3-2, palmtop computers currently provide the broadest range of functions for EMA studies.

Devices for collecting physiological data may not need capabilities to present self-report assessments or capture self-report data, but many do include inherent functions for scheduling assessments at regular intervals and for checking the validity of recordings. Specialized devices may record certain events; for example, there are instrumented medication devices that make a time-stamped record every time they are activated (Berg, Dunbar-Jacob, & Rohay, 1998). In studies that collect biological samples via EMA protocols (e.g., Van Eck, Berkhof, Nicolson, et al., 1996), there is an unsolved need for time-stamping to ensure timeliness and for a method to assess the adequacy of the sample.

Portability is an essential feature of EMA devices when the aim is to capture data at representative moments, since the device should travel with the subjects in the environments they typically inhabit. This limits the applicability of otherwise capable devices like laptops and web-based systems. To state the obvious, cost and logistics weigh into selecting a method for data collection. Each investigator

Table 3-2. Devices used for collection of EMA data

Device/technology	Recording, Prompting, or both	Self-report	Manage assessment logic[1]	Record data	Time-stamp[2]	Manage scheduling			Portable
						Predefined[4]	Responsive[5]	Prompting[3]	
Paper	r	Y	×	✓	×	×	×	×	✓
Tape recorder	r	Y	×	✓	×	×	×	×	✓
Web	r	Y	✓	✓	✓	✓/×[6]	×	×	×
Physiological monitor	r	N	✓	✓	✓	×	×	×	✓
Event recorders[7]	r	N	✓	✓	✓	×	×	×	✓
Biological sample[8]	r	N	×	✓	×	×	×	×	✓
Beeper	p	–	×	×	×	✓	×	✓	✓
Watch	p	–	×	×	×	✓	×	✓	✓
IVR inbound	r	Y	✓	✓	✓	✓	×	×	×/✓[9]
IVR with outbound	p+r	Y	✓	✓	✓	✓	✓[10]	✓	×/✓[7]
Laptop computer	p+r	Y	✓	✓	✓	✓	✓	✓	×
Palmtop computer	p+r	Y	✓	✓	✓	✓	✓	✓	✓

✓ Function is supported

× Function is not supported

– Not applicable: device does not record data

1 Includes enforcing skip patterns and ensuring in-range and formally correct data

2 Data records are stamped with date and time of completion

3 Includes ability to proactively prompt the user (e.g., by "beeping")

4 For example, random scheduling or other, arbitrary, schedule that can be predefined

5 Allowing for change in scheduling in response to data received

6 Usually handle only fixed time schedules

7 For example, instrumented medication containers

8 Devices for collecting biological sample (e.g., saliva, breath, etc.)

9 If use cell phone

10 Requires connection between database, programming, and outbound calling

must decide the appropriate trade-off of cost and burden for capability, data quality, and validity. Cost considerations need to encompass the entire research process. High-tech devices often require substantially upfront expense. However, paper diaries often incur high costs at later steps such as data entry and validation.

Conceptualizing EMA Studies and the Role of Time

The EMA data can be used to address a variety of research hypotheses. It is important that the investigator carefully formulate the study objectives and hypotheses as a starting point for developing an EMA protocol (see Bolger et al., 2003, for a useful discussion and framework). Since they sample the person repeatedly over time, EMA data are particularly well suited to addressing hypotheses about within-person variation in behavior or experience over time. Nevertheless, EMA data can be fruitfully used to address "atemporal" between-person differences, such as differences between patients who are given one treatment versus another (e.g., Shiffman et al., 2000). In this instance, the use of EMA methods is not intended to focus on variation over time, but to improve the reliability and validity of measurement.

The aggregation of repeated assessments damps out the noisiness of single assessments, thereby improving reliability and enhancing study sensitivity or power (see, for example, McKenzie et al., 2004). The benefit of increased sensitivity and power is enormous: it enables the investigator to detect smaller effects or, conversely, allows the study to proceed with a much smaller sample size. The validity of assessment is improved by minimizing bias due to retrospective recall and other biases inherent in global assessment. Because behavior and experience vary over time (even if time is not the central interest), the reliability and validity of assessment are improved by achieving a representative sampling of experience or behavior over time.

In some studies, events rather than persons are of central interest, but variation over time is still regarded as unimportant. People may be studied over time merely to allow for specific events to be observed and described; for example, the investigator may wish to describe the phenomenology of symptom episodes such as panic attacks. A special case occurs when the investigator seeks data on events that are unique rather than recurrent (e.g., the very first cigarette ever smoked; Eissenberg & Balster, 2000). In this instance, individuals at risk for the event may need to be observed for long periods in order to observe these singular events. In these instances, time is not an important part of the design or analysis; it is simply what passes as one waits for the target events to occur.

More often, EMA methods are applied in studies where the within-subject variation over time is of central interest. In some studies, time itself is the variable of interest. EMA methods can be used to analyze temporal patterns in experience, such as cyclical patterns, where time is seen as reflecting some underlying cyclical process (e.g., circadian rhythms, menstrual rhythms). In some cases, the investigator may not be focused on such systematic patterns of variation in the target phenomenon, but simply is establishing the degree of variation over time.

For such time-based hypotheses, it does not matter what period of time is sampled; any time will do. In other instances, the investigator is not interested in variation over time, per se, but in the time course of experience following a particular event or starting point. In the simplest case, one might assess a change in behavior between baseline and intervention periods (e.g., McKenzie et al., 2004); here "time" effects capture the effects of the intervention or experimental manipulation. Investigators might also be interested in the trajectory of experience following onset of disease, in the natural history of the phenomenon under study, or in response to an event, which can either be an externally imposed event (e.g., the course of symptoms after an episode of chemotherapy; Basen-Engquist, Chapter 12, this volume) or a naturally occurring event captured by EMA data (e.g., a bout of drinking; Collins, Chapter 10, this volume). In these instances, the timeline under investigation is rooted in a triggering event or milestone.

In many EMA studies, the linear passage of time, per se, is not of interest, but variation over time simply provides opportunities to observe variation and covariation in relevant events or experiences. Thus, an investigator might be interested in how mood differs when subjects are smoking versus when they are not (e.g., Mermelstein, Chapter 6, this volume). "Time" is not an element in these hypotheses or the analyses, which organize the observations collected over time according to their attributes (smoking or not smoking). Similarly, an investigator might be interested in the covariation of continuous phenomena over time (e.g., whether psychosocial stress is associated with concurrent heart rate or blood pressure; for example, Kamarck, Chapter 14, this volume).

An extension of this "covariation" approach may use lagged observations (e.g., to evaluate how today's fatigue affects tomorrow's mood) to address the limitation in interpreting concurrent phenomena. This approach reintroduces time into the equation, but only in the sense of being sensitive to temporal sequence (i.e., whether changes in fatigue precede changes in mood). In any case, in most EMA studies, the sampling of behavior and experience over time is crucial to the research question, even if time, per se, is not an element of the hypotheses or analyses.

Limitations on Inferences from EMA Data

EMA data often yield richly detailed data sets that provide a vast number of observations for analysis (with concomitant statistical power) and rich insights into the participants' behavior. EMA methods also can help eliminate several confounds that plague global self-report data. However, the EMA investigator must stay aware of the usual limits and caveats that may limit interpretation of the data. EMA studies are often correlational in design, relating variation on one variable (e.g., stress) with variation in another (e.g., blood pressure). Such observed associations among variables in EMA data are correlational and may not imply causation. For example, stress and blood pressure could covary because participants are stressed at work, where they engage in physical movement and drink coffee, which in turn raises blood pressure. It is important to consider a priori possible confounding variables that may account for observed correlations and, where possible, to collect data about the confounding variables, so that they can be statistically controlled in the analysis (e.g., Kamarck, Chapter 14, this volume, controls for physical activity and coffee drinking in assessing effects of stress on blood pressure). Some of the confounds (but not all) that undermine inferences from concurrent correlational data can also be addressed by providing for time-lagged or prospective analyses.

Common sources of confounding influence in ecological data include the effects of time of day (e.g., drinking tends to occur in the evening and therefore is associated with low arousal), day of week (e.g., weekend vs. weekday), and concurrent activities or states (see example above about blood pressure). These confounds can be statistically controlled if the necessary observations are available. Ideally, such analyses are considered when the EMA study is designed, so that the protocol can ensure adequate data for these statistical controls. However, it is not possible to assess all confounding variables or assess them perfectly, so investigators must exercise appropriate caution in making causal inferences from correlational EMA data.

Some confounds that may infect EMA data cannot be addressed in the analysis because the relevant data are missing. Nonresponse and missing diary entries are often a source of bias. In event-based recording, participants may fail to record some events, and participants engaged in time-based recording may fail to complete entries at the appointed time. It cannot be assumed that the occasions that elicit nonresponse are random. For example, participants may fail to note an episode when the symptoms are mild, or may fail to respond to prompting when they are emotionally upset or when symptoms are particularly intense, thus biasing the sample of occasions that is available for analysis. For this reason, achieving high compliance with EMA monitoring is crucial to the integrity of the design. Steps to achieve this, including participant training and monitoring, compliance feedback and prompting, and careful diary design, are very important.

EMA investigators must also be sensitive to the possibility that the demands of an EMA protocol could limit the range of participants who can be recruited into a trial, and thus reduce the representativeness of the subject sample. For example, participants in certain jobs (e.g., assembly-line workers, surgeons) may be unable to accommodate being beeped or completing assessments during the working day. Technology used in the study may also limit the sample, if some people are unwilling to be "wired" or others are intimidated by or unable to use the technology. However, concerns about these issues should not be based on mere intuition or prejudice; for example, evidence suggests that older adults are able to effectively use electronic diaries (Kamarck, Chapter 14, this volume). Conversely, certain conditions (e.g., blindness, deafness) would obviously affect the kind of methodology that could be used.

EMA methods also do not eliminate all of the difficulties that attend interpretation of self-report data. While recall bias is minimized, other factors can still undermine the validity of self-report. For example, participants may lie about their state or may have limited access to or insight into their condition.

Again, awareness of method limitations and appropriate circumspection in one's inferences and conclusions are indicated. EMA methods can substantially improve the reliability and validity of data, but when interpreting such data, it is important to still bear in mind the limits of self-report and the potential of other influences on the data.

Conclusions

Much as investigators must thoughtfully consider research design and interpretation of data in any study, EMA investigators must give careful attention to the design of EMA protocols. Because EMA studies aim to sample participants' experience in highly variable real-world settings, issues of representative sampling become paramount. In this chapter I have outlined some of the issues EMA investigators must consider and some examples of EMA designs that investigators can choose. These by no means exhaust the possible design options, and EMA investigators will undoubtedly develop yet-unthought-of designs to creatively answer new research questions.

EMA is not a series of fixed protocols, but an approach to understanding real-world experience and behavior by sampling it repeatedly over time. Accordingly, the EMA protocol must, first and foremost, be dictated by the investigator's research question and by the structure of the phenomenon being studied. With good design, EMA studies can yield new insights into behaviors and experiences that influence health.

References

Benowitz, N. L. (1983). The use of biologic fluid samples in assessing tobacco smoke consumption. *NIDA Research Monograph, 48*, 6–26.

Berg, J., Dunbar-Jacob, J., & Rohay, J. M. (1998). Compliance with inhaled medications: The relationship between diary and electronic monitor. *Annals of Behavioral Medicine, 20*, 36–38.

Bolger, N., Davis, A., & Rafaeli, E. (2003). Diary methods: Capturing life as it is lived. *Annual Review of Psychology, 54*, 579–616.

Bradburn, N. M., Rips, U., & Shevell, S. K. (1987). Answering autobiographical questions: The impact of memory and inference on surveys. *Science, 236*, 157–161.

Broderick, J. E., Schwartz, J. E., Shiffman, S., Hufford, M. R., & Stone, A. A. (2003). Signaling does not adequately improve diary compliance. *Annals of Behavioral Medicine, 26*, 139–148.

Checkoway, H. (2004). Case-crossover designs in occupational health. *Occupational and Environmental Medicine, 61*, 953–954.

Clark, D. M., & Teasdale, J. D. (1982). Diurnal variation in clinical depression and accessibility of memories of positive and negative experiences. *Journal of Abnormal Psychology, 91*, 87–95.

Collins, R. L., Kashdan, T. B., & Gollnisch, G. (2003). The feasibility of using cellular phones to collect ecological momentary assessment data: Application to alcohol consumption. *Experimental and Clinical Psychopharmacology, 11*, 73–78.

Cramer, J. A., Mattson, R. H., Prevey, M. L., Scheyer, R. D., & Ouellette, V. L. (1989). How often is medication taken as prescribed? A novel assessment technique. *JAMA, 261,* 3273–3277.

Csikszentmihalyi, M., & Larson, R. (1987). Validity and reliability of the experience-sampling method. *Journal of Nervous and Mental Disease, 175,* 509–513.

Duncan, E., & Grazzani-Gavazzi, I. (2004). Positive emotional experiences in Scottish and Italian young adults: A diary study. *Journal of Happiness Studies, 5,* 359–384.

Eissenberg, T., & Balster, R. L. (2000). Initial tobacco use episodes in children and adolescents: Current knowledge, future directions. *Drug & Alcohol Dependence, 59,* S41–S60.

Freeman, L. M. Y., & Gil, K. M. (2004). Daily stress, coping, and dietary restraint in binge eating. *International Journal of Eating Disorders, 36,* 204–212.

Glanz, K., Shigaki, D., Farzanfar, R., Pinto, B., Kaplan, B., & Friedman, R. H. (2003). Participant reactions to a computerized telephone system for nutrition and exercise counseling. *Patient Education & Counseling, 49,* 157–163.

Gwaltney, C. J., Shiffman, S., & Sayette, M. A. (2005). Situational correlates of abstinence self-efficacy. *Journal of Abnormal Psychology, 114,* 649–660.

Huttenlocher, J., Hedges, L. V., & Bradburn, N. M. (1990). Reports of elapsed time: Bounding and rounding processes in estimation. *Journal of Experimental Psychology: Learning, Memory, & Cognition, 16,* 196–213.

Litt, M. D., Cooney, N. L., & Morse, P. (1998). Ecological momentary assessment (EMA) with treated alcoholics: Methodological problems and potential solutions. *Health Psychology, 17,* 48–52.

Maclure, M. (1991). The case-crossover design: A method for studying transient effects on the risk of acute events. *American Journal of Epidemiology, 133,* 144–153.

McDonald, D. A., & Almeida, D. M. (2004). The interweave of fathers' daily work experiences and fathering behaviors. *Fathering, 2,* 235–251.

McFall, R. M. (1977). Parameters of self-monitoring. In R. B. Stuart (Ed.), *Behavioral self-management: Strategies, techniques, and outcome* (pp. 196–214). New York: Brunner/Mazel.

McKenzie, S., Paty, J. A., Grogan, D., Rossano, M., Curry, L., Sciarappa, K., & Hufford, M. (2004). Proving the eDiary dividend. *Applied Clinical Trials, 13*(6), 54–58.

Park, C. L., Armeli, S., & Tennen, H. (2004). Appraisal-coping goodness of fit: A daily Internet study. *Personality & Social Psychology Bulletin, 30,* 558–569.

Paty, J. A., Kassel, J. D., & Shiffman, S. (1992). The importance of assessing base rates for clinical studies: An example of stimulus control of smoking. In M. DeVries (Ed.), *The experience of psychopathology* (pp. 347–352). Cambridge, England: Cambridge University Press.

Quinn, P., Goka, J., & Richardson, H. (2003). Assessment of an electronic daily diary in patients with overactive bladder. *British Journal of Urology, 91,* 647.

Rathbun, S., Shiffman, S., & Gwaltney, C. (2005). Point process models for the social sciences. In Walls, T. A., & Schafer, J. S. (Eds.), *Models for intensive longitudinal data.* New York: Oxford University Press.

Shiffman, S. (2000). Comments on craving. *Addiction, 95* (Supplement 2), S171–S175.

Shiffman, S., Engberg, J., Paty, J. A., Perz, W., Gnys, M., Kassel, J. D., & Hickcox, M. (1997). A day at a time: Predicting smoking lapse from daily urge. *Journal of Abnormal Psychology, 106,* 104–116.

Shiffman, S., Gwaltney, C. J., Balabanis, M., Liu, K. S., Paty, J. A., Kassel, J. D., Hickcox, M., & Gnys, M. (2002). Immediate antecedents of cigarette smoking: An analysis from ecological momentary assessment. *Journal of Abnormal Psychology, 111,* 531–545.

Shiffman, S., Hickcox, M., Paty, J. A., Gnys, M., Kassel, J. D., & Richards, T. (1996). Progression from a smoking lapse to relapse: Prediction from abstinence violation effects and nicotine dependence. *Journal of Consulting and Clinical Psychology, 64,* 993–1002.

Shiffman, S., Elash, C. A., Paton, S., Gwaltney, C. J., Paty, J. A., Clark, D. B., Liu, K. S., & Di Marino, M. E. (2000). Comparative efficacy of 24-hour and 16-hour transdermal nicotine patch for relief of craving and withdrawal. *Addiction, 95*(8), 1185–1195.

Shiffman, S., & Paty, J. A. (2003). Using an electronic diary to capture frequent events. In Poster presented at a meeting entitled, *From quality of life to patient outcomes assessment: research agenda for a paradigm shift.* Drug Information Association.

Shiffman, S., & Paty, J. A. (2006). Smoking patterns of non-dependent smokers: Contrasting chippers and dependent smokers. *Journal of Abnormal Psychology, 115,* 509–523.

Shiffman, S., Paty, J. A., Gnys, M., Kassel, J. D., & Hickcox, M. (1996). First lapses to smoking: Within-subjects analyses of real-time reports. *Journal of Consulting and Clinical Psychology, 64,* 366–379.

Shiffman, S., & Waters, A. J. (2004). Negative affect and smoking lapses: A prospective analysis. *Journal of Consulting and Clinical Psychology, 72*(2), 192–201.

Stone, A. A., & Shiffman, S. (1994). Ecological momentary assessment (EMA) in behavioral medicine. *Annals of Behavioral Medicine, 16,* 199–202.

Stone, A. A., Shiffman, S., Schwartz, J. E., Broderick, J. E., & Hufford, M. R. (2002). Patient non-compliance with paper diaries. *British Medical Journal, 324,* 1193–1194.

Teasdale, J. D., & Fogarty, S. J. (1979). Differential effects of induced mood on retrieval of pleasant and unpleasant events from episodic memory. *Journal of Abnormal Psychology, 88,* 248–257.

Tiffany, S. T. (1990). A cognitive model of drug urges and drug use behavior: Role of automatic and non-automatic processes. *Psychological Review, 97,* 147–168.

van Eck, M. M., Berkhof, H., Nicolson, N. A., & Sulon, J. (1996). The effects of perceived stress, traits, mood states, and stressful events on salivary cortisol. *Psychosomatic Medicine, 58,* 447–458.

Wheeler, L., & Reis, H. T. (1991). Self-recording of everyday life events: Origins, types, and uses. *Journal of Personality, 59,* 339–354.

Yip, T., & Cross, W. E. Jr. (2004). A daily diary study of mental health and community involvement outcomes for three Chinese American social identities. *Cultural Diversity and Ethnic Minority Psychology, 10,* 394–408.

4

Special Methodological Challenges and Opportunities in Ecological Momentary Assessment

Michael R. Hufford

Ecological Momentary Assessment (EMA) methods have the potential to dramatically enhance the ecological validity of research findings by helping researchers move their assessments out of the laboratory and into the daily lives of their subjects. For EMA to be successful—both in terms of researchers' ability to implement these methods and having the resulting data inform research programs—a variety of unique methodological issues raised by these methods must be considered and addressed.

This chapter presents a brief overview of the rationale for real-time data collection, especially as it places a premium on subject compliance with the EMA protocols. The empirical literature that has examined subject compliance with field-based data collection is then reviewed. Several specific methodological issues are then discussed, including subject reactivity to EMA methods, how to achieve a reasonable sampling burden for subjects, subjects' own evaluations of different EMA reporting platforms in terms of their ease of use, and psychometric issues to be considered when moving from paper to electronic data collection methods.

Real-Time Data Collection

> "The palest ink is better than the best memory."
> —Chinese proverb

The value of EMA data rests on a fundamental proposition—by overcoming recall inaccuracies and biases that affect patient-reported outcome (PRO) data, we can better understand subjects' experiences. That is, if it were possible for subjects to accurately recall details of their daily lives—days, weeks, or months after they have occurred—researchers could simply rely on subjects' recall of events, saving the time and energy involved in using real-time data collection methods. Unfortunately, a large body of empirical research has shown that recall is both inaccurate and systematically biased (Stone, Shiffman, & DeVries, 2000). The net result of this literature is to undermine what has been called the "reappearance hypothesis;" that is, the belief that a faithful copy of experience is kept in the mind, which can then be recalled at a later time (Schacter, 1996).

We now know that the process of recall relies on a variety of mental shortcuts, or heuristic strategies, to reconstruct past events. This retrospective reconstruction of experience is imperfect and vulnerable to a range of biases. Each step in the recall process has the potential to introduce inaccuracy and bias into PRO data. For example, in order for any memory content to be available for later recall, it must first be encoded into memory. Encoding is always incomplete and imperfect and is influenced by a variety of processes (Tourangeau, 2000). Whether something is encoded at all is influenced by its perceived salience at the time, which may be a function of the person's subjective state at the time of the event (Erickson & Jemison, 1991; Linton, 1991). Thus, subjects' memories of symptoms and events do not start with an objective, accurate record, but are both error- and bias-prone from the start of the encoding process.

When subjects are asked by researchers to subsequently recall an encoded experience, they do not simple retrieve and "replay" the experience in question, as the reappearance hypothesis suggests. Rather, a variety of heuristics are used to actively reconstruct the information. As outlined in Table 4-1, a variety of heuristics are known to affect the recall of PRO data.

Table 4-1. Recall biases affecting PRO datas

Type of heuristic	Explanation
Availability	More salient (e.g., severe symptoms), recent, or unusual events are more likely to influence recall than other events (Joffe et al., 1989; Wagenaar, 1986).
Recency	More recent events are more accessible to memory and, as a result, have a disproportionate impact on the recall of PRO data (Shiffman et al., 1997).
State biases	Like setting effects, state biases affect PRO data by virtue of making certain content more accessible than others. For example, people are more likely to retrieve negatively valenced information when they are in a negative mood, thus introducing substantial bias (Clark & Teasdale, 1982, 1985).
Saliency	The personal relevance of an experience can affect encoding and retrieval, as salient, more intense experiences are more likely to be encoded and subsequently recalled (Menon & Yorkton, 2000).

(Continued)

Table 4-1. (Continued)

Type of heuristic	Explanation
Effort after meaning	People's natural and unconscious tendency is to recon-strue events so as to make them consistent with subsequent events (Brown & Harris, 1978; Eich et al., 1985; Means et al., 1994; Ross, 1989). For example, one study found that the degree of fatigue retrospectively reported by radiation therapy subjects prior to treatment was actually influenced by whether their fatigue increased or decreased following the radiation treatment. In other words, when recalling their pretreatment fatigue, some subjects overestimated and others underestimated it in light of their subsequent reaction to treatment (Sprangers et al., 1999).
Instruction set	One often overlooked source of error in retrospective reports is participants' misunderstanding of questionnaire instruction sets that require them to aggregate and summa-rize their experience in the recent past. For example, Bailey and Martin (2000) analyzed subjects' understanding of what time interval "past month" referred to during completion of quality of life questionnaires across 11 studies. If participants were asked on the 15th of a month to recall the past month, only 64% correctly interpreted "past month" to refer to the period from the 15th of the current month to the 15th of the previous month. In other words, 36% of participants used an incorrect interval as the basis of their recall (for example, some participants used the past 2 weeks only, the entire month previous to the current month, or a 6-week period as the basis for their recall).
Aggregation	The aggregation of experiences, once recalled, is a source of bias. This type of cognitive processing is necessary to respond to questions about the occurrence or frequency of events ("*How many headaches did you have this week?*") or their average or typical characteristics ("*How much gastric discomfort did you have this week?*"). For example, research shows that subjects' recall of their "average" pain is heavily influenced by the saliency (peak pain) and recency (pain intensity at the end of the episode) of their pain experience during the recall interval (Eich et al., 1985; Redelmeier & Kahneman, 1996; Stone et al., 2000).

Subject Compliance and EMA

The empirical literature supporting the inaccuracies and biases resulting from a reliance on recall is one of the key reasons that researchers began using diary methods in the first place (Hufford & Shiffman, 2002; Verbrugge, 1980). The move to field-based data collection carried with it the promise of avoiding recall biases and capturing data closer in time to events and symptoms of interest. However, EMA methods also shift the burden of remembering to make timely entries onto the participants. For example, if they routinely fail to complete their diaries in a timely way—by hoarding and backfilling them in what some researchers euphemistically refer to as "parking lot compliance"—then the data are vulnerable to the very recall biases that motivated the transition to EMA from in-clinic research in the first place. In short, EMA fundamentally relies on participants to be compliant with the data collection protocol.

There is a rich—although by no means celebrated—history of subjects being noncompliant with almost all aspects of research protocols, from scheduled site visits (Gendreau, Hufford, & Stone, 2003), to medication taking (e.g., Boudes, 1998; Urquhart, 1994) and diary compliance (Stone, Shiffman, Schwartz, et al., 2002). A common assumption is that subject noncompliance is bothersome at worst, and it will not meaningfully affect the conclusions of a study. This is a questionable assumption on several levels.

Subject noncompliance with research protocols is not necessarily random. As a result, the impact of noncompliance is not simply "noise" in the data, but systematic bias. For example, a study among type I diabetics by Mazze and colleagues (1984) found that not only did the electronic monitoring of glucose levels fail to correspond to paper diary entries, but also the errors were systematic. Fully two thirds of subjects reported glucose values in their paper diaries so as to obscure hyper- and hypoglycemia, leading to biased clinical impressions of their glycemic control. In other words, they adjusted their glucose readings up or down, most likely in an attempt to appear to have their glycemia under better control than was actually the case. This is a sobering finding— noncompliance can obscure a clear picture of subjects' true disease state. The implications of these sorts of biases as a function of noncompliance can be serious for both researchers and clinicians. For example, in severe cases of urinary incontinence, diary data are used to establish the baseline severity of voiding to help decide whether surgery is needed. If subjects overestimate their symptom severity by backfilling many diary entries immediately before a site visit, the potential exists for recall bias to lead to an inappropriate surgical intervention.

The application of EMA methods to the collection of PRO data has been historically grounded in four potential advantages that they offer to clinical research (Stone & Shiffman, 1994; Verbrugge, 1980). First, recall problems are avoided if subjects make their entries in real time. Second, the repeated completion of assessments in a diary potentially adds to the reliability of the data by allowing aggregation of multiple assessments over time. Aggregation of multiple measures reduces noise in data (i.e., unreliability), making the measurement more sensitive to treatment effects (Nived, Sturfelt, Eckernas, et al., 1994). Third, EMA data are more representative of subject experience in everyday life, because subjects repeatedly provide data in real-world settings. This increase in "ecological validity" ensures that the data represent actual real-life experience and are generalizable to clinical application (Shiffman, 2000; Stone, Shiffman, & DeVries, 2000). Finally, the richness of momentary diary data potentially allows for a more detailed analysis of treatment effects, particularly with regard to processes that exert their influence over time. Thus, it is possible to examine trends in PRO data over time (e.g., assessing speed of pain relief as well as overall efficacy), the relationship of medication effects to adherence, or their relationship to other variables (e.g., stress, diet, workload). Studies confirm that diaries can detect treatment-related effects in PRO data that otherwise would have been missed if the data were collected only during research site visits (e.g., Houpt, McMillan, Wein, et al., 1999; Norman, McFarlane, Streiner, et al., 1982).

Of these four potential advantages of EMA methods, the issue of compliance with the intensive sampling schemes has recently received the most empirical attention. Subject noncompliance to EMA protocols can potentially undermine the validity and sensitivity of the data. Many researchers can testify to having caught more than one subject diligently backfilling a week's worth of diary cards before a site visit. Indeed, the pattern of increased subject compliance with medication administration that occurs immediately before a research site visit is so common that it has its own name—white coat compliance (Urquhart, 1994; Urquhart & De Klerk, 1998).

Diary compliance has been objectively, though indirectly, assessed in eight studies that used various instrumented devices (e.g., inhalers, blood glucose monitors) to track the actual time and date of events recorded in the diary (Chmelik & Doughty, 1994; Jonasson, Carlsen, Sodal, et al., 1999; Mazze et al., 1984; Milgrom, Bender, Akcerson, et al., 1996; Simmons, Nides, Rand, et al., 2000; Spector, Kinsman, Mawhinney, et al., 1986; Straka, Fish, Benson, et al., 1997; Verschelden, Cartier, L'Archeveque, et al., 1996). The correspondence between these data from the instrumented devices and the paper diary entries were then compared to one another. A dramatic difference between subjects' reported versus actual compliance was observed across the studies. Whereas the paper diaries appeared to indicate high rates of compliance (88%), the objectively validated actual rates of compliance with usage of the instrumented medical device were significantly lower (54%). In other words, almost 40 percent of the paper diaries were false, due to a mix of subject data entry errors and outright backfilling and falsification of data.

A study published in the *British Medical Journal* directly measured compliance to both paper and electronic diaries (Stone et al., 2002). The study was designed to document actual subject compliance with paper diaries. Subject compliance was assessed using a newly developed instrumented paper diary (IPD) that electronically tracked diary use unobtrusively. Photosensors built into the paper diary triggered an electronic record of the date and time of each diary opening and closing. Compliance rates from this IPD were compared with those achieved using a compliance-enhanced electronic diary (ED). The primary objective of the study was to quantify compliance with paper diaries.

Eighty chronic pain subjects were assigned to use the IPD or the ED to record their pain over a 3-week period. All subjects were asked to complete a pain assessment thrice daily (10 a.m., 4 p.m., and 8 p.m.). Two types of compliance were analyzed: reported compliance (based on the time and date handwritten on completed diary cards) and actual compliance (based on the time and date record that was automatically recorded by the diary devices). The EDs allowed entries to be made only during a window of ±15 minutes around the scheduled assessment times and incorporated features to enhance compliance, such as sounding an alarm at the time of assessment and on-screen feedback if an assessment was missed (Shiffman, Paty, Gnys, et al., 1996). The diary data were collected from the IPD and ED participants at weekly clinic visits, and they were given feedback and instructions based on their evident performance. For participants using the IPDs, feedback was given regarding their submitted diary cards. For participants using the EDs, feedback was given regarding their actual compliance with timely completion of the diary.

The reported compliance in the IPD group was very high: participants submitted paper diary cards with handwritten dates and times corresponding to an average of 90 percent of assessment occasions. The objective record told a different story, however: actual compliance with the paper diaries was much lower, averaging only 11 percent (95% confidence interval [CI]: 8%–14%). Thus, 79 percent of paper diary cards were falsified. The pattern of noncompliance was informative. On 32 percent of study days, the IPD had not been opened at all, so participants had neglected their task for the entire day. However, they submitted 94 percent of the required cards for those days. More disturbing still, several participants also showed evidence of forward-filling their paper diary cards in advance of the actual time (Stone, Shiffman, Schwartz, et al., 2003).

In the ED group, actual compliance was 94 percent (95% CI: 91%–96%). In other words, subjects completed each pain report within the required 30-minute window 94 percent of the time. These high rates of subject compliance are consistent with findings from several peer-reviewed studies using a compliance-enhancing ED system (Shiffman et al., 1996; Tiplady, Crompton, Dewar, et al., 1997; Kamarck, Shiffman, Smithline, et al., 1998).

In a follow-on study, Broderick and colleagues (2003) tried to understand what factors of the ED system were responsible for the observed differences in actual compliance rates (Broderick, Schwartz, Shiffman, et al., 2003). A group of 27 chronic pain subjects were recruited and asked to complete the same diary protocol as in the earlier study, except that this time, participants were given programmable wristwatches to help remind them when to complete their paper diary cards. Once again, reported compliance was quite good, ranging from 85 to 91 percent. However, actual participant compliance with the paper diaries was 29 percent for the 30-minute compliance window and 39 percent for the 90-minute compliance window. Moreover, actual compliance dropped significantly during the 3-week study.

The unique IPD used by Stone and colleagues (2002, 2003) allowed for an objective assessment of paper diary compliance for the first time. The compliance findings from this study showed that participants were very noncompliant with the protocol when using paper diaries. Further, it demonstrated that compliance is often faked by participants using paper diaries, giving the false impression of good compliance. In contrast, the ED system delivered very high rates of compliance, demonstrating that the poor compliance seen in the paper diary group was not a function of the study sample.

Similar results suggesting participant noncompliance with paper diaries, focusing on the characteristics of the resulting diary data, have also been reported (Innocenti, Lauritsen, Hendel, et al., 2003). In a sample of 177 heartburn subjects, a significantly higher autocorrelation of symptoms was found among participants who used a paper diary to record their symptoms compared to those who used an electronic diary or interactive voice response systems (IVRS) to record their symptoms. The authors conclude that much of the paper diary data was entered after the fact, producing the observed artificially high rates of autocorrelation among the paper diary data.

Reasons for Subject Noncompliance

Why do so many participants fail to comply with data collection protocols? It is not because they are bad people. In volunteering for research projects, most participants are acting on a genuine desire to help researchers. But the hassles of everyday life and natural human forgetfulness can serve to dramatically compromise subject compliance if steps are not taken to help them adhere to the daily data collection.

The empirical literature on noncompliance, both with medication taking and diary completion, has not found any consistent relationship between noncompliance and demographic characteristics or disease severity (Chmelik & Doughty, 1994; Jonasson et al., 1999; Mazze et al., 1984; Milgrom et al., 1996; Simmons et al., 2000). As outlined in Table 4-2, a number of general factors likely play a role in producing subject noncompliance.

Promoting Compliance

As has been reviewed in detail elsewhere (Hufford & Shiffman, 2003), an examination of the medication and diary compliance literatures suggests that seven behavioral science principles can be used to enhance subject compliance to EMA protocols (Table 4-3).

The empirical literature shows that EMA studies using these principles tend to generate high rates of participant compliance across a variety of different protocols and therapeutic areas (e.g., Kamarck et al., 1998; Shiffman et al., 1996; Stone et al., 2002; Tiplady et al., 1997).

Compliance and EMA Reporting Platforms

Although it is possible to design a study that relies solely on participants to remember to make timed entries and record events as they occur, recent advances in EMA reporting platforms make it possible to help them to be compliant. EMA can be

Table 4-2. Reasons for subject noncompliance

Desire to please. A subject's desire to participate in clinical research and be a "good subject" may create motivation to retrospectively complete missed diary entries. Empirical evidence confirms that subjects' noncompliance can be related to whether they are aware that the researcher is tracking their compliance (Simmons et al., 2000).

Forgetting. Subjects are sometimes asked to make entries at varying intervals, requiring them to faithfully remember when to make diary entries. For complex diary protocols, or those that require multiple entries per day, the demand on working memory is even greater. Given the vagaries of human memory and the demands of daily living, it is not surprising that many subjects simply forget to make diary entries.

Monitoring burden. When diary entries are supposed to be cued by events, such as symptom flareups, the subject's diary burden becomes proportional to symptom severity or event frequency—that is, an increasing rate of symptoms can overwhelm subjects as they try to complete an assessment for each occurrence. Increasing subject burden as a result of an inflexible diary protocol can introduce systematic bias into the data because subjects may systematically stop entering symptoms because of reporting fatigue.

Lack of feedback. Like the rest of us, research subjects respond to incentives and cues. Some types of PRO data collection methods, such as paper diaries, make it difficult to comply and easy to be noncompliant with the data collection protocol. More broadly, paper diaries offer the subject no feedback regarding compliance. Without cues to structure subject behavior and incentives to establish and reward it, good and consistent compliance is difficult to achieve and maintain in the field.

---

implemented in a variety ways, including paper diaries, pager systems to cue paper-based recordings, electronic diaries, and IVRS.

The peer-reviewed literature suggests that subject compliance varies considerably depending on the EMA platform used to capture the data. It should be noted that any review of research methods collapsing across various studies risks highlighting certain findings about a reporting platform (e.g., mean rates of compliance) while ignoring other factors that may predict compliance (e.g., how well the platform was implemented by the research team). With that caveat, compliance findings from four different reporting platforms are reviewed—pager-based system, IVRS, paper diaries, and electronic diaries.

Radio-signaled pagers were frequently used in early experience sampling studies (Csikszentmihalyi & Larson, 1987). "Smart" wristwatches also have been used as the signaling device. These pager-based systems allow for individualized scheduling and have been frequently used in psychiatric studies in particular. Both pagers and "smart" wristwatches often have to limit their data collection to specific windows during the day, often between 8 a.m. and 8 p.m., to avoid waking subjects with varying sleep habits. This is far from trivial, as studies have found that up to 26 percent of randomly scheduled assessments during the waking day fell outside an 8 a.m. to 8 p.m. time window and assessments outside of this window differed significantly from assessments within the window (Shiffman, 2000). A very substantial

Table 4-3. Helping subjects to be compliant with EMA protocols

---

Build compliance into the protocol. Adherence considerations must be part of design, execution, and writeup of a research program (Stone & Shiffman, 2002). The EMA protocol should be structured so as to facilitate and reward subject compliance.

Subject training. To be adherent with the EMA protocol, subjects must be adequately trained by site personnel so that they understand what, exactly, is being asked of them (Verbrugge, 1980). Any diary or other PRO data collection method should be extremely simple and intuitive and therefore require little training regarding the system's basic functions.

User interface issues. Diaries and other methods of PRO data collection should be easy for subjects to use (Hufford et al., 2002). Ensuring that the user interface is friendly and intuitive is essential to enhance diary or other PRO data collection compliance.

"Drive" the protocol. Programmed reminders have consistently been found to improve adherence rates in clinical research (Hufford & Shields, 2002), though they are by no means a guarantee of high rates of compliance (Broderick et al., 2003). Real-time compliance reminders can be built into some PRO methods of data collection, such as electronic diaries, to prompt subjects to complete entries. Moreover, by providing subjects with timely, real-time compliance reminders, electronic diaries can encourage the type of habit-forming interactions with the data collection device that are characteristic of effective computer interfaces (Raskin, 2000).

Guide subjects through assessments. PRO data collection methods should easily handle complex branching within assessments. Rather than forcing participants to decide whether they should complete certain assessment items depending on their answers to other items, electronic EMA systems can be programmed to administer the correct items in the correct logical sequence.

"Livability" functions. Collecting real-time, real-world PRO data requires that participants incorporate the data collection system into their daily lives. As a result, field-based data collection systems should include a number of "livability" functions that help participants be compliant with the protocol. For example, functions allowing them to suspend any active "beeping" for sleeping at night, napping during the day, and when programmed reminders might be inappropriate (e.g., at church), all help participants remain adherent with the protocol. Empirically, it has been shown that the inclusion of these "livability" functions does not result in participants abusing them to avoid monitoring (Shiffman, 2000).

Create a sense of accountability. Participants are more compliant with protocols if they feel a sense of accountability for the data (Rabin et al., 1996; Urquhart, 1994). If they know that their compliance with the data collection protocol is being tracked, and they receive real-time feedback regarding their compliance, they tend to report feeling engaged in the study protocol. In other words, if participants know that they will be held accountable for their data, they tend to be more vigilant regarding their data entry (Simmons et al., 2000).

---

limitation of these signaling devices is that although issuance of the signal can be controlled or confirmed, timely compliance with assessments cannot.

Interactive voice response systems have been used for many years in surveys and business/administrative applications (see Corkrey & Parkinson, 2002, for a review).

These systems typically rely on participants to remember to make incoming calls to a central call center where they can electronically record answers to scripted questions using the telephone touchpad. More recently, IVRS applications have been developed that allow researchers to use cellular technology to actively place outgoing calls to participants to more dynamically sample their experiences. Rates of compliance in the IVRS literature vary from outstanding (e.g., 93%–96%; Mundt, Perrine, Searles, et al., 1995; Searles, Perrine, Mundt, et al., 1995; Weiler, Christ, Woodworth, et al., 2004) to very poor (e.g., 40%; Shiffman, Dresler, Hajek, et al., 2002).

As outlined above, several recent publications have directly assessed and contrasted participants' reported versus actual compliance with paper diaries (Stone et al., 2002, 2003). The findings are sobering. While reported compliance is outstanding, objective compliance appears to be much lower. In short, these data suggest that any claim of adequate compliance using paper diaries should be verified using some objective indicator of compliance.

Many researchers have successfully used daily mailing of paper diaries to help to ensure compliance on at least a daily basis with paper diaries. This is not a trivial enhancement. At the same time, for EMA protocols requiring more intensive or carefully timed assessments (vs. once-daily assessments), even these safeguards may not ensure timely compliance with the protocol.

Hufford and Shields (2002) published a comprehensive review of the peer-reviewed publications using electronic diaries. Of the 76 published papers available in 2002, only 44 percent reported compliance rates. This finding supports the call from other researchers that compliance rates be a mandatory part of reporting requirements in the peer-reviewed literature (Stone & Shiffman, 2002). Of the 30-plus papers that did report compliance, the vast majority reported rates in excess of 80 percent. Studies that fell below 80 percent primarily experienced technical failures from early hardware and software problems, resulting in a high rate of noncompliance.

Interestingly, there is good evidence that, given the opportunity, participants will electronically backfill their diary data just as they will their paper diary data. A study by Johannes and colleagues (2000) found that allowing participants to change the date and time on the ED resulted in 100 percent of them electronically backfilling at least some data. This points to an important principle—there is nothing inherent about the technology that makes participants comply with ED protocols. Rather, it is the thoughtful application of this technology, using some of the principles outlined above, that helps participants to comply with the study protocol (Hufford & Shiffman, 2003).

Choosing an EMA reporting platform is inevitably driven by many factors, not just anticipated rates of subject compliance. Once the hypotheses for a research program have been established, the density of sampling can be determined, which in turn informs how important timely compliance will be to the EMA protocol. A host of other considerations inevitably affect which reporting platform will be used. As Delespaul (1992) has noted, these considerations include the size of the reporting device, reliability, expense, flexibility, and verifiability (i.e., data security) of the reporting platform.

Reactivity to EMA

It is no small irony that, by successfully achieving high rates of compliance with EMA protocols, researchers must confront the specter of another potential methodological concern—reactivity. Nearly 30 years ago, Nelson (1977) defined a reactive effect as describing the degree to which self-report data could be affected by the act of assessing them.

Reactivity may affect EMA data in at least two ways. First, participants may react to the effects of self-monitoring. Self-monitoring refers to a two-stage process in which participants first identify that a target event or behavior has occurred and then record their responses (Nelson, 1977). EMA researchers often ask participants to report on antecedents, momentary experiences, or consequences of specific events. In this way, participants are acting as a proxy for the researcher, recording details of specific events (e.g., migraine headaches) or behaviors (e.g., smoking). If participants reported engaging in specific behaviors less frequently while self-monitoring in EMA protocols, reactivity could be to blame.

Second, participants may be reactive to the prompted assessments that are characteristic of many EMA protocols. That is, by virtue of stopping what they are doing in the course of their daily life and reflecting and reporting on their experiences, prompting for assessment completion could change the very data that are being sampled. This type of reactivity could manifest itself by participants reporting increased levels of frustration during randomly prompted assessments during the day compared to other structured assessments during the day. If this were the case, and participants confirmed being burdened by the random prompts themselves, then reactivity could explain that pattern of data.

Several studies have examined reactivity to EMA and found little or no evidence of reactive effects (Cruise, Broderick, Porter, et al., 1996; Hufford, Shields, Shiffman, et al., 2002; Litt, Cooney, & Morse, 1998). In the most controlled study of reactivity to EMA, Stone and colleagues (2003) assigned pain subjects to complete either no EMA monitoring or sampling of their daily pain using electronic diaries 3, 6, or 12 times daily. No evidence was found that the pain ratings were systematically reactive to the EMA monitoring.

In many ways, these findings of little reactivity to EMA are surprising and counterintuitive. Why shouldn't the assessment of subjects in real time affect their PRO data? Part of the answer may lie in the inherent limitations of reactive effects. For example, if one is using EMA to better understand the time of onset of a new treatment for acute pain, it would be surprising if the simple act of asking participants about their pain would significantly affect it. This begs an issue that has not received much empirical attention—to what extent does reactivity vary not as a function of the monitoring per se, but rather as a function of the type of data that are being recorded? Recent research has begun to look at different targets of potential reactive effects, from how the PRO data can be affected by reactive effects, to how subjects' motivation for treatment may be affected by reactivity to EMA (Hufford et al., 2002). To date, little evidence has been found to support the hypothesis that EMA engenders either type of reactivity.

Subject Burden

Most researchers focus on novel applications of EMA study designs as they inform old hypotheses and enable the formulation of new ones (Bolger, Davis, & Rafaeli, 2003). In addition to the conceptual and statistical issues raised by EMA designs, researchers have their hands full implementing these methods. As a general rule of thumb, the greater insights that EMA can provide often appear directly proportional to the research infrastructure needed to support these types of studies. The technical preparation of many EMA reporting platforms (especially EDs and IVRS), as well as their maintenance and upkeep in the field, can place a very real, tangible drain on research teams. Along with all of the new conceptual and operational concerns inherent in running EMA studies, another set of concerns deals with how EMA affects the subject.

EMA places novel demands on the subject. People who may work hard to avoid computers in their daily life find themselves being asked to interact with a cellular telephone or use a palmtop computer, possibly for the first time in their lives. Many EMA designs rely on multiple assessments per day, often in the midst of a disease episode, requiring their time and attention to be compliant with the data collection protocol. These demands that are placed on subjects in EMA research require that researchers carefully examine how their protocol and reporting platform will affect participants in their research.

At least six different aspects of an EMA study affect participant burden: the density of sampling (90% of published ED studies sample subjects more than once per day; Hufford & Shields, 2002), the length of the PRO assessments, the user interface of the reporting platform, the complexity of the PRO assessments (i.e., the cognitive load, or effort, required to complete the assessments; Hufford & Shiffman, 2002), duration of monitoring, and stability of the reporting platform. Of these various aspects of EMA study design, the importance of a good user interface has recently received some systematic attention in the literature.

Good User Interface Design

Bias can be introduced into research in many different ways. For example, if participants, because of specific visual limitations or lack of familiarity with computers, are unable to use an EMA reporting platform, the conclusions of the research may be affected by that recruitment bias. Over the past 15 years, the costs of palmtop computers have dropped considerably, while the hardware and software foundations for these systems have matured considerably. In the rush to apply these technologies to clinical research, some painful lessons have been learned about what makes an electronic assessment platform usable to participants.

Palmblad and Tiplady (2004) recently summarized their experience using these systems in clinical research and set out a number of user interface principles that are applicable to EMA researchers. For example, they discuss the importance of having an inclusive design mindset; that is, the system should be designed for the participant who is likely to find the system the most challenging to use. To date, most palmtop computers have had fairly small screen sizes. While the text can be made as large as is typically used in paper diary research, it is recommended that it be made as large as possible—ideally at least 12-point font (about 4.2 mm from the bottom of the lowest descender to the top of the highest ascender). Also, screen layouts should not rely on a Microsoft Windows-based understanding of computing. That is, scrollbars and similar tools used often in a variety of operating systems may introduce artificial ceiling or floor effects in the data among participants unaccustomed to using them to "scroll" to see additional text. In other words, put the entire question text and responses on a single screen whenever possible.

What may seem like a trivial attention to these aspects of user interface design can dramatically affect both the end users' experience of the EMA reporting platform and the resulting data. In the studies reviewed below, subjects were debriefed regarding their experiences using various EMA reporting platforms.

Subject Evaluations of EMA Reporting Platforms

One question that often arises regarding the application of EMA to clinical research is whether subjects will reject the reporting platform outright, or at a minimum find it difficult to use. At this point, there are literally hundreds of studies involving tens of thousands of subjects using paper diaries, EDs, and IVRS to expect good adoption of these methods.

Several studies have directly contrasted subjects' evaluations of different types of EMA reporting platforms. Weiler and colleagues (2004) compared subjects' evaluations of IVRS and paper diaries in a crossover trial among a sample of 87 adults with allergic rhinitis. They found that the vast majority of subjects, 85 percent, preferred the paper diary to the IVRS system. Drummond and colleagues (1995) reported that 57 percent of their gastrointestinally disordered subjects preferred the electronic assessment, while only 13 percent preferred the paper versions (30% expressed no preference). Further, neither age, gender, comfort with technology nor the use of computers was found to be associated with subjects' assessment preferences. Tiplady and colleagues (1997) compared electronic and paper diaries in 22 respiratory clinic outpatients who were monitored with both methods for 4 weeks. Fifty-nine percent preferred the electronic diary over the paper diary, while 18 percent preferred paper (23% expressed no preference). Again, the subjects' age, gender, and comfort/familiarity with technology were not associated with their diary preference.

Rabin and colleagues (1996) also explored subject preference for EDs relative to paper diaries after allowing urinary incontinence subjects to self-monitor with each method for 1 week. Over 98 percent of their subjects and over 80 percent of their control group explicitly expressed preference of the ED over the paper diary. Furthermore, both groups more positively evaluated the ED versus the paper diary on a variety of attributes (e.g., "fun," "easy to use," and "feel involved"). Finally, Johannes and colleagues (2000) found that approximately 70 percent of their all-female sample ($n = 23$) preferred an electronic menstrual diary to a paper menstrual diary.

Two other studies examined whether previous computer experience was a prerequisite to participate and be compliant with EDs. Gaertner and colleagues (2004) contrasted paper and electronic pain diaries among 24 subjects suffering from either cancer- or noncancer-related pain. This 4-week counterbalanced design found that 83 percent of subjects reported preferring the ED to the paper diary. An additional notable finding was that 67 percent of these subjects had either never or rarely used a computer before. Finkelstein and colleagues (2000) examined a sample of asthma subjects from a low socioeconomic urban community without previous computer experience ($n = 17$). Over 3 weeks, the subjects were required to interact with the electronic diary at least twice daily. Results were that the vast majority (82%) found the procedures "not difficult at all." This suggests that previous computer experience is not necessary for subject compliance with electronic PRO data collection systems.

In sum, a small literature has begun to examine subjects' preferences for different EMA reporting platforms. The data outlined above need to be supported by additional studies examining the impact of auditory and visual impairments on PRO data collection, how proxy reporting by significant others or caregivers affects EMA data, and what specific changes need to be made to EMA reporting platforms to deal with specific disease states, such as Parkinson's disease (Nyholm, Kowalski, & Aquilonius, 2004).

Psychometric Issues

The administration of PRO measures using EMA raises some unique psychometric issues. For example, will capturing data in real time affect the accuracy of PRO data? If a questionnaire had been developed to assess a symptom weekly, how will the psychometric properties of that measure change if it is now administered repeatedly throughout the day? How do paper versus electronic versions of scales compare to one another? The psychometric issues raised by EMA can be lumped into two broad categories: (1) How do real-time EMA data compare to PRO data that have traditionally been captured relying on recall and aggregation, and (2) How does the assessment method (paper vs. electronic) affect the data? These questions are gaining increased attention as the United States Food and Drug Administration (FDA) has become concerned with the consistent application of PRO assessments in clinical trials (Scott, 2004).

Real-time Versus Recall: Different Views of the Same Construct?

To date, little systematic research has examined how real-time data compare to recall-based data on the same construct or endpoint. Indeed, it is often unclear, a priori, what the relationship should be behind real-time and recall-based measures of the same construct. For instance, should momentary measures of quality of life correlate highly to quality-of-life measures asking about well-being over the past 4 weeks? One inherent aspect of much PRO data is its evaluative component (e.g., well-being reports). In contrast, asking subjects how they are feeling in the moment is a very different question, one that appears to rely on a different memory mechanism in the generation of the answer.

Robinson and Clore (2002) have suggested that real-time PRO data rely on episodic memory, characterized by a specific memory tied to a particular event. Episodic memories tend to decay rapidly, to be autobiographical in nature, and to be very time-dependent or prone to forgetting. In contrast, recall-based PRO reports rely on semantic memory, characterized by symbolic and conceptual thought. Data generated relying on semantic memory tend to be less time-dependent, conceptual in nature, and less prone to forgetting than episodic-based memories. This distinction is important because it suggests that the same event may be recalled using a very different set of mental heuristics, depending in part on when a subject is asked about the experience—right as it is happening, or days or weeks later. This analysis suggests that we should not always expect a close correspondence between real-time and recall-based data of the same endpoint. Importantly, more research is needed to better understand the mechanism of these differences and to clearly predict under what circumstance we should, and should not, expect a high degree of correspondence between real-time and recall data of the same symptom or event.

From a methodological point of view, if recall and real-time data produce the same conclusion, either the measure or the phenomenon under observation may be responsible. A measure may fail to reveal a change in a construct, say negative affectivity, because it was not implemented in such a way as to be sensitive to moment-to-moment or day-to-day fluctuations. Most PRO measures were developed to assess constructs in aggregate, over time. Instruction sets such as "On average . . .," "Over the past 7 days . . ." or "Over the past 4 weeks . . ." are often used to frame subjects' recall of the experience in question. As such, the norms and properties of many traditional PRO measures are oriented such that their instructions, items, and response options rely on detecting changes that exert themselves over time. For example, many measures of adult attention-deficit disorder symptomatology ask about the frequency of certain events occurring over the past 12 months (e.g., Adler, Spencer, Faraone, et al., 2003). Some of these assessment items make perfect sense when administered relying on recall: *"How often do you have trouble keeping your attention when you are doing boring or repetitive work?"* This same item may receive a very different response when administered in an EMA protocol. For example, a negative response could reflect either that the participant was not having trouble paying attention to a boring task or had not yet engaged in any boring tasks that day. In other words, sampling events in real time requires that the researcher understand the base rate of the experience under study, so that the wrong conclusion is not drawn because one infers from absence of evidence that there is evidence of absence, so to speak.

On the other hand, the experience or event of interest may have a time course that is not amenable to EMA. For example, some stable traits, like temperament, may not be expected to show moment-to-moment fluctuations. It is also possible that an experience or event could be so fleeting that even a dense sampling scheme may fail to detect its occurrence. In either case, just as it is important that the EMA measure be sensitive to change, it is also important that the construct itself be amenable to the sampling density of an EMA protocol.

Psychometric Correspondence

A much larger body of empirical work has examined the psychometric correspondence between paper and electronic versions of the same PRO measure. These studies hold the assessment content itself relatively constant and examine the impact of changing a reporting platform, or assessment method, on the resulting data. Changes in an assessment can potentially take many forms, from changing the instruction set (e.g., period of recall), to the wording of an individual item, to changing the length of a visual analog scale, to changing the font of the letters. In general, these psychometric equivalency studies seek to understand whether, by virtue of asking a question electronically, you get a different answer.

In this literature, it is critically important to clarify what changes to PRO measures do, and do not, affect their psychometric properties. For example, Schwarz (1999) summarized a rich literature from cognitive science and psychometrics showing that properties of measures, such as their wording and response options (e.g., rating scales going from –5 to 5 vs. 0 to 10), can and do affect PRO data. In general, this literature suggests that changing the wording of assessments, anchors, or response options to specific items and the layout of PRO measures (e.g., horizontal vs. vertical scales) can affect the properties of the data (Schwarz, Grayson, & Knapuer, 1998; Sriwatanakul, Kelvie, Lasagna, et al., 1983; Wewers & Lowe, 1990).

Some research on psychometric equivalency has examined changes to the Visual Analog Scale (VAS), a widely used assessment format that allows subjects to rate a variety of subjective symptoms on a continuous scale. The typical implementation of a VAS question is a 100-mm line anchored on both ends with verbal descriptors representing different extremes of subject experience (e.g., "Not at all" and "Extremely"). The implementation of hand-held technology to the collection of subject diary data (Shiffman, Hufford, & Paty, 2001; Stone & Shiffman, 1994) has introduced a new variant of the traditional paper-based VAS. Because current handhelds have screens less than 100 mm in width or height, VASs on these devices are shorter than 10 cm, which could affect their psychometric properties. Several validation studies have examined the correspondence between paper and electronic versions of the same VAS scales and found them to be both statistically (Jamison et al., 2001) and functionally equivalent (Stubbs et al., 2000).

Another line of research has shown that electronic and paper-based versions of the same assessment can produce different data when implemented in different platforms, although these differences speak to validity more than reliability. For example, research has shown that subjects perceive that their electronic data, which typically disappear from view, are more confidential than reporting data using paper forms, where someone else can view the handwritten responses. This perception can have a direct impact on the validity of the data. Turner and colleagues (1998) found that the computer administration of a survey sampling sexual behavior, violence, and drug use among 1,690 adolescents revealed that subjects randomly assigned to the electronic PRO survey reported more rates of aberrant sexual behavior compared to subjects randomly assigned to the paper form by factors of three or more. In other cases, differences have been found between paper and electronic versions of the same measure because subjects reported frequently forgetting to complete the paper diaries (Rabin et al., 1996). In this case, the lack of psychometric correspondence throws doubt on the validity of the old paper version of the measure, not the new electronic one.

The evolving literature on psychometric equivalence makes two clear points. First, changing the wording of items, especially in regard to item anchors and recall periods, can affect the psychometric properties of the data. Conversely, it is also clear that not every aspect of a paper measure is sacred. Some researchers have suggested that unless electronic versions of paper-based measures retain the same white space, font type, screen or paper color, and line breaks, the measure must be revalidated. In fact, many studies have directly examined electronic versus paper administration of the same measure and found that these characteristics do not affect the properties of PRO data in terms of mean scores, dispersion measures, or reliability scores (e.g., Gaertner et al., 2004; Hank & Schwenkmezger, 1996; Jansen, 1985; Ryan, Corry, Attewell, et al., 2002; Schwarz et al., 1998). This should not come as too surprising; it is hard to imagine how a subject experiencing severe dental pain would somehow rate his or her pain differently based on whether the font of the question was in Arial or Times New Roman.

Empirical studies of the correspondence between paper and electronic assessment methods need to continue to examine how these methods affect the construct validity of the data. As electronic means of capturing real-time data become more common and measures are developed for and validated on electronic reporting platforms in the first place, there may come a time when the question is not whether an electronically administered real-time assessment matches its paper counterpart, but rather what evidence there is that a paper-based measure, with no verification of when it was completed by the subject in the field, corresponds to its validated electronic counterpart.

Summary

This chapter has reviewed a number of methodological challenges associated with the collection of EMA data. These methods impose some unique burdens both on the researchers who use them as well as on their research subjects. These challenges can be overcome. Researchers have successfully applied a variety of assessment platforms to the collection of real-time data in EMA studies.

The subsequent chapters of this text show that the methodological challenges inherent in implementing EMA pale in comparison to the opportunities that these methods provide to researchers. EMA is providing novel insights into the mechanism of drug addiction and factors associated with cardiovascular morbidity and is helping researchers provide a better test of their clinical trial endpoints, to name only a few recent applications. As the implementation of EMA becomes more ubiquitous across the psychological, social, and medical sciences, researchers will increasingly be able to take their research out of the lab and into the natural environment of their subjects' daily lives.

REFERENCES

Adler, L. A., Spencer, T., Faraone, S. V., Kessler, R., Howes, M., Biederman, J., & Secnik, K. (October, 2003). Poster presented at The American Academy of Child and Adolescent Psychiatry, Miami, FL.

Bailey, A. S., & Martin, M. L. (October, 2000). In *Quality of Life Questionnaires, What Do Subjects Understand "Past Month" to Mean?* Poster presented at the International Society for Quality of Life Research conference, Vancouver, Canada.

Bolger, N., Davis, A., & Rafaeli, E. (2003). Diary methods: Capturing life as it is lived. *Annual Review of Psychology, 54,* 579–616.

Boudes, P. (1998). Drug compliance in therapeutic trials: a review. *Controlled Clinical Trials, 19,* 257–168.

Broderick, J. E., Schwartz, J., Shiffman, S., Hufford, M. R., & Stone, A. A. (2003). Signaling does not adequately improve diary compliance. *Annals of Behavioral Medicine, 26,* 139–148.

Brown, G. W., & Harris, T. (1978). *Social origins of depression.* London: Tavistock.

Chmelik, F., & Doughty, A. (1994). Objective measurements of compliance in asthma treatment. *Annals of Allergy, 73,* 527–532.

Clark, D. M., & Teasdale, J. D. (1982). Diurnal variation in clinical depression and accessibility of memories of positive and negative experiences. *Journal of Abnormal Psychology, 91,* 87–95.

Clark, D. M., & Teasdale, J. D. (1985). Constraints on effects of mood on memory. *Journal of Personality and Social Psychology, 48,* 1595–1608.

Corkrey, R., & Parkinson, L. (2002). Interactive voice response: Review of studies 1989–2000. *Behavior Research Methods, Instruments, and Computers, 34,* 342–353.

Cruise, C. E., Broderick, J., Porter, L., Kaell, A. T., & Stone, A. A. (1996). Reactive effects of diary self-assessment in chronic pain subjects. *Pain, 67,* 253–258.

Csikszentmihalyi, M., & Larson, R. (1987). Validity and reliability of the Experience Sampling Method. *Journal of Nervous and Mental Disease, 175,* 526–536.

Delespaul, P. A. E. G. (1992). Technical note: devices and time sampling procedures. In M. W. deVries (Eds.), *The experience of psychopathology* (pp. 363–376). Cambridge, UK: Cambridge University Press.

Drummond, H. E., Ghosh, S., Ferguson, A., Brackenridge, D., & Tiplady, B. (1995). Electronic quality of life questionnaires: A comparison of pen-based electronic questionnaires with convention paper in a gastrointestinal study. *Quality of Life Research, 4,* 21–26.

Eich, E., Reeves, J. L., Jaeger, B., & Graff-Radford, S. B. (1985). Memory for pain: Relation between past and present pain intensity. *Pain, 23,* 375–379.

Erickson, J. R., & Jemison, C. R. (1991). Relations among measures of autobiographical memory. *Bulletin of the Psychonomic Society, 29,* 233–236.

Finkelstein, J., Cabrera, M. R., & Hripcsak, G. (2000). Internet-based home asthma telemonitoring. *Chest, 117,* 148–155.

Gaertner, J., Elsner, F., Pollmann-Dahmen, K., Radbruch, L., & Sabatowski, R. (2004). Electronic pain diary: A randomized crossover study. *Journal of Pain and Symptom Management, 28,* 259–267.

Gendreau, M., Hufford, M. R., & Stone, A. A. (2003). Measuring clinical pain in chronic widespread pain: Selected methodological issues. *Best Practice and Research in Clinical Rheumatology, 17,* 575–592.

Hank, P., & Schwenkmezger, P. (1996). Computer-assisted versus paper-and-pencil based self-monitoring: An analysis of experiential and psychometric equivalence. In J. Fahrenberg & M. Myrtek (Eds.), *Ambulatory assessment* (pp. 85–99). Seattle, WA: Hogrefe & Huber.

Houpt, J. B., McMillan, R., Wein, C., & Paget-Dellio, S. D. (1999). Effect of glucosamine hydrochloride in the treatment of pain of osteoarthritis of the knee. *Journal of Rheumatology, 26,* 2423–2430.

Hufford, M. R., & Shields, A. L. (2002). Electronic diaries: An examination of applications and what works in the field. *Applied Clinical Trials, 11*(4), 46–56.

Hufford, M. R., Shields, A. L., Shiffman, S., Paty, J., & Balabanis, M. (2002). Reactivity to Ecological Momentary Assessment: An example using undergraduate problem drinkers. *Psychology of Addictive Behaviors, 16,* 205–211.

Hufford, M. R., & Shiffman, S. (2003). Subject-reported outcomes: assessment methods. *Disease Management and Health Outcomes, 11,* 77–86.

Hufford, M. R., & Shiffman, S. S. (2002). Methodological issues affecting the value of subject-reported outcomes data. *Expert Review of Pharmacoeconomics and Health Outcomes, 2*(2), 119–128.

Hufford, M. R., Shiffman, S., Paty, J., & Stone, A. A. (2001). Ecological Momentary Assessment: real-world, real-time measurement of subject experience. In J. Fahrenberg & M. Myrtek (Eds.), *Progress in Ambulatory Assessment* (pp. 69–92). Seattle, WA: Hogrefe and Huber Publishers.

Innocenti, A., Lauritsen K., Hendel L., Praest J., Lytje M. F., Clemmensen-Rotne K., & Wiklund, I. (October, 2003). *Symptom recording in a randomised clinical trial: Paper diaries vs. electronic or telephone data capture.* Poster presented at the Drug Information Association conference Electronic Subject Diaries and the Regulatory Process: What's Going On? Washington, DC.

Jamison, et al. (2001). Electronic vs. paper VAS Ratings: A randomized, crossover, comparative study utilizing healthy volunteers. *Journal of Pain (Suppl.), 2,* 7.

Jansen, J. H. (1985). Effect of questionnaire layout and size and issue-involvement on response rate in mail surveys. *Perceptual and Motor Skills, 61,* 139–142.

Joffe, R. T., MacDonald, C., & Kutcher, S. P. (1989). Life events and mania: A case-controlled study. *Psychiatry Research, 30,* 213–216.

Johannes, C. B., Crawford, S. L., Woods, J., Goldstein, R. B., Tran, D., Mehrotra, S., Johnson, K. B., & Santoro, N. (2000). An electronic menstrual cycle calendar: Comparison of data quality with a paper version. *Menopause, 7,* 200–208.

Jonasson, G., Carlsen, K., Sodal, A., Jonasson, C., & Mowinckel, P. (1999). Subject compliance in a clinical trial with inhaled budesonide in children with mild asthma. *European Respiratory Journal, 14,* 150–154.

Kamarck, T. W., Shiffman, S., Smithline, L., Goodie, J. L., Paty, J. A., Gnys, M., & Jong, J. Y. (1998). Effects of task strain, social conflict, and emotional activation on ambulatory cardiovascular activity: Daily life consequences of recurring stress in a multiethnic adult sample. *Health Psychology, 17,* 17–29.

Linton, S. J. (1991). Memory for chronic pain intensity: Correlates of accuracy. *Perceptual and Motor Skills, 72,* 1091–1095.

Litt, M. D., Cooney, N. L., & Morse, P. (1998). Ecological momentary assessment (EMA) with treated alcoholics: Methodological problems and potential solutions. *Health Psychology, 17*, 48–52.

Mazze, R. S., Shamoon, H., Pasmantier, R., Lucido, D., Murphy, J., Hartmann, K., Kuykendall, V., & Lopatin, W. (1984). Reliability of blood glucose monitoring by subjects with diabetes mellitus. *American Journal of Medicine, 77*, 211–217.

Means, B., Swan, G. E., Jobe, J. B., & Esposito, J. L. (1994). The effects of estimation strategies on the accuracy of respondents' reports of cigarette smoking. In N. Schwartz & S. Sudman (Eds.), *Autobiographical memory and the validity of retrospective reports* (pp. 107–119). New York: Springer-Verlag.

Menon, G., & Yorkton, E. A. (2000). The use of memory and contextual cues in the formation of behavioral frequency judgments. In A. A. Stone et al. (Eds.), *The science of self-report: implications for research and practice* (pp. 63–80). Mahwah, NJ: Lawrence Erlbaum Associates, Publishers.

Milgrom, H., Bender, B., Ackerson, L., Bowry, P., Smith, B., & Rand, C. (1996). Noncompliance and treatment failure in children with asthma. *Journal of Allergy and Clinical Immunology, 98*, 1051–1057.

Mundt, J. C., Perrine, M. W., Searles, J. S., & Walter, D. (1995). An application of interactive voice response (IVR) technology to longitudinal studies of daily behavior. *Behavior Research Methods, Instruments, and Computers, 27*, 351–357.

Nelson, R. O. (1977). Assessment and therapeutic functions of self-monitoring. In M. Hersen, R. M. Eisler, and P. Miller (Eds.), *Progress in behavioral modification* (pp. 3–41). New York: Academic Press.

Nived, O., Sturfelt, G., Eckernas, S. A., & Singer, P. (1994). A comparison of 6 months' compliance of subjects with rheumatoid arthritis treated with Tenoxicam and Naproxen. Use of subject computer data to assess response to treatment. *Journal of Rheumatology, 21*, 1537–1541.

Norman, G. R., McFarlane, A. H., Streiner, D. L., & Neale, K. (1982). Health diaries: strategies for compliance and relation to other measures. *Medical Care, 20*, 623–629.

Nyholm, D., Kowalski, J., & Aquilonius, S. M. (2004). Wireless real-time electronic data capture for self-assessment of motor function and quality of life in Parkinson's disease. *Movement Disorders, 19*, 446–451.

Palmblad, M., & Tiplady, B. (2004). Electronic diaries and questionnaires: Designing user interfaces that are easy for subjects to use. *Quality of Life Research, 13*, 1199–1207.

Rabin, J. M., McNett, J., & Badlani, G. H. (1996). "Compu-voiding II": The computerized voiding diary. *Journal of Medical Systems, 20*, 19–34.

Raskin, J. (2000). *The humane interface: new directions for designing interactive systems.* Reading, MA: Addison Wesley Longman, Inc.

Redelmeier, D., & Kahneman, D. (1996). Subjects' memories of painful medical treatments: Real-time and retrospective evaluations of two minimally invasive procedures. *Pain, 66*, 3–8.

Robinson, M. D., & Clore, G. L. (2002). Belief and feeling: Evidence for an accessibility model of emotional self-report. *Psychological Bulletin, 128*, 934–960.

Ross, M. (1989). Relation of implicit theories to the construction of personal histories. *Psychological Review, 96*, 341–357.

Ryan, J. M., Corry, J. R., Attewell, R. & Smithson, M. J. (2002). A comparison of an electronic version of the SF-36 General Health Questionnaire to the standard paper version. *Quality of Life Research, 11*, 19–26.

Schacter, D. L. (1996). *Searching for memory: The brain, the mind, and the past.* New York: Basic Books.

Schwarz, N. (1999). Self-reports: How the questions shape the answers. *American Psychologist, 54,* 93-105.

Schwarz, N., Grayson, C., & Knauper, B. (1998). Formal features of rating scales and the interpretation of question meaning. *International Journal of Public Opinion Research, 10,* 177–183.

Scott, J. (June, 2004). J. A. *Validation of electronic patient reported outcomes (ePROs): An endpoint review perspective.* Poster presented at the Drug Information Association Annual Meeting, Washington, DC.

Searles, J. S., Perrine, M. W., Mundt, J. C., & Helzer, J. E. (1995). Self-reports of drinking using touch-tone telephone: extending the limits of reliable daily contact. *Journal of Studies on Alcohol, 56,* 375–382.

Shiffman, S. (2000). Real-time self-report of momentary states in the natural environment: Computerized ecological momentary assessment. In A. A. Stone, J.S. Turkkan, C. A. Bachrach, J. E. Jobe, H. S. Kurtzman, & V. S. Cain (Eds.), *The science of self-report: implications for research and practice.* (pp. 277–296). Mahwah, NJ: Lawrence Erlbaum Associates, Publishers.

Shiffman, S., Dresler, C. M., Hajek, P., Gilburt, S. J. A., Targett, D. A., & Strahs, K. R. (2002). Efficacy of a nicotine lozenge for smoking cessation. *Archives of Internal Medicine, 162,* 1267–1276.

Shiffman, S., Hufford, M., Hickox, M., et al. (1997). Remember that? A comparison of real-time versus retrospective recall of smoking lapses. *Journal of Consulting and Clinical Psychology, 65,* 292–300.

Shiffman, S., Hufford, M. R., & Paty, J. (2001). Subject experience diaries in clinical research, Part 1: The subject experience movement. *Applied Clinical Trials, 10,* 46–56.

Shiffman, S., Paty, J. A., Gnys, M., Kassel J. A., & Hickcox, M. (1996). First lapses to smoking: Within-subjects analysis of real-time reports. *Journal of Consulting and Clinical Psychology, 64,* 366–379.

Simmons, M. S., Nides, M. A., Rand, C. S., Wise, R. A., & Tashkin, D. P. (2000). Unpredictability of deception in compliance with physician-prescribed bronchodilator inhaler use in a clinical trial. *Chest, 118,* 290–295.

Spector, S., Kinsman, R., Mawhinney, H., Siegel, S., Rachelefsky, G., Katz, R., & Rohr, A. (1986). Compliance of subjects with asthma with an experimental aerosolized medication: Implications for controlled clinical trials. *Journal of Allergy and Clinical Immunology, 77,* 65–70.

Sprangers, M. A. G., Van Dam, F. S., Broersen, J., Lodder, L., Wever, L., Visser, M. R., Oosterveld, P., & Smets, E. M. (1999). Revealing response shift in longitudinal research on fatigue: The use of the thentest approach. *Acta Oncology,* 38, 709–718.

Sriwatanakul, K., Kelvie, W., Lasagna, L., Calimlim, J. F., Weis, O. F., & Mehta, G. (August, 1983). Studies with different types of visual analog scales for measurement of pain. *Clinical Pharmacology and Therapeutics,* 234–239.

Stone, A. A., Broderick, J. B., Kaell, A. T., Delespaul, P., & Porter, L. (2000). Does the peak-end phenomenon observed in laboratory pain studies apply to real-world pain in rheumatoid arthritics? *Journal of Pain, 1,* 203–218.

Stone, A. A., Broderick, J. E., Schwartz, J. E., Shiffman, S., Litcher-Kelly, L., & Calvanese, P. (2003). Intensive momentary reporting of pain with an electronic diary: Reactivity, compliance, and subject satisfaction. *Pain, 104,* 343–351.

Stone, A. A., & Shiffman, S. (1994). Ecological momentary assessment: Measuring real world processes in behavioral medicine. *Annals of Behavioral Medicine, 16,* 199–202.

Stone, A. A., & Shiffman, S. (2002). Capturing momentary, self-report data: A proposal for reporting guidelines. *Annals of Behavioral Medicine, 24*, 236–243.

Stone, A. A., Shiffman, S., & DeVries, M. W. (2000). Ecological Momentary Assessment. In D. Kahneman et al. (Eds.), *Well-being: the foundations of hedonic psychology* (pp. 26–39). New York: Russell Sage Foundation.

Stone, A. A., Shiffman, S., Schwartz, J. E., Broderick, J. E., & Hufford, M. R. (2002). Subject noncompliance with paper diaries. *British Medical Journal, 324*, 1193–1194.

Stone, A. A., Shiffman, S., Schwartz, J., Broderick, J. E., & Hufford, M. R. (2003). Subject compliance with electronic and paper diaries. *Controlled Clinical Trials, 24*, 182–199.

Straka, R., Fish, J., Benson, S., & Suh, J. (1997). Subject self-reporting of compliance does not correspond with electronic monitoring: An evaluation using isosorbide dinitrate as a model drug. *Pharmacotherapy, 17*, 126–132.

Stubbs, R. J. et al. (2000). The use of visual analogue scales to assess motivation to eat in human subjects: A review of their reliability and validity with an evaluation of new hand-held computerized systems for temporal tracking of appetite ratings. *British Journal of Nutrition, 84*, 405–415.

Tiplady, B., Crompton, G. K., Dewar, M. H., et al. (1997). The use of electronic diaries in respiratory studies. *Drug Information Journal, 31*, 759–764.

Tourangeau, R. (2000). Remembering what happened: Memory errors and survey reports. In A. A. Stone, J. S. Turkkan, C. A. Bachrach, J. B. Jobe, H. S. Kurtzman, & V. S. Cain (Eds.), *The science of self-report: implications for research and practice* (pp. 29–48). Mahwah, NJ: Lawrence Erlbaum Associates, Publishers.

Turner, C. F., Ku, L., Rogers, S. M., Lindberg, L. D., Pleck, J. H., & Sonenstein, F. L. (1998). Adolescent sexual behavior, drug use, and violence: Increased reporting with computer survey technology. *Science, 280*, 847–848.

Urquhart, J. (1994). Role of subject compliance in clinical pharmacokinetics: A review of recent research. *Clinical Pharmacokinetics, 27*, 202–215.

Urquhart, J., & De Klerk, E. (1998). Contending paradigms for the interpretation of data on subject compliance with therapeutic drug regimens. *Statistics in Medicine, 17*, 251–267.

Verbrugge, L. M. (1980). Health diaries. *Medical Care, 18*, 73–95.

Verschelden, P., Cartier, A., L'Archeveque, A., Trudeau, C., & Malo, J. L. (1996). Compliance with and accuracy of daily assessment of peak expiratory flows (PEF) in asthmatic subjects over a three-month period. *European Respiratory Journal, 9*, 880–885.

Wagenaar, W. A. (1986). My memory: A study of autobiographical memory over six years. *Cognitive Psychology, 18*, 225–252.

Weiler, K., Christ, A. M., Woodworth, G. G., Weiler, R. L., & Weiler, J. M. (2004). Quality of subject-reported outcome data captured using paper and interactive voice response diaries in an allergic rhinitis study: Is electronic data capture really better? *Annals of Allergy, Asthma, and Immunology, 92*, 335–339.

Wewers, M. E., & Lowe, N. K. (1990). A critical review of visual analog scales in the measurement of clinical phenomena. *Research in Nursing and Health, 13*, 227–236.

5

The Analysis of Real-Time Momentary Data: A Practical Guide

Joseph E. Schwartz and Arthur A. Stone

Collecting real-time momentary data enables researchers to address a variety of questions, including some that are difficult, if not impossible, to address with traditional retrospective questionnaires. This chapter is intended to be a practical guide for analyzing real-time data. By necessity, it begins with a somewhat formal presentation of the general statistical model that is the basis for all of the subsequent analyses. The structure of momentary data is complex and, as might be expected, so are the analyses. The benefit of mastering the analytic concepts is the ability to address, with appropriate statistical techniques, numerous fascinating questions about daily life experience. Although the use of symbols and equations in the chapter may be intimidating, taking the time to decipher them will provide the necessary background for understanding the analyses. The symbols will take on concrete meaning as they are replaced with actual variables in the application sections of the chapter.

Next, we describe the momentary data that are used illustratively throughout the chapter, including person-level (e.g., age, sex, personality) and moment-level (e.g., location, mood) variables. The main section of the chapter illustrates the analyses of seven types of questions that could be addressed with these data. We use the conceptual structure described in the first section to direct how computer code for analyzing the data is generated. As the reader will see, there are many decisions that the researcher faces, and we have attempted to discuss many of the most important ones, providing specific decisions for the illustrative data set.

Before jumping into the complex issues and unfamiliar nomenclature associated with the analyses of data sets generated by real-time data capture protocols, the reader may feel a tad more comfortable to know that a frequently used data analysis technique in the social and behavioral sciences is actually a special case of the hierarchical linear modeling that follows. Most readers will be familiar with repeated measures analysis of variance (RM-ANOVA), a well-known technique for analyzing data collected over time. There are certain types of data structures that are appropriate for RM-ANOVA, and they usually include data that were collected at a few/several fixed time points, have no missing values (or else a person's entire data will be excluded from the analysis), and have covariates that do not change over time. Although not explicitly specified by the user, other assumptions about the variances and correlations of the residuals are incorporated into RM-ANOVA analysis programs. The point is that RM-ANOVA is just a special case of the kinds of data that can be handled with multilevel models, also known as hierarchical linear models, and the results of such analyses, using the default autocorrelation and error structures built into RM-ANOVA, would yield exactly the same findings.[1]

However, for the analysis of most real-time data, like those generated by the studies discussed in this volume, the assumptions underlying the strict data structure required by RM-ANOVA are almost never met. Three examples of this are the following: (1) real-time data are usually not equally spaced in time, as is the case with random prompting of real-time reports, (2) some predictor variables are usually moment-level (not person-level) variables, and (3) real-time data almost always have instances of missing data, times when participants were supposed to make a report but did not. These and many other characteristics of real-time data are easily handled by multilevel models.

There are other considerations for analyzing real-time data. First, the sheer size of the resulting data sets can be quite daunting to the novice. Second, as in other repeated-measures data, the nested structure of the data is more complex than the familiar cross-sectional (person-by-variable) type of data. There are typically many momentary assessments for each individual. Both the large number of observations per person and the likelihood that the number of observations varies across persons differentiate most real-time momentary data from traditional repeated measures data. As mentioned above, the timing of observations can vary both within persons (uneven spacing of assessments) and between persons. This, as well as the usual presence of moment-level predictor variables, causes the data to be "unbalanced" such that the moment-level factors are rarely orthogonal to the person-level factors. Finally, like traditional time series data, real-time momentary data tend to exhibit serial autocorrelation such that repeated observations from the same person collected over a relatively short interval tend to be more similar to each other than observations separated by a longer time interval. This chapter describes and illustrates how one broad class of statistical models, known as multilevel models, can be used to address a variety of questions that researchers might seek to answer with real-time momentary data.

Theoretical Considerations

The General Multilevel Model

Formal presentations of the general two-level statistical model can be found in multiple sources (e.g., Bryk & Raudenbush, 1992; Bryk, Raudenbush, & Congdon, 1996;

Laird & Ware, 1982; Singer & Willett, 2003; Walls, Jung, & Schwartz, 2006). While we ultimately express the model as a single equation, it is easier to understand if it is initially presented as a set of separate equations. In the following presentation, we assume that there is an outcome variable, y_{it} (with i indexing persons and t indexing the momentary assessments of the ith person), J person-level predictor variables, x_{ji}, and K moment-level predictor variables, z_{kit}. At the core of the model, there is the "Level 1" equation describing the within-person relationship of y_{it} to the z_{kit}:

Level 1: Momentary Outcome is Predicted by Momentary Predictors

$$y_{it} = \pi_{0i} + \pi_{1i}z_{1it} + \pi_{2i}z_{2it} + \pi_{3i}z_{3it} + \ldots + \pi_{Ki}z_{Kit} + \varepsilon_{it}$$

$$\text{or, } y_{it} = \pi_{0i} + \sum_{k=1}^{K} \pi_{ki}z_{kit} + \varepsilon_{it}$$

[1]

The π_k's are regression coefficients and, importantly, the "i" subscript in each of the coefficients indicates that each coefficient is free to vary from person to person and thus each person has his/her own equation. If we were to drop the "i" subscript from any of the π_k's, it would imply that the coefficient was the same for all people (i.e., that it was "fixed)." Heuristically, though not in practice, the Level 1 equation is estimated separately for each person. The usual assumptions are made about the distribution of the ε_{it}; that they are independent, normally distributed with mean zero and constant variance σ^2, and uncorrelated with each of the predictors, z_k. The variance-covariance matrix, "Σ_R", of the T_i residuals, $\{\varepsilon_{it}\}$, for person i is sometimes called the "R-matrix." With the just-stated assumptions, the R-matrix has the value σ^2 in all diagonal cells and zero in all off-diagonal cells. (The assumption of independence is relaxed, below, to allow for serial autocorrelation [non-zero off-diagonal cells], and although we will not discuss such extensions, it is possible to estimate models that allow for some forms of heteroskedastic variances.) The reader will note that none of the person-level variables (e.g., sex, age, personality) are included in Equation 1 because they are constant (have no variance) across the T_i momentary observations of the ith person.

We now move to the next higher order, person-level, equation(s). Here, each of the regression coefficients in the Level 1 equation (the π_k's) becomes the dependent variable of a "Level 2" equation.[2] It is here that the person-level predictors enter the analysis. Of particular significance is the Level 2 equation for π_0, the intercept in the Level 1 equation:

Level 2: People's Intercepts are Predicted by Person-Level Predictors

$$\pi_{0i} = \beta_{00} + \beta_{01}x_{1i} + \beta_{02}x_{2i} + \beta_{03}x_{3i} + \ldots + \beta_{0J}x_{Ji} + \delta_{0i}$$

$$\text{or, } \pi_{0i} = \beta_{00} + \sum_{j=1}^{J} \beta_{0j}x_{ji} + \delta_{0i}$$

[2a]

It states that the set of intercepts from the within-person (Level 1) equations can be expressed as a linear function of the person-level predictors plus a residual term, δ_{0i}. The residual term is included to account for that portion of the individual differences in intercepts that cannot be accounted for by the measured person-level variables. It is Equation [2a] that incorporates the "main effects" of the person-level predictors on the outcome variable, y_{it}. Each of the other Level 1 coefficients, π_k, is also treated as the dependent variable in a Level 2 equation:

Individual differences in the effect of z_k on the outcome are predicted by person-level predictors

Level 2

$$\pi_{ki} = \beta_{k0} + \beta_{k1}x_{1i} + \beta_{k2}x_{2i} + \beta_{k3}x_{3i} + \ldots + \beta_{kJ}x_{Ji} + \delta_{ki}$$

$$\text{or, } \pi_{ki} = \beta_{k0} + \sum_{j=1}^{J} \beta_{kj}x_{ji} + \delta_{ki}$$

[2b]

Note that, whenever $\beta_{kj} \neq 0$ when $k > 0$ and $j > 0$, it implies that the individual differences in the within-person effect of momentary variable z_k on y are related to person-level variable x_j. There are several special cases of the Level 2 equations. First, if $\beta_{kj} = 0$ for all $j > 0$, then none of the person-level variables, x_j, are related to the within-person effect of momentary variable z_k on y.

RANDOM VERSUS FIXED EFFECTS

One of the major decisions in performing multilevel analyses is whether to treat the effects of moment-level predictors as "fixed" or "random." When B_k is treated as a fixed effect, then one is assuming either (1) that the effect of the predictor on the outcome is identical for all persons or (2) that any differences in the effect are entirely accounted for by measured person-level variables, x_j, in the Level 2 equation. Mathematically, treating π_k as a fixed effect implies that the residual term in its Level 2 equation (δ_k) is 0 for all persons, and hence $Var(\delta_k)$ is also 0. Usually when π_k is treated as a fixed effect, there are no x_j in its Level 2 equation, in which case $\pi_{ki} = \beta_{k0}$ and the effect of z_k on y is (assumed to be) the same for all persons. In contrast, when π_k is treated as a random effect, one allows for unexplained individual differences in the effect of z_k on the outcome measure.

While it is usually easier to estimate models in which the coefficients of moment-level variables are treated as fixed effects, we strongly recommend empirically examining the extent to which the effects of one's primary moment-level predictors vary across individuals before treating them as fixed effects. Treating as fixed a coefficient that actually varies considerably among persons, $Var(\delta_k) > 0$, does not usually have much impact on the estimate of β_{k0} or other β_{kj}, but it can result in grossly underestimating their standard errors and hence overestimating their statistical significance. In contrast, we usually treat the effect of moment-level "control variables" as fixed effects, both because this simplifies the model and because our goal is to statistically control for the average effects that these variables have on the outcome.[3]

Fixed Versus Random Effects: Although models in which the coefficients of the moment-level predictors are treated as fixed effects are easier to specify and estimate, one should be skeptical of the standard errors and resulting significance tests for these coefficients unless one has determined that there is little or no variability in these coefficients based on analyses in which these same predictors are treated as random effects.

Choice of a Covariance Structure for the Residuals, δ_K, of the Level 2 Equations

In addition to specifying the form of the variance–covariance matrix of the Level 1 equation residuals (the R-matrix, described above), the structure of the variance–covariance matrix for the set of residual terms of the Level 2 equations, "Σ_G", must also be specified. In general, the variance of the residuals for one Level 2 equation will differ from the variance of the residuals for a different Level 2 equation. Furthermore, there is usually no rationale for assuming that the covariance of the residuals for two equations will be zero, or any other particular value. Accordingly, except in special cases, one should not impose any constraints on Σ_G, also known as the G-matrix, other than the standard distributional assumptions that the residual terms {all δ_k, including δ_0} have a multivariate normal distribution with each δ_k having a mean of zero. In addition, each δ_k is assumed to be uncorrelated with all person-level predictor variables, x_j, all momentary predictor variables, z_k, and the within-person residuals, ε.

Combining the Level 1 and Level 2 Equations into a Single Equation

By replacing each π_k in the Level 1 equation with the corresponding Level 2 equation, one can arrive at a single equation that incorporates the effects of both the person-level and the momentary predictors:

$$
\begin{aligned}
y_{it} = \beta_{00} &+ \beta_{01}x_{1i} + \beta_{02}x_{2i} + \beta_{03}x_{3i} + \ldots + \beta_{0J}x_{Ji} + \delta_{0i} \\
&+ (\beta_{10} + \beta_{11}x_{1i} + \beta_{12}x_{2i} + \beta_{13}x_{3i} + \ldots + \beta_{1J}x_{Ji} + \delta_{1i})\, z_{1it} \\
&+ (\beta_{20} + \beta_{21}x_{1i} + \beta_{22}x_{2i} + \beta_{23}x_{3i} + \ldots + \beta_{2J}x_{Ji} + \delta_{2i})\, z_{2it} \\
&+ (\beta_{30} + \beta_{31}x_{1i} + \beta_{32}x_{2i} + \beta_{33}x_{3i} + \ldots + \beta_{3J}x_{Ji} + \delta_{3i})\, z_{3it} \\
&+ \ldots + (\beta_{K0} + \beta_{K1}x_{1i} + \beta_{K2}x_{2i} + \beta_{K3}x_{3i} + \ldots + \beta_{KJ}x_{Ji} + \delta_{Ki})\, z_{Kit} + \varepsilon_{it}
\end{aligned}
$$

$$
\text{or,}\ y_{it} = \beta_{00} + \sum_{j=1}^{J}\beta_{0j}x_{ji} + \sum_{k=1}^{K}\beta_{k0}z_{kit} + \sum_{j=1}^{J}\sum_{k=1}^{K}\beta_{kj}x_{ji}z_{kit} + \delta_{0i} + \sum_{k=1}^{K}\delta_{ki}z_{kit} + \varepsilon_{it}
$$

In this last equation, β_{00} is the overall intercept, the β_{0j} coefficients in the first summation correspond to the main effects of the person-level variables, the β_{k0}

coefficients in the second summation correspond to the main effects of the moment-level variables, and the β_{kj} coefficients in the double summation correspond to the cross-level interaction effects. Each interaction term coefficient reflects the extent to which individual differences in the effect on y of one of the momentary variables, z_k, are related to one of the person-level variable, x_j. As before, each δ_k represents that portion of the individual differences in the π_{ki} that cannot be predicted from the person-level predictor variables and ε_{it} represents that portion of y_{it} that cannot be predicted from the moment-level predictor variables.

Application of Multilevel Models

Model Estimation Using SAS's Proc MIXED

The MIXED procedure in SAS (Littell, Milliken, Stroup, & Wolfinger, 1996; Singer, 1998) provides estimates of models having the general form of Equation [3]. In addition to a choice of the method of estimation (see below), it is quite flexible in terms of allowing the user to specify a variety of structures for the variance–covariance matrix of the $\{\delta_k\}$ (i.e., Σ_G) and the T_i-by-T_i variance-covariance matrix (Σ_R) of the within-person residuals, ε_{it}. The β coefficients of Equation [3] are typical regression coefficients and are sometimes referred to as the "fixed parameters" of the model. The parameters of the G-matrix and the R-matrix are collectively known as the "random parameters" of the model. The MIXED procedure generates estimates of both sets of parameters,[4] as well as estimates of their asymptotic standard errors, Wald tests of significance, and measures of overall model fit. (Recently, SPSS has added a procedure to estimate multilevel models.)

Rather than describe, in the abstract, the syntax and available options for specifying a Proc MIXED analysis, we will present this material in the context of a set of illustrative analyses. But first, we briefly describe the data that will be analyzed.

The Data Set

The data used in this chapter come from a study of self-reported momentary pain in rheumatological patients. Several analyses addressing the relationship between aggregated momentary pain and weekly recall of pain have already been reported (Stone, Broderick, Schwartz, et al., 2003; Stone, Broderick, Shiffman, et al., 2004). Briefly, 68 participants were diagnosed with one of four disorders: fibromyalgia, rheumatoid arthritis, osteoarthritis (hip or knee), or ankylosing spondylitis. Momentary data were collected multiple times per day for 2 weeks (labeled Weeks 1 and 2 of the study), using an electronic diary (ED) that was programmed to prompt individuals 3, 6, or 12 times per day; participants were randomly assigned to one of the three sampling intensity subgroups. At each prompt, they reported their location, mood, and pain, answering 11 to 21 questions, depending on skip-outs.

Overall, participants responded to 94 percent of the prompts (range: 63%–99%), for a total of 5,321 momentary assessments. They also completed a demographic questionnaire at enrollment and completed 1-week retrospective recall reports at the end of each week of monitoring. The protocol was approved by the Stony Brook University's Committee on Research Involving Human Subjects and all participants signed an informed consent form.

Our focus in the illustrations presented below is on respondents' momentary assessment of their frustration levels. We felt that this variable had many of the characteristics of variables generated by real-time data capture studies, such as having the capability to fluctuate over relatively brief periods of time, of being potentially reactive to the immediate psychosocial environment, and of potentially having a "trait" component for each respondent (i.e., a stable level that represents an individual's average level of frustration). We note that this is a continuous variable given that it was rated on a 100-point visual analogue scale (VAS) as opposed to categorical or nominal scales. Many other momentary variables such as pain, fatigue, symptom intensity, mood, and craving have similar qualities, and thus the illustrations presented below will be especially relevant for the analyses of such variables. Some alterations in the analyses would be required for nominal and categorical variables, but the general analytic scheme and the issues discussed also apply to those variables.

Table 5-1 shows a small portion of the data set to be analyzed. It contains variables at three levels of analysis: the person level, the week level, and the momentary level. The person-level variables are the same for all observations of a given person and include ID (a unique 3-digit identifier for each participant), EMAgroup (indicating whether the participant is in the 3-, 6-, or 12-assessments-per-day sampling intensity group), EduLevel (a categorical variable indicating the participant's educational attainment), and Income (a categorical variable indicating the participant's income during the previous year).

The week-level variables are constant for all observations of a person that were made during a given week and include Week (coded 1 for the first week of momentary assessments and 2 for the second week), Frust71 and Frust72 (the 7-day recall of frustration level for the preceding week reported on a 10-cm VAS scale at the end of each week), and FrustN1 and FrustN2 (the current frustration level reported on a 10-cm VAS scale at the end of each week). The moment-level variables include RecDate and RecTime (date and time of the assessment, automatically recorded by the electronic diary), ContTime[5] (a computed continuous measure of time, measured in hours, since the participant's first assessment), PainVAS0 (the participant's VAS rating, 0 to 100, of current pain at each assessment), and Frust (the participant's VAS rating, 0 to 100, of current frustration, a mood item, at each assessment).

Analyses Illustrating the Use of Multilevel Models to Address Several Potential Research Questions

This is the core section of this chapter. Each illustration begins with the statement of a research question. We then briefly specify a multilevel model, in the form of Equation 3, whose estimates address the question. Next we present the

Table 5-1. Data to be analyzed (all records for ID = 403, some for ID = 407)

Obs	ID	EMAgroup	Week	RECDATE	RECTIME	Conttime	EDULEVEL	Inc	FRUST71	FRUSTN1	FRUST72	FRUSTN2	Painvas0	Frust
1	403	3	1	01/14/02	20:35	0.00	5	1	65	7	62	38	93	13
2	403	3	1	01/15/02	14:15	17.67	5	1	65	7	62	38	56	48
3	403	3	1	01/15/02	19:57	23.37	5	1	65	7	62	38	54	0
4	403	3	1	01/16/02	7:43	35.13	5	1	65	7	62	38	88	18
5	403	3	1	01/16/02	14:45	42.17	5	1	65	7	62	38	85	67
6	403	3	1	01/16/02	22:00	49.42	5	1	65	7	62	38	86	84
7	403	3	1	01/17/02	9:10	60.58	5	1	65	7	62	38	62	63
8	403	3	1	01/17/02	20:52	72.28	5	1	65	7	62	38	90	79
9	403	3	1	01/18/02	11:27	86.87	5	1	65	7	62	38	87	81
10	403	3	1	01/18/02	13:35	89.00	5	1	65	7	62	38	73	81
11	403	3	1	01/18/02	15:53	91.30	5	1	65	7	62	38	82	86
12	403	3	1	01/18/02	21:57	97.37	5	1	65	7	62	38	68	44
13	403	3	1	01/19/02	13:10	112.58	5	1	65	7	62	38	65	63
14	403	3	1	01/19/02	19:03	118.47	5	1	65	7	62	38	72	63
15	403	3	1	01/20/02	0:40	124.08	5	1	65	7	62	38	60	60
16	403	3	1	01/20/02	10:32	133.95	5	1	65	7	62	38	62	56
17	403	3	1	01/20/02	21:39	145.07	5	1	65	7	62	38	74	0
18	403	3	2	01/21/02	20:33	167.97	5	1	65	7	62	38	59	24
19	403	3	2	01/22/02	8:39	180.07	5	1	65	7	62	38	55	22
20	403	3	2	01/22/02	13:35	185.00	5	1	65	7	62	38	61	49
21	403	3	2	01/22/02	20:58	192.38	5	1	65	7	62	38	56	32
22	403	3	2	01/22/02	23:04	194.48	5	1	65	7	62	38	63	67
23	403	3	2	01/23/02	9:12	204.62	5	1	65	7	62	38	85	84
24	403	3	2	01/23/02	17:26	212.85	5	1	65	7	62	38	67	62
25	403	3	2	01/23/02	21:42	217.12	5	1	65	7	62	38	63	32
26	403	3	2	01/24/02	10:07	229.53	5	1	65	7	62	38	55	30
27	403	3	2	01/24/02	16:58	236.38	5	1	65	7	62	38	54	31
28	403	3	2	01/24/02	20:11	239.60	5	1	65	7	62	38	57	38
29	403	3	2	01/25/02	20:03	263.47	5	1	65	7	62	38	86	67
30	403	3	2	01/26/02	15:58	283.38	5	1	65	7	62	38	57	43
31	403	3	2	01/26/02	19:20	286.75	5	1	65	7	62	38	61	56
32	403	3	2	01/27/02	9:36	301.02	5	1	65	7	62	38	55	48
33	403	3	2	01/27/02	14:59	306.40	5	1	65	7	62	38	55	60
34	403	3	2	01/28/02	1:56	317.35	5	1	65	7	62	38	79	73
35	403	3	2	01/28/02	9:41	325.10	5	1	65	7	62	38	51	49
(next subject)														
36	407	3	1	01/14/02	17:37	0.00	4	5	37	30	30	6	0	0
37	407	3	1	01/15/02	10:43	17.10	4	5	37	30	30	6	21	59
38	407	3	1	01/15/02	13:34	19.95	4	5	37	30	30	6	11	11
39	407	3	1	01/15/02	16:56	23.32	4	5	37	30	30	6	17	0
40	407	3	1	01/15/02	19:29	25.87	4	5	37	30	30	6	0	58

SAS syntax to estimate the model, summarize key aspects of the resulting output, and provisionally answer the question based on the resulting estimates for our data. In some of what follows, we will be describing the results of the analyses and the conclusions that could be drawn. For those interested in the details of how these results were abstracted from the SAS printout, an annotated copy of this printout is available from the first author. In addition, copies of the dataset used in these analyses and the SAS syntax are also available by request.

The first research question is one that is not often asked. However, we think that it is not only a "natural" first question to ask about momentary outcome measures, but one that also provides a good context for examining the pattern of autocorrelations of the within-person responses. The results of this examination can then be incorporated into all subsequent analyses. The discussion of this first question is by far the lengthiest, because it is here that we describe the general code for programming analyses using SAS's Proc MIXED, and all subsequent analyses depend upon understanding the structure of this programming code.

Question 1. *Do people differ in their average levels of reported momentary frustration? If so, how much?*

This is in some respects an odd question, because the form of the question does not address hypotheses that are generally of great concern to researchers. It is, though, the basis for examining individual differences (person-level variables), and that is evident if one imagines that the answer to the question is "No." In this case, we would conclude that individuals' average frustration levels do not differ, apart from chance factors inherent in the measurement instruments and the specific sample of moments that were assessed, which would imply that exploring individual differences in average levels of frustration would turn out, in essence, to be a frustrating endeavor. A positive answer to the question justifies the examination of variability among persons in average frustration levels. The exception to these general statements is when there is an a priori hypothesis to be tested: this should be examined regardless of the answer to Question 1, because the statistical power to test a specific a priori hypothesis is substantially greater than that of the global test of "any" individual differences.

Model 1:   Level 1 equation: $\quad \text{Frust}_{it} = \pi_{0i} + \varepsilon_{it} = \quad$ Person's mean + Deviation from Person's mean

Level 2 equation: $\quad \pi_{0i} = \beta_{00} + \delta_{0i} \quad = \quad$ Grand mean (of person means) + Deviation of person's mean from Grand mean

integrated equation: $\text{Frust}_{it} = \beta_{00} + \delta_{0i} + \varepsilon_{it}$

Frust_{it} is the ith person's t^{th} momentary report of frustration. In the Level 1 equation of this specification, π_{0i} represents the ith person's mean level of reported momentary frustration for the 2-week monitoring period, and the ε_{it} are the within-person deviations from this mean. In the Level 2 equation, β_{00} is the grand mean, the mean of the person means, and δ_{0i} corresponds to the deviation of the ith person's mean from the grand mean. This model is equivalent to a traditional nested analysis of variance with unequal numbers of observations per person and implies a decomposition of variance. The variance of the δ_{0i}, $Var(\delta_{0i})$, equals the between-person variance, the variance in persons' mean levels of frustration, while $Var(\varepsilon_{it})$ equals the within-person variance, assumed constant across persons. From the "trait-state" perspective, the between-person variance is attributable to stable (over the 2-week monitoring period) trait-like differences in frustration, while the within-person variance reflects the "state" component of frustration (including any random measurement error). The ratio of the between-person variance to the total variance (sum of between- and within-person variances) is the intraclass correlation coefficient (ICC).

SPECIFICATION OF THE MODEL IN SAS

SAS users will be familiar with the title and libname statements at the beginning of this syntax file, as well as the comment lines describing the variables. In terms of the Proc MIXED syntax, the PROC statement specifies the data file to be analyzed, the method of estimation (either ML for full-information maximum likelihood or REML for restricted maximum likelihood),[6] and COVTEST in order to obtain tests of significance for the random parameters of the model, in this case the estimate of the between-person variance. The CLASS statement lists the categorical variables that will be used in the analysis and must include any variable that is used in the SUB = subcommand of the RANDOM and REPEATED statements (see below).

The MODEL statement specifies the dependent variable and the fixed parameters of the model. Unless one specifically states otherwise (see analysis for Question 6), the intercept β_{00} is assumed to be part of the model. In this example there are no predictor variables and, therefore, the right side of the equation is left blank. For the printout to report the estimate of the intercept, we specify "solution" as an option on the MODEL statement.

At this point, there are two, essentially equivalent, ways to specify a traditional decomposition of variance. The RANDOM statement is used to specify the structure of the variance–covariance matrix for the random coefficients (the G-matrix) and the REPEATED statement is used to specify the structure of the variance–covariance matrix of the within-person residuals (R-matrix). In the first approach, the RANDOM statement is used to specify that the intercept, π_{0i}, in the Level 1 equation may vary across individuals in ways that are not accounted for by any of the explanatory variables (of which there are none). This variability corresponds to $VAR(\delta_{0i})$. Except in very unusual cases, at least in our experience, the "TYPE" of the G-matrix should be specified as "UN" (i.e., unstructured), which implies that there are no constraints imposed.

The "SUB" subcommand is used to specify a variable that uniquely identifies the Level 2 unit of analysis; in all our examples, this is the subject ID variable. Given that no REPEATED statement is included, Proc MIXED assumes that the

ε_{it} are all independent (uncorrelated) and identically distributed with mean zero and $\mathrm{Var}(\varepsilon_{it})$; this implies that R_i is a diagonal T_i-by-T_i matrix with diagonal elements all equal to $\mathrm{Var}(\varepsilon_{it})$. The software will thus produce estimates of fixed parameter β_{00} and random parameters $\mathrm{VAR}(\delta_{0i})$ and $\mathrm{Var}(\varepsilon_{it})$.

The alternative specification of a traditional decomposition of variance comes out of repeated measures ANOVA. In that framework, $\delta_{0i} + \varepsilon_{it}$ is treated as a single residual term, call it λ_{it}. These λ_{it} are uncorrelated across persons, but are now correlated within persons. The resulting R_i-matrix for λ_{it} has all diagonal elements equal to "$\mathrm{VAR}(\delta_{0i}) + \mathrm{Var}(\varepsilon_{it})$" and all off-diagonal elements equal to $\mathrm{VAR}(\delta_{0i})$. This specification of the R_i-matrix has two parameters and is known in the repeated measures ANOVA literature as "compound symmetry" (hence TYPE=CS on the REPEATED statement). The "SUB" subcommand serves the same purpose on the REPEATED statement as on the RANDOM statement.

```
title 'FRUST1.SAS: Decomposition of Variance';
title2 'QUESTION 1: DO PEOPLE DIFFER IN THEIR AVERAGE LEVELS
                OF FRUSTRATION';

libname pain 'E:\NCI\STUDY1';


/*

LIST OF VARIABLES USED IN THIS ANALYSIS
ID: unique person identifier
FRUST: momentary report of frustration (dependent variable)
CONTTIME: a measure of continuous time since subject's first report of
                the study (unit = 1 hour, but includes fractions of hours)

*/

proc mixed data=pain.alldemo2 noclprint method=ml covtest;
  class id;
  model frust= / solution;
  random intercept / type=un sub=id;
  title3 'Multilevel Model with different error structures';
  title4 'MODEL 1a: Compound symmetry - specification most consistent
                w/ multilevel model';
proc mixed data=pain.alldemo2 method=ml covtest;
  class id;
  model frust= / solution;
  repeated / type=cs sub=id;
  title4 'MODEL 1b: Compound symmetry - alternative specification';
```

SPECIFICATION OF AUTOCORRELATED RESIDUALS

Thus far we have assumed that the within-person residuals are uncorrelated with each other. As suggested earlier, this is probably an implausible assumption for most real-time momentary data. It is likely that two reports of frustration, including their residual terms, will be more similar if the interval between them was relatively short (e.g., 1 to 2 hours) than if the reports were made many hours or even days apart.

A first-order autoregressive model is often used to model serial autocorrelation. It assumes that the correlation between two assessments decreases exponentially as a function of the time interval between them. In addition to $Var(\varepsilon_{it})$, this specification of R_i has only one parameter, ρ, the correlation between the residuals of two observations obtained 1 hour (the unit of measurement for our continuous time variable, ContTime) apart.[7] The within-person residuals of assessments obtained at times τ_t and $\tau_{t'}$ are assumed to be correlated $\rho^{|\tau_t - \tau_{t'}|}$. Thus, as the interval approaches zero, the correlation approaches 1.0, implying that frustration changes very little from one instant to the next as long as the situational factors, z_k, remain unchanged. Given that ρ must be less than 1.0, the correlation between observations approaches zero for sufficiently large intervals between assessments.

The Proc MIXED software allows one to specify that the within-person residuals are serially correlated, consistent with a first-order autoregressive pattern. To implement this, and continue to allow for between-person variability in average frustration levels, one must modify the first of the two previous specifications, adding a REPEATED statement. This statement should specify TYPE=SP(POW) (conttime), where "conttime" is the name of a variable that measures time on a continuous scale. In the present data, conttime is measured in hours, with the time of each participant's first assessment arbitrarily set to zero. (The absolute levels of this variable are irrelevant since the model depends only on the time differences between assessments.)[8]

```
proc mixed data=pain.alldemo2 noclprint method=ml covtest;
   class id;
   model frust= / solution;
   random intercept / type=un sub=id;
   repeated / type=sp(pow)(conttime) sub=id;
   title4 'MODEL 1c: Compound symmetry plus serial autocorrelation
                  [SP(POW)]';
```

In nearly every set of real-time momentary data that we have analyzed, the estimated autocorrelation of residuals has been significantly greater than zero, resulting in a substantial improvement in the overall fit of the model to the data (see below).

There is an extension to the first-order autoregressive specification that frequently results in substantial further improvement in the model. In the appendix to this chapter we describe the "toeplitz model" of autocorrelated within-person residuals and how it can be used to estimate how the correlation between residuals actually varies in relation to the time interval between the assessments—that is, whether it actually declines exponentially. The results can be used to construct a graph of this relationship, known as a "variogram," over which one can superimpose a plot of the predicted relationship based on the estimates from the first-order autoregressive specification.

In several data sets, especially those with many assessments per participant, the results from the toeplitz model suggest that the autocorrelation does not approach 1.0 as the time interval shrinks toward zero and that the autocorrelation of residuals declines more gradually than the exponential rate assumed by the first-order autoregressive specification. This is consistent with the pattern that would be expected if each assessment of the outcome variable was subject to some degree of random measurement error. By adding the keyword "LOCAL" to the preceding REPEATED statement, we modify the model to assume that ε_{it} is the sum of two orthogonal components, μ_{it} and v_{it}, where only μ_{it} exhibits first-order autoregressive serial correlation, while the v_{it} are uncorrelated across assessments. We call this the "modified first-order autoregressive" or "AR(1) + noise" specification.

One interpretation of v_{it} is that it corresponds to random measurement error.[9] The assumption of orthogonality implies that $\text{Var}(\varepsilon_{it}) = \text{Var}(\mu_{it}) + \text{Var}(v_{it})$. In the majority of analyses we have conducted applying this model to momentary data, the estimates of $\text{Var}(\mu_{it})$ and $\text{Var}(v_{it})$ are of roughly similar magnitude while the estimate of the autocorrelation parameter for μ_{it} is substantially higher than the corresponding parameter for ε_{it} in the preceding model.

```
proc mixed data=pain.alldemo2 noclprint method=ml covtest;
   class id;
   model frust= / solution;
   random intercept / type=un sub=id;
   repeated / type=sp(pow)(conttime) sub=id local;
   parms 450 220 .77 220;
   title4 'MODEL 1d:  Compound symmetry plus SP(POW) and LOCAL';
```

With this specification, the SAS software often has difficulty converging to a valid solution. This can be handled by providing reasonable initial estimates for the random parameters of the model on a PARMS statement. Based on our experience, we typically use the estimates of $\text{VAR}(\delta_{0i})$, ρ, and $\text{Var}(\varepsilon_{it})$ from the (unmodified) first-order autoregressive specification (450, .54, and 441, respectively; Table 5-2) to generate starting values around $\text{VAR}(\delta_{0i})$, $\text{Var}(\varepsilon_{it})/2$, $(1+\rho)/2$, and $\text{Var}(\varepsilon_{it})/2$ for the modified first-order autoregressive specification {450, 220, .77, and 220 for $\text{VAR}(\delta_{0i})$, $\text{Var}(\mu_{it})$, ρ, and $\text{Var}(v_{it})$, respectively}.

Table 5-2 contains estimates of the nested ANOVA model for the three specifications described above: uncorrelated within-person residuals (column 1), first-order autoregressively correlated residuals (column 2), and first-order autoregressively correlated residuals with uncorrelated "measurement error" (column 3). The estimated pattern of serial autocorrelation of the within-person fluctuations for the modified and unmodified first-order autoregressive specifications are graphed in Figure 5-1. Table 5-3 compares the fit of the three models. The three models are nested since the first model is a constrained variant of the second (under the constraint that $\rho = 0$) and the second is a constrained variant of the third (under the constraint that $\text{Var}(v_{it}) = 0$). Therefore, we can test the significance of the improvement in fit using the change in the log-likelihood (LL) ratio.

Table 5-2. Decomposition of variance for frustration ($n = 5321$ observations from 68 participants)

Source of variance	Compound symmetry	+ AR(1)	+ "noise"
Between-person	458[1]	450[1]	436[1]
Within-person	424	441	445
Autocorrelated	—	441[1]	257[1]
Autocorrelation (1 hr)		0.54[a]	0.86[1]
Uncorrelated	424[1]	—	187[1]
Percent between-person[2]	52%	50%	50%
-2 LL	47589	46905	46686

[1] $p < 0.0001$
[2] intraclass correlation (ICC) = Var(Between-person) / {Var(Between-person) + Var(Within-person)}

Under the null hypothesis that the constrained model is correct, the change in −2 LL has a chi-square distribution with degrees of freedom equal to the difference in the number of parameters in the two models. As shown in Table 5-3, the modified first-order autoregressive specification fits the data much better than either of the other two models, and hence it will be used in all subsequent analyses.

According to the estimates of this best-fitting model, 50 percent of the total variance (sum of the three components) over the 2-week period is attributable to trait-like individual differences ($p < 0.0001$) in average levels of frustration, and the remaining 50 percent is due to fluctuations in frustration within persons. These fluctuations can be further decomposed into a state component (29%, $p < 0.0001$) that exhibits quite high serial autocorrelation (1-hour correlation = .86, $p < 0.0001$, implying that the 2-hour, 3-hour, and 4-hour correlations are .74, .64, and .55) and a remaining component (21%) that exhibits no autocorrelation and may reflect random measurement error. Of note, the estimate of β_{00}, the mean of the person means, is 34.5 (se = 2.6, $p < 0.0001$), suggesting that this sample of chronic pain patients tends to experience/report considerable frustration. The large amount of between-person variance suggests that demographic characteristics, individual attributes, differences among people in their rheumatological condition, and/or environmental characteristics might affect frustration. Similarly, the extensive within-person fluctuations in frustration suggest that situational factors also affect frustration. To the extent that the non-autocorrelated component of the within-person variance does reflect random measurement error, we would not expect this component of variance to shrink very much as explanatory variables are added to the model.

ANSWER TO QUESTION 1

There are substantial differences among people in their average levels of frustration. Approximately 50 percent of the total variance in momentary reports of

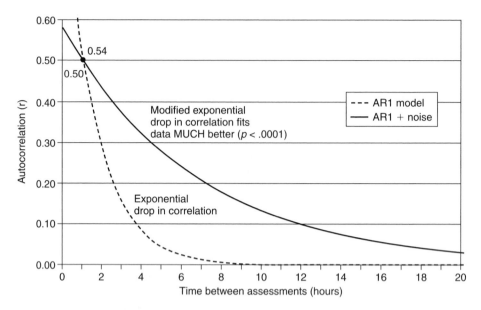

Figure 5-1. Predicted correlations of within-person fluctuations in self-reports of frustration according to estimates of AR(1) and "AR(1) + noise" specifications of autocorrelation pattern.

frustration is due to differences between participants in average frustration. Our best estimate, taken from the final model, is that the standard deviation of people's average frustration is about 21, the square root of 436. Similarly, the within-person fluctuations in momentary frustration levels have a standard deviation of about 21 (the square root of 445). Given a 100-point VAS item, it appears that study participants used the full range of the scale.

Note to the reader. If you have made it this far, you have survived the most difficult material. Though this first example may not address an important

Table 5-3. Comparison of fit among models

Model	−2 LL	Change (−2 LL)	Change (*df*)	*p*
Compound symmetry	47589.1			
+ AR(1)	46904.7	684.6	1	<0.0001
+ "noise"	46685.8	218.9	1	<0.0001

Since each model adds one parameter to the preceding model, the change in -2LL should be referred to a χ^2 distribution with $df = 1$ (critical value for $\alpha = .05$ is 3.84). While there may be even better fitting specifications for the pattern of autocorrelation among the within-person residuals, clearly the third of these three specifications fits much better than the other two.

substantive question, it sets the ground for all subsequent analyses by focusing directly on the distinction between relative amounts of between-person and within-person variance. It also provides an opportunity to examine the within-person pattern of autocorrelation and to arrive at a specification of this that can be used in all subsequent analyses of this outcome variable.

Question 2. *Does frustration vary by socioeconomic status (education and/or income)?*

The form of this question is similar to many analyses researchers seek to conduct. Socioeconomic status (SES) is just one of many person-level factors that index characteristics of individuals (e.g., age, sex, race) or of the treatments to which individuals are exposed (control vs. experimental status in a non-crossover design, for example). Since person-level characteristics cannot explain within-person fluctuations in an outcome, this type of question implicitly asks whether people's average level of frustration (for the 2-week monitoring period) is predicted by their SES.

Model 2:   Level 1 equation: $Frust_{it} = \pi_{0i} + \varepsilon_{it}$
           Level 2 equation: $\pi_{0i} = \beta_{00} + \beta_{01} SES_i + \delta_{0i}$
           Integrated equation: $Frust_{it} = \beta_{00} + \beta_{01} SES_i + \delta_{0i} + \varepsilon_{it}$

This data set contains two measures of SES, a four-category measure of education (high school graduate, 1 to 3 years of college, a college degree, postgraduate training) and a five-category measure of family income (<\$20K, \$20K to 34K, \$35K to 49K, \$50K to 74K, >\$75K). In separate analyses, each variable was treated categorically (analogous to a one-way ANOVA) in order to obtain (1) a global test of whether mean frustration levels differed among categories and (2) estimates of the category means and their standard errors. The syntax for these two analyses appears below and the results are graphed in Figure 5-2 (the point estimates for each category, with thin bars portraying the 95% confidence intervals). For both predictors, it appears that there is a threshold effect, such that people's average frustration levels are lower for those above some level of SES (those with at least some college and those with family incomes of \$50K or more). Based on this observation, we performed post hoc analyses to determine whether dichotomous measures of education and income adequately capture the differences among the multiple categories. As illustrated by the solid lines in both figures, the dichotomous measures parsimoniously summarize the relationships of education and income to frustration.

Syntax for analysis of income as a predictor of frustration:

title 'FRUST2.SAS: Relationship of FRUSTRATION to SES';
title2 'QUESTION 2: DOES FRUSTRATION VARY BY SES';

options ls=110 ps=80 nocenter nofmterr;
libname pain 'E:\NCI\STUDY1';

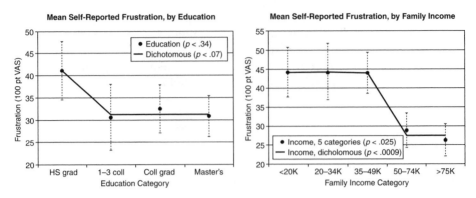

Figure 5-2. The relationship of frustration to education and family income (person-level predictors).

```
/*
LIST OF VARIABLES USED IN THIS ANALYSIS
ID:          unique person identifier
FRUST:       momentary report of frustration (dependent variable)
CONTTIME:    a measure of continuous time since subject's first report
             of the study (unit = 1 hour, but includes fractions of hours)
INCOME:      income measured in 5 categories (<20K, 20–34, 35–49,
             50–74, 75+)
INCOME2:     dichotomous measure of income (0=<50K, 1=50+)
*/
proc mixed data=pain.alldemo2 noclprint noinfo method=ml covtest;
  class id income;
  model frust=income / solution;
  random intercept / type=un sub=id;
  lsmeans income;
  repeated / type=sp(pow)(conttime) sub=id local;
  parms 435 255 .85 185;
  title3 'Error Model: Compound symmetry plus SP(POW) and LOCAL';
  title4 'Between-person predictor: Income (5 categories)';
  title5 'Income Treated as a Categorical Variable (in CLASS statement)';
proc mixed data=pain.alldemo2 noclprint noinfo method=ml covtest;
  class id income2;
  model frust=income2 / solution;
  random intercept / type=un sub=id;
  lsmeans income2;
  repeated / type=sp(pow)(conttime) sub=id local;
  parms 435 255 .85 185;
  title4 'Between-person predictors: Income - dichotomous (>=$50,000)';
```

The inclusion of "income" on the CLASS statement ensures that it is treated as a categorical, rather than interval-level, measure. The LSMEANS statement, which can be used only for categorical predictor variables, requests estimates of the predicted mean frustration level and its standard error for each income category. The starting values for the PARMS statement are taken from the last column of Table 5-2.

ANSWER TO QUESTION 2

Individuals' mean levels of frustration differ significantly by income. Those whose family income is $50K or more have average frustration levels that are, on average, 17 points below those with lower family incomes. The estimate of unexplained between-person variance in this model, $Var(\delta_{0i})$, is 368, compared to 436 in the model without income, indicating that the dichotomous measure of income accounts for 16 percent ($= 1–368/436$) of the between-person variance. For the parallel analysis of education, the test of differences among the four categories of education was not statistically significant. Nevertheless, the data suggest that those who have not attended college have higher average frustration levels than those with at least some college education.

A SIMPLE BUT INADEQUATE ALTERNATIVE STRATEGY FOR QUESTION 2

Those who are unfamiliar with multilevel modeling might analyze the relationship between SES and frustration by computing the mean of frustration separately for each person and then performing a traditional one-way ANOVA to test for SES-related differences in these means. While this approach has the virtue of simplicity, and often leads to the same conclusion vis-à-vis whether the relationship is statistically significant, the multilevel modeling approach is generally superior.[10] This is because sample means (of frustration) are only estimates of individuals' "true" means; each mean is subject to sampling variability that is the equivalent of random measurement error in traditional psychometric theory. Furthermore, this measurement error variance (estimated by the squared standard error of the mean) is likely to vary from person to person, due primarily to differences in the number of momentary assessments, which can then result in the violation of the homoskedasticity of residuals assumption of ANOVA. This unreliability also results in an overestimation of the amount of total variance in the person means and a downwardly biased estimate of the percentage of between-person variance in frustration that can be accounted for by SES. In contrast, multilevel modeling treats the person means as a latent variable (i.e., corrected for unreliability), providing a "better" estimate of between-person variance and the percentage that is accounted for. In addition to this argument for its theoretical superiority, multilevel modeling allows one to easily include or control for moment-level covariate(s) such as location (work, home, elsewhere) or pain (see analysis for Question 5).

Question 3. *Is frustration related to pain?*

This question shifts the focus of the analysis to understanding the within-person associations among momentary variables. Real-time data collection studies have the unique ability to address these sorts of questions; thus, we imagine that the analyses described below will be quite common in real-time studies. Pain is a momentary variable, like frustration, and therefore a more precise statement of this question would be, *"Does a person's frustration tend to be higher when his/her pain is higher?"* Or, *"Are changes in a person's frustration level related to (correlated with) changes in pain?"* We begin by treating the slope of the relationship between frustration and pain as a fixed effect, thereby assuming that it is the same for everyone; if this were a causal relationship, we would be assuming that pain has the same effect on frustration for everyone.

Model 3: Level 1 equation: $\text{Frust}_{it} = \pi_{0i} + \pi_{1i} \text{Pain}_{it} + \varepsilon_{it}$

Level 2 equations: $\pi_{0i} = \beta_{00} + \delta_{0i}$

$\pi_{1i} = \beta_{10}$

integrated equation: $\text{Frust}_{it} = \beta_{00} + \beta_{10} \text{Pain}_{it} + \delta_{0i} + \varepsilon_{it}$

Syntax:

```
title 'FRUST3.SAS:   Relationship of FRUSTRATION to PAIN';
title2 'QUESTION 3:   IS FRUSTRATION RELATED TO (CURRENT)
              PAIN?';

options ls=108 ps=80 nocenter;

libname pain 'E:\NCI\STUDY1';

/*
LIST OF VARIABLES USED IN THIS ANALYSIS
ID:      unique person identifier
FRUST:   momentary report of frustration (dependent variable)
CONTTIME:  a measure of continuous time since subject's first report
           of the study (unit = 1 hour, but includes fractions of
           hours)
PAINVAS0:  momentary report of pain (100-point VAS)
INCOME:    income measured in 5 categories (<20K, 20–34, 35–49,
           50–74, 75+)
INCOME2:   dichotomous measure of income (0=<50K, 1=50+)
EDUC2:     dichotomous measure of education (0=High School,
           1=some college+)
*/

proc mixed data=pain.alldemo2 noclprint noinfo method=ml covtest;
  class id;
  model frust=painvas0 / solution;
```

random intercept / type=un sub=id;
repeated / type=sp(pow)(conttime) sub=id local;
parms 435 255 .85 185;
title5 'Compound symmetry plus SP(POW) and LOCAL';
title6 'Model 3: PAINVAS0 treated as a fixed effect';

Answer to Question 3

The results (not shown) indicate a very substantial positive relationship between pain and frustration. The regression coefficient indicates that a 10-point increase on the 100-point VAS pain scale is associated with a 2.1-point increase in frustration (B_{10} = .21, se = .013, t = 16.3, $p < 0.0001$). The addition of pain to the final version of Model 1 (see Question 1) reduces the unexplained within-person variance (sum of autocorrelated and non-autocorrelated) by 5.7 percent. Furthermore, because people differ in their average levels of pain, and pain is related to frustration, momentary pain also reduces the unexplained between-person variance by 10.6 percent. Thus, we can say that momentary pain accounts for 10.6 percent of the between-person variability in average levels of frustration and 5.7 percent of the within-person variability in frustration. However, the estimate of the standard error of B_{10} and the significance test are premised on the assumption that the relationship of frustration to pain is the same for all persons. What if this assumption is incorrect?

Question 4. *Does the relationship between frustration and pain vary across individuals?*

The prior analysis assumed that the relationship of frustration to pain was the same for all individuals. As noted earlier, if this assumption is false, the standard error of the pain coefficient will be underestimated and the significance may be exaggerated. Therefore, before concluding that fluctuations in frustration are related to fluctuations in pain, it is important to investigate the possibility, perhaps likelihood, of individual differences in this relationship.[11] To address this question, we treat the coefficient of pain in the Level 1 equation as a random effect or random coefficient.

Model 4:   Level 1 equation: $Frust_{it} = \pi_{0i} + \pi_{1i} Pain_{it} + \varepsilon_{it}$
Level 2 equations: $B_{0i} = \beta_{00} + \delta_{0i}$
$B_{1i} = \beta_{10} + \delta_{1i}$
Integrated equation: $Frust_{it} = \beta_{00} + \beta_{10} Pain_{it} + \delta_{0i}$
$+ \delta_{1i} Pain_{it} + \varepsilon_{it}$

To estimate this model, the momentary pain variable needs to be listed on the RANDOM statement. By specifying "GCORR" on this statement, the printout will include the estimate of the correlation between the intercepts and the slopes—that is, between δ_{0i} and δ_{1i}.[12]

Syntax:
title3 'QUESTION 4: DOES RELATIONSHIP VARY ACROSS
INDIVIDUALS?';
proc mixed data=pain.alldemo2 noclprint noinfo method=ml covtest;
class id;
model frust=painvas0 / solution;
random intercept painvas0 / type=un sub=id gcorr;
repeated / type=sp(pow)(conttime) sub=id local;
parms 435 0 1 245 .85 200;
title6 'PAINVAS0 treated as a random effect';

In terms of the question being posed, our initial interest is in the estimate of the variability in the pain coefficients, $Var(\delta_{1i})$. If it is close to zero, then the differences among individuals in the relationship of frustration to pain are minimal or nonexistent, justifying the treatment of the effect as fixed. [13] Otherwise, there is empirical evidence of individual differences. Those who find standard deviations easier to interpret than variances can calculate the square root of $Var(\delta_{1i})$. If $Var(\delta_{1i}) > 0$, then β_{10} is no longer the coefficient of pain; rather, it is the average of people's pain coefficients. In this case, the test of the hypothesis that frustration is related to momentary pain (i.e., that $\beta_{10} \neq 0$) depends on the random variability among persons in this relationship. Specifically, the standard error of β_{10} increases relative to the fixed effect model, because it must take the $Var(\delta_{1i})$ into account, and the degrees of freedom will depend on the number of individuals in the analysis rather than the total number of momentary assessments. Both of these adjustments reduce the statistical power of the test compared to the previous analysis where the coefficient of pain was treated as a fixed effect.

Thus, if nonnegligible individual differences exist, it can happen that the estimate of the effect of pain on frustration is statistically significant when it is treated as a fixed effect, but nonsignificant when it is treated as a random effect. This would indicate that there is a positive relationship for some individuals and a negative relationship for others. In this situation, it is tempting to report the statistically significant coefficient from the fixed effects model. Is there anything wrong with this? The answer is, "Probably." If, as in most cases, one wishes to generalize from the participants in the present study to other potential participants from the same population, then one's test of the effect of pain on frustration should adjust for individual differences in this effect if they exist.

ANSWER TO QUESTION 4

In the present study, the estimated variance of the pain coefficients is 0.034 (se = .009, $p < 0.0001$), making the standard deviation 0.183. Clearly, there are significant individual differences in the relationship of frustration to pain. The estimate of β_{10}, the average of people's pain coefficients, is 0.239 (se = .028, $p < 0.0001$), quite similar to when the effect of pain was treated as fixed. Assuming the coefficients of pain have a normal distribution, $N(.239,.183)$, we estimate that 90 percent of individuals have positive coefficients, and that 95 percent of people's coefficients are between -0.120 and $+0.599$. Consistent with the previous paragraph, the standard error of the average coefficient, $.028$, is more than twice the magnitude of the standard error when the coefficient of pain was treated as a fixed effect ($.013$). Taking into account the individual differences in slopes, the percent of within-person variance in frustration that is accounted for by pain increases from 5.7 percent for the fixed effect model to 9.1 percent. As noted in footnote 12, the $\text{Var}(\delta_{0i})$ is no longer a measure of unexplained between-person variance; it will change if one adds or subtracts a constant from the pain variable.

At this point, we can confidently conclude that current frustration is related to current pain (for most people). This within-person relationship implies that changes in pain are correlated with changes in frustration, which is much stronger evidence for a causal relationship between these two constructs than that provided by traditional cross-sectional (between-person) studies. This said, the analyses presented here cannot reveal the causal direction, if any, of the relationship—only that increases in one variable tend to be associated with increases (or decreases) in the other.[14]

Question 5. *Are the individual differences in the relationship of frustration to pain associated with SES?*

The question we now address puts together several of the prior analyses in order to determine if within-person associations are reliably related to stable person factors. Specifically, we ask, is the change in frustration associated with a 10-point increase in pain different for those with more education or higher incomes than for others? This question requires us to evaluate a cross-level interaction effect— that is, the interaction of a person-level characteristic with a momentary measure. As in traditional regression analysis, it is usually advisable to compare the interaction model to an additive model that includes both momentary pain and SES as predictors. The following syntax is used to estimate (1) the additive model with pain and the dichotomous family income (or education) measure, and (2) the interaction model for pain and income.

Additive	Level 1 equation:	$\text{Frust}_{it} = \pi_{0i} + \pi_{1i}\,\text{Pain}_{it} + \varepsilon_{it}$
Model 5a:	Level 2 equations:	$\pi_{0i} = \beta_{00} + \beta_{01}\,\text{SES}_i + \delta_{0i}$
		$\pi_{1i} = \beta_{10} + \delta_{1i}$

	Integrated equation:	$\text{Frust}_{it} = \beta_{00} + \beta_{01}\,\text{SES}_i + \beta_{10}\,\text{Pain}_{it}$ $+ \delta_{0i} + \delta_{1i}\,\text{Pain}_{it} + \varepsilon_{it}$

Interaction	Level 1 equation:	$\text{Frust}_{it} = \pi_{0i} + \pi_{1i}\,\text{Pain}_{it} + \varepsilon_{it}$
Model 5b:	Level 2 equations:	$\pi_{0i} = \beta_{00} + \beta_{01}\,\text{SES}_i + \delta_{0i}$
		$\pi_{1i} = \beta_{10} + \beta_{11}\,\text{SES}_i + \delta_{1i}$

	Integrated equation:	$\text{Frust}_{it} = \beta_{00} + \beta_{01}\,\text{SES}_i + \beta_{10}\,\text{Pain}_{it}$ $+ \beta_{11}\,(\text{SES}_i \times \text{Pain}_{it}) + \delta_{0i}$ $+ \delta_{1i}\,\text{Pain}_{it} + \varepsilon_{it}$

Syntax:

```
title4 'QUESTION 5:  DOES FRUSTRATION-PAIN RELATIONSHIP
                     VARY BY SES?';
proc mixed data=pain.alldemo2 noclprint noinfo method=ml covtest;
  class id;
  model frust=income2 painvas0 / solution;
  random intercept painvas0 / type=un sub=id gcorr;
  repeated / type=sp(pow)(conttime) sub=id local;
  parms 435 0 1 245 .85 185;
  title7 'Income treated as a dichotomous variable (main effects)';

proc mixed data=pain.alldemo2 noclprint noinfo method=ml covtest;
  class id;
  model frust=income2 painvas0 income2*painvas0 / solution;
  random intercept painvas0 / type=un sub=id gcorr;
  repeated / type=sp(pow)(conttime) sub=id local;
  parms 435 0 1 245 .85 185;
  title8 'Interaction of income2 w/ PainVAS0';
```

ANSWER TO QUESTION 5

In the first of these analyses, both income and pain are significant predictors of frustration (both $p < 0.005$), with coefficients similar to the previous models. The estimated relationships are shown in Figure 5-3A. In the second analysis, the interaction of income and pain is not at all significant ($p > 0.50$), suggesting that the additive model is a parsimonious representation of the relationships of pain and income to frustration (Figure 5-3B). Thus, at any given level of momentary pain, those with family incomes of at least $50K are, on average, less frustrated than those with lower family incomes, but income does not account for individual differences in the pain–frustration relationship; the lines are nearly parallel. However, the results are somewhat different if we use our dichotomous measure of education as the measure of SES. While the additive effect of education is not statistically significant (Figure 5-3), there is a significant interaction effect ($p < 0.01$), indicating that increases in pain are associated with greater increases in frustration in those with no college experience than for those with at least some college. The graph of this interaction pattern (Figure 5-3D) indicates that, at low levels of pain, those with and without some college have similar levels of frustration, but at higher levels of pain, those with no college report substantially higher levels of pain than those with some college. The unexplained (between-person) variance in the coefficients of pain [$\text{Var}(\delta_{1i})$] in the interaction model is 84.2 percent of its value in the additive model. This can be interpreted as indicating that the dichotomous education variable can account for 15.8 percent of the individual differences in the relationship of pain to frustration.

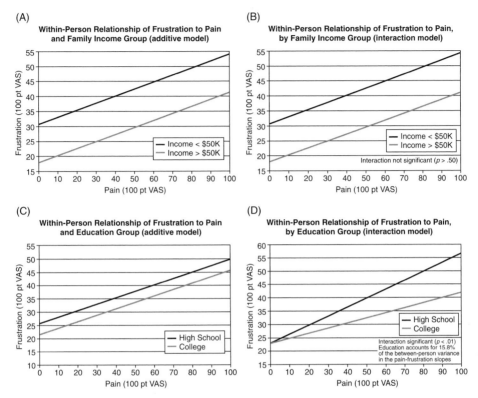

Figure 5-3. Additive and interactive models of the relationship of SES and momentary pain to frustration.

Question 6: *How reproducible/stable are individual differences from week to week?*

In the earlier decomposition of variance (Question 1), we estimated the percentage of variance that was attributable to stable individual differences across the 2-week period. Here, we break the 2-week period into separate 1-week periods, estimate each person's mean for each week, and examine the correlation of the week 1 means with the week 2 means. There are two reasons for raising this question. Pragmatically, a very high correlation would suggest that 1 week of monitoring could provide a very good estimate of a person's 2-week average frustration level. At a more conceptual level, the distinction between trait and state components of frustration is somewhat relative. From the perspective of the earlier analysis, trait differences referred to differences that were stable for 2 weeks, and week-to-week variability in people's average frustration levels was implicitly treated as part of state variance. To date, few researchers have asked questions like, *"Over what period of time do people's moods remain stable (or change)?"* By breaking the total monitoring period into subperiods, we can begin to address this question empirically.

Model 6:   Level 1 equation: $Frust_{it} = \pi_{1i} Week_{1it} + \pi_{2i} Week_{2it} + \varepsilon_{it}$

Level 2 equations: $\pi_{1i} = \beta_{10} + \delta_{1i}$
$\pi_{2i} = \beta_{20} + \delta_{2i}$

Integrated equation: $Frust_{it} = \beta_{10} Week_{1it} + \beta_{20} Week_{2it}$
$+ \delta_{1i} Week_{1it} + \delta_{2i} Week_{2it} + \varepsilon_{it}$

where, $Week_{1it}$ = 1 for all week 1 assessments and 0 for all week 2 assessments, and
$Week_{2it}$ = 1 for all week 2 assessments and 0 for all week 1 assessments.

This model differs from all of the previous models in that neither the Level 1 equation nor the integrated equation includes an intercept term. With this specification, π_{1i} equals the ith person's mean frustration level during the first week and π_{2i} equals his or her mean during the second week. β_{10} and β_{20} equal the mean of the person means for weeks 1 and 2 and δ_{1i} and δ_{2i} equal the deviations of the weekly person means from β_{10} and β_{20}, respectively.

It is interesting to contrast this model with a more traditional analysis in which one simply computes individuals' average frustration levels for each week and correlates the two sets of means. This "empirical" correlation will generally be smaller (attenuated) than the correlation obtained from the multilevel analysis because of the unreliability, due to sampling variability, of the computed averages. In contrast, π_{1i} and π_{2i} in the multilevel model are latent variables, and the estimate of the correlation between them (the correlation between δ_{1i} and δ_{2i}) implicitly adjusts for the effects of sampling variability. In the following syntax, we compute the weekly averages for each person and their correlation, and then estimate the corresponding multilevel model.

Syntax:

```
title2 'QUESTION 6: Reproducibility of average frustration levels from
Week 1 to Week 2';
* First computing empirical correlation between CALCULATED weekly means;

* Calculates weekly mean levels of frustration for each subject;
* (data already sorted by id and week);
proc means data=pain.alldemo2 noprint; by id week;
  var frust;
  output out=means_wk mean=frust;

* Transforms 136 weekly means into 68 pairs of weekly means;
data repeated; set;  by id week;
  retain frust1 frust2;
  array frus frust1 frust2;
  if first.id then do;  frust1=.;  frust2=.;  end;
  frus[week]=frust;
  if last.id then output;
```

```
proc corr; var frust1 frust2;
title3 'Correlations of computed weekly averages of frustration';

proc mixed data=pain.alldemo2 noclprint noinfo method=ml covtest;
    class id week;
    model frust=week / noint solution;
    random week / type=un sub=id gcorr;
    lsmeans week / pdiff;
    repeated / type=sp(pow)(conttime) sub=id local;
    parms 440 360 440 245 .85 200;
    title3 'Compound symmetry plus SP(POW) and LOCAL';
    title4 'Correlation of Weeks 3 and 4 Mean Frustration';
```

The analysis of the computed person averages for each week yields estimated means and standard deviations (of the weekly person means) of 34.8 and 22.1 for week 1 and 34.5 and 22.5 for week 2. The week 1/week 2 test–retest correlation is .895. This is certainly a strong correlation, which will undoubtedly lead some to wonder why they should worry about its being attenuated and underestimating the true week-to-week stability of average frustration levels.

ANSWER TO QUESTION 6

The analogous estimates from the multilevel model are that the means (of person means) for the 2 weeks are 34.8 and 34.4 and the variances are 444.33 and 460.20, making the standard deviations 21.8 and 21.5. The LSMEANS statement generates a significance test for the change in means ($t = .34$, $p > 0.50$). As anticipated, the standard deviations in the previous paragraph are somewhat larger due to sampling variability. The multilevel estimates of variances are adjusted for this. As a result, the estimated week 1/week 2 test–retest correlation, reported in the printout, is .943. While .943 might not be considered "much higher" than .895, this result from the multilevel model indicates that only half of the variance of the week-to-week change in computed mean frustration levels [Var(change in calculated means) $= 22.1^2 + 22.5^2 - 22.1*22.5*.895 = 103.7$] reflects true change [Var(change in "true" means) $= 21.8^2 + 21.5^2 - 21.8*21.5*.943 = 52.1$; $52.1/103.7 = .50$] and the other half is due to sampling variability in the estimates of each week's averages. Stated differently, it appears that the computed weekly averages would be adequate for analyzing the relationship of person-level factors to average frustration levels, but not for analyzing factors that might account for week-to-week changes in average frustration levels.

If one were interested in testing whether the standard deviations of the week 1 and week 2 averages were equal, one could modify the TYPE= subcommand on the RANDOM statement to be TYPE=TOEP(2), thereby imposing the equality constraint, and then use the change in the −2 LL to test whether the fit of the former model was significantly better than that of this constrained model.

Question 7. *Are there temporal patterns to frustration? Is there a diurnal pattern to frustration? If so, can we model it? Does frustration tend to be higher on weekdays than weekends?*

Each of these questions concerns whether frustration is related to time, be it time of day, day of week, or day of monitoring. From one perspective, time is just another moment-level factor. But from another perspective, time is conceptually quite different. For example, time is not subjective and with electronic diaries it need not even be self-reported; electronic diaries typically time- and date-stamp each momentary report. Second, time is exogenous. Frustration cannot affect time (unless people self-select when they will complete momentary assessments). On the other hand, the existence of a relationship between the two may reflect either an underlying biological process (such as a circadian rhythm) or, perhaps more likely, the existence of third factors that exhibit similar temporal patterns (such as engagement in work vs. non-work activities) and influence frustration. Models in which time is the primary moment-level predictor are also known as "growth curve models," highlighting their focus on temporal patterns.

We first consider three models examining the diurnal pattern of frustration. The first divides the 24-hour day into 1-hour blocks, for the purpose of estimating the average diurnal pattern at a fairly micro level. The second model is similar, but uses eight 3-hour time blocks. These two models are nonparametric representations of the diurnal pattern in that they do not assume any underlying functional form. The third model fits a sinusoidal curve to the diurnal pattern to assess how well this smooth two-parameter equation captures/represents the diurnal pattern. For ease of estimation, we treat the effects of time as fixed, ignoring for the moment the possibility/likelihood that individuals' diurnal patterns may differ.

Model 7a: Level 1 equation:

$$y_{it} = \sum_{k=1}^{24} \pi_{ki} \, \text{Hour}_{kit} + \varepsilon_{it}$$

Model 7b: Level 1 equation:

$$y_{it} = \sum_{k=1}^{8} \pi_{ki} \, \text{Hr\_block}_{kit} + \varepsilon_{it}$$

Model 7c: Level 1 equation:

$$\text{Frust}_{it} = \pi_{0i} + \pi_{1i} \, \text{Sine}(\text{TOD}_{1it}/4) + \pi_{2i} \, \text{Cosine}(\text{TOD}_{2it}/4) + \varepsilon_{it}$$

where, TOD is time of day, measured in minutes past midnight. It is divided by 4 in order to translate the 1440 minutes in a day into the 360° of a circle, thereby making the periodicity of the effect equal to 24 hours.

ANSWER TO QUESTION 7

In the following SAS code, the LSMEANS statement in the first analysis provides estimates of mean frustration levels and their standard errors for each hour of the day. The code for the second model is the same, replacing the variable "hour" by one in which hour is collapsed into eight 3-hour blocks. Figure 5-4A shows a

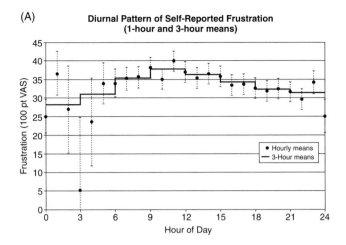

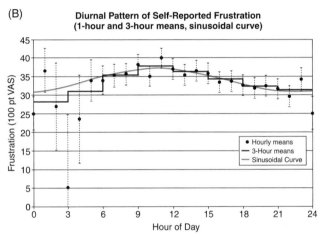

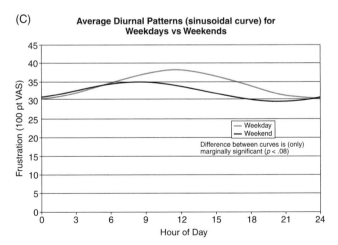

Figure 5-4. Diurnal pattern of frustration.

plot of the mean levels of frustration (± 1 standard error). The large standard errors for the early morning hours, 1 to 5 a.m., are due to the small number of momentary assessments made at these times and indicate that the means for these hours are not very precisely estimated. While the differences across the day may not look large, a test of the null hypothesis that there is no diurnal pattern (i.e., that the mean is constant across the 24 hours) is easily rejected ($F_{23,5230} =$ 3.69, $p < 0.0001$). Figure 5-4A superimposes the means of the 3-hour blocks and shows that this more gross analysis captures the diurnal pattern fairly well. Using reduction in the –2 LL from the null model (one that assumes no diurnal pattern) to assess improvement in fit, the model with the 8-category time variable captures almost two thirds of the improvement in fit of the 24-category time variable, while the former uses less than one-third the degrees of freedom. Nonetheless, the more detailed analysis does provide a significantly better fit ($\chi^2 = 28.7$, $df = 16$, $p < 0.03$). Figure 5-4B superimposes the estimates of the sinusoidal diurnal pattern model. Using only 2 degrees of freedom, this model fits the data nearly as well as the nonparametric 7-*df* model ($\chi^2 = 2.6$, $df = 5$, $p > 0.50$), and only marginally worse than the 23-*df* model ($\chi^2 = 31.3$, $df = 21$, $p < 0.07$).[15]

Syntax:

title 'FRUST7.SAS: temporal patterns of FRUSTRATION';
title2 'QUESTION 7: ARE THERE TEMPORAL PATTERNS TO
                FRUSTRATION?';

/*

LIST OF VARIABLES USED IN THIS ANALYSIS
ID: unique person identifier
FRUST: momentary report of frustration (dependent variable)
CONTTIME: a measure of continuous time since subject's first report of
                 the study (unit = 1 hour, but includes fractions of hours)
HOUR: a 24-category measure (e.g., 8 = 8:00 – 8:59am)
To fit a sinusoidal curve to the diurnal pattern of frustration, we use
COSINE: cosine(2*PI * time-of-day/1440), where PI=3.1415...., and
SINE: sine(2*PI * time-of-day/1440)
WEEKEND: 0 = Mon thru Fri, 1 = Sat or Sun

*/

proc mixed data=pain.alldemo2 noclprint noinfo method=ml covtest;
  class id hour;
  model frust=hour / solution;
  lsmeans hour;
  random intercept / type=un sub=id;
  repeated / type=sp(pow)(conttime) sub=id local;
  parms 440 245 .85 200;
  title3 'Compound symmetry plus SP(POW) and LOCAL';

```
title4 'Mean hourly levels of frust (FIXED EFFECT)';
proc mixed data=pain.alldemo2 noclprint noinfo method=ml covtest;
  class id;
  model frust=sine cosine / solution;
  random intercept / type=un sub=id;
  repeated / type=sp(pow)(conttime) sub=id local;
  parms 440 245 .85 200;
  title4 'Sinusoidal model of diurnal cycle of frust (FIXED EFFECT)';
```

Day-of-week effects can be analyzed in a similar manner. Consider two models, one in which we estimate a separate mean level of frustration for each day of the week, and one in which we assume that Monday through Friday have the same mean level and Saturday and Sunday have the same mean (that is, a weekend vs. weekday effect). We note that if the predominant temporal pattern across days is due to a weekend/weekday effect, then the analysis examining differences among all 7 days will be less powerful to detect the pattern. This appears to be the case. The 6-*df* test for any day-of-week effects in the first analysis is of only borderline significance ($p < 0.07$), while the 1-*df* test of the weekend/weekday difference is highly significant ($p < 0.002$).

Figure 5-5 shows the predicted levels of frustration for both models and clearly illustrates that the means are similar for Monday through Friday and for Saturday and Sunday.

We went on to examine the diurnal pattern (sinusoidal model) and day-of-week (weekday vs. weekend) effects in one model by estimating a model in which

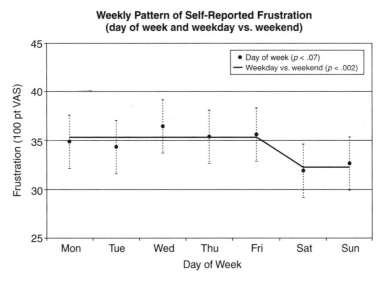

Figure 5-5. Weekly pattern of self-reported frustration (day of week and weekday vs. weekend).

separate sinusoidal curves are fit for weekdays and for weekend days. The syntax for both an additive model and an interaction model appears below, and the results of the interaction model are illustrated in Figure 5-4C. They suggest that the amplitude of the diurnal cycle is greater for weekdays than weekends and that the largest differences between weekdays and weekends occur during the middle of the day, between 9 a.m. and 7 p.m.

```
proc mixed data=pain.alldemo2 noclprint noinfo method=ml covtest;
  class id;
  model frust=weekend sine cosine / solution;
  random intercept sine cosine / type=un sub=id;
  repeated / type=sp(pow)(conttime) sub=id local;
  parms 400 0 20 0 0 20 220 .90 210;
  title4 'Sinusoidal model of diurnal cycle of frust (RANDOM EFFECT)';
  title5 'Main effect of weekday vs weekend';

proc mixed data=pain.alldemo2 noclprint noinfo method=ml covtest;
  class id;
  model frust=weekend sine cosine weekend*sine weekend*cosine /solution;
  random intercept sine cosine / type=un sub=id;
  repeated / type=sp(pow)(conttime) sub=id local;
  parms 400 0 20 0 0 20 220 .90 210;
  title5 'Differences between weekday and weekend';
```

Conclusion

Our goal in writing this chapter has been to provide readers with a practical guide for analyzing real-time, momentary data. Developments in technology, combined with researchers' interest in collecting ecologically valid data about peoples' daily experiences, are making the collection of real-time data feasible for most investigators. The promise of these data is their ability to allow us to peek into the complexities of experiences in order to achieve a more comprehensive description of daily life and to quantitatively test theories with a finer-grain resolution than has hitherto been possible. The chapter has, we think, demonstrated that extraordinarily relevant questions can be rigorously addressed with multilevel statistical models. However, it is obvious that a great deal of thought, understanding, and patience is necessary when using these methods to analyze real-time data. We were not able to provide a simple cookbook of analytic recipes for every scenario; instead, we sought to present examples of many of the basic questions one faces with momentary data and an understanding of the basic analytic principles required for analyses.

Appendix: Use of the Toeplitz Specification to Examine the Pattern of Autocorrelation

In this chapter we considered three possible patterns of autocorrelation for the within-person residuals: (1) no autocorrelation, (2) a first-order autoregressive specification, and (3) a modified first-order autoregressive (modified AR1) specification that also allows for an uncorrelated component of variance (perhaps random measurement error). We saw that while the second specification was substantially better than the first, the third specification provided a better fit to the data than either of the first two. However, we did not investigate the extent to which the modified AR1 specification provides a "good" fit to the data. To do this, one must examine how the correlation between two residuals varies in relation to the time interval between them. After a little manipulation of the data, the toeplitz error structure can be used to address this issue.

The desirable property of the toeplitz specification is its flexibility in terms of not making strong assumptions about the rate at which the correlation between residuals of two momentary reports, by the same individual, decreases as the time interval increases. Instead, it estimates a separate parameter for each time interval up to some maximum interval, and then assumes that there is no correlation between residuals separated by more than this maximum interval. The generic form of the toeplitz specification is illustrated below. Its weaknesses are that (1) the timing of the momentary reports, an inherently continuous variable, must be collapsed into discrete categories with no more than one report per category (per individual) and (2) it typically requires numerous parameters to adequately represent the pattern of serial correlation, which in turn may necessitate that starting values be estimated through a set of iterative analyses. In addition, estimation of models with a large number of random parameters is computationally intensive, requiring substantially more computer time to reach a solution.

$$
\begin{array}{l}
\text{Toeplitz}(5) \\
\text{specification} \\
\\
R_i =
\end{array}
\begin{bmatrix}
1 & \rho_2 & \rho_3 & \rho_4 & \rho_5 & 0 & 0 & 0 \\
\rho_2 & 1 & \rho_2 & \rho_3 & \rho_4 & \rho_5 & 0 & 0 \\
\rho_3 & \rho_2 & 1 & \rho_2 & \rho_3 & \rho_4 & \rho_5 & 0 \\
\rho_4 & \rho_3 & \rho_2 & 1 & \rho_2 & \rho_3 & \rho_4 & \rho_5 \\
\rho_5 & \rho_4 & \rho_3 & \rho_2 & 1 & \rho_2 & \rho_3 & \rho_4 \\
0 & \rho_5 & \rho_4 & \rho_3 & \rho_2 & 1 & \rho_2 & \rho_3 \\
0 & 0 & \rho_5 & \rho_4 & \rho_3 & \rho_2 & 1 & \rho_2 \\
0 & 0 & 0 & \rho_5 & \rho_4 & \rho_3 & \rho_2 & 1
\end{bmatrix} Var(\varepsilon_{it})
$$

Implementing the toeplitz specification

For the present data, we took the existing continuous time variable (time since the first assessment) and rounded it to the nearest half-hour. This meant that every person had an observation for time category 0. The highest value was 358, corresponding to 14 days and 22 hours after the first assessment. Since the data set does not contain an observation for every half-hour category between 0 and 358, it is important to add observations to the data set for time categories that do not already exist. These added observations will have missing data for the core variables and will not enter into the estimation process but are needed in order for the categorical time variable to correctly represent the approximate time interval between observations. The next step is to ensure that no subject has two observations with the same time category. Of the 5,321 assessments in our data, 14 pairs had the same time category; we arbitrarily kept the first and deleted the second.

SAS Syntax:

```
title 'TOEP0.SAS:  Decomposition of Variance - Toeplitz Model';
options ls=108 ps=80 nocenter nofmterr noxwait;
libname pain 'E:\NCI\CONF\WORKSHOP';

/*

LIST OF VARIABLES USED IN THIS ANALYSIS
ID: unique person identifier
FRUST: momentary report of frustration (dependent variable)
CONTTIME: a measure of continuous time since midnight of the first day
          of the study (unit = 1 hour, but includes fractions of hours)

*/

data frust;  set pain.frust;  by id;
  retain lag_time lag_time2;
  if first.id then do;  lag_time=.;  lag_time2=.;  end;
  if lag_time ne . then time_dif=round(conttime-lag_time,.0001);
  if lag_time2 ne . then time_dif2=round(conttime-lag_time2,.0001);
  conttime_cat=round(conttime,.5);
  output;
  if lag_time ne . then lag_time2=lag_time;
  lag_time=conttime;

proc freq;  table time_dif time_dif2;  where time_dif<2;
title2 'Distribution of time differences (in hours) between consecutive reports';
title3 '(used to determine that very few observations were < 30 minutes apart)';

proc means;
title2 'Need to determine maximum number of intervals (should be
~14×24×2)';

data x (drop=i); id=401;  do i=0 to 716;  conttime_cat=i/2;  output;  end;
  * creating a mini dataset with all possible time categories from 0 to 358;
  * choosing an ID for which minimum value of time_dif>.5;
```

```
data frust;  merge frust x;  by id conttime_cat;

data frust dup;  set frust;  by id conttime_cat;
* dropping reports w/ same conttime_cat as previous report;
  if first.conttime_cat then output frust;
  if not (first.conttime_cat and last.conttime_cat) then output dup;

proc print data=dup;  var id conttime conttime_cat frust;
title2 'Listing of 14 pairs of observations that have same conttime_cat';

proc mixed data=frust noclprint method=ml covtest;
  class id conttime_cat;
  model frust= / solution;
  random intercept / type=un sub=id;
  repeated conttime_cat / type=toep(4) sub=id;
  title2 'Multilevel Model with different error structures';
  title3 'MODEL 1d:  Bet-person Component + W/in-person Toeplitz (4)';
```

We began by estimating a toeplitz(4) specification (distinct correlations for assessments obtained approximately 30, 60, and 90 minutes apart, but assuming

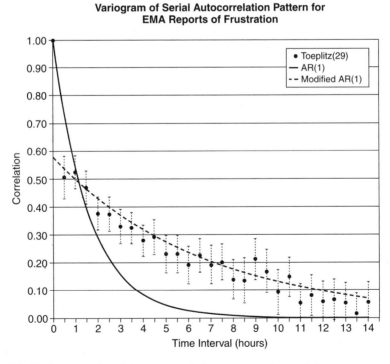

Figure 5-6. Variogram of serial autocorrelation pattern for real-time reports of frustration.

a correlation of 0 for assessments obtained more than 105 minutes apart). We used these estimates as starting values to next estimate a toeplitz(8), followed by a toeplitz(12), toeplitz(16), toeplitz(21), toeplitz(25), and finally a toeplitz(29) specification. Each successive model except the last provided a statistically significantly better fit to the data than the preceding one, albeit with diminishing marginal improvements. The difference in -2 LL between the toeplitz(29) and toeplitz(25) specifications was 6.2 with $df = 4$ ($p < 0.19$), suggesting that there is little reason to estimate toeplitz models with even more parameters.

The toeplitz(29) model yields estimates of correlations for each half-hour interval from 0.5 through 14 hours, assuming zero autocorrelation for observations obtained more than 14 hours apart. These correlations and their approximate 95 percent confidence intervals are shown in the variogram in Figure 5.6. This graph also includes the predicted correlations based on the AR(1) and modified AR(1) specifications (estimated using TYPE=SP(POW)). It is readily apparent that the modified AR(1) specification with its three parameters provides a very good approximation to the 29-parameter toeplitz specification.

ACKNOWLEDGMENTS

We thank the participants in the momentary pain study for their cooperation and acknowledge the efforts of our collaborators (Joan Broderick, Pamela Calvanese, and Steven Grossman) and staff who were involved in the collection of data used in this chapter. Support of this research NIH (CA85819 and HL47540) is gratefully acknowledged.

Notes

1. Another special case, perhaps less familiar to behavioral scientists, is time series analysis, typically applied to many repeated observations obtained from a single "subject" at equally spaced intervals.

2. For those familiar with structural equation modeling, the π_k's can be conceptualized as (unobserved) latent variables that are regressed, in the Level 2 equations, on measured person-level variables.

3. Instead of "fixed effects" and "random effects," the statistical literature on multilevel models sometimes refers to "fixed coefficients" and "random coefficients" (e.g., Longford, 1993). These terms are interchangeable.

4. Unfortunately, the SAS printout lists the estimates of the fixed parameters (all the β's in Equations [2a], [2b], and [3]) under the heading of "Solution for fixed effects," a subtly different use of the term "fixed effect" than that described earlier. In our presentation, as well as other presentations of multilevel models, the distinction between fixed and random effects pertains to the π coefficients of the within-person equations, specifically whether their Level 2 equations include δ-terms for unmeasured individual differences. SAS displays the estimates of the random parameters and associated statistics under the heading "Covariance Parameter Estimates."

5. ContTime contains information about the time interval between any two assessments and, as described below, is used to specify models that allow/adjust for serial autocorrelation of the within-person residuals.

6. There are pros and cons to each of these two methods. ML defines the likelihood function in terms of all the parameters, both fixed and random, to be estimated. It generates estimates that are most consistent with the data. However, the estimates of the random parameters will typically be slightly biased toward zero because they do not adjust for the loss in degrees of freedom caused by using the estimates of the fixed parameters to estimate the random parameters. (This is the same issue that, in ordinary statistics, causes the denominator of the usual [unbiased] estimate of the sample variance to be N-1 rather than N.)

REML conditions the estimates of the random parameters on the estimates of the fixed parameters in the model. While this improves the estimates of the random parameters (Snijders & Bosker, 1999), it means that the estimates and fit statistics of two models that have different fixed parameters cannot be compared. Of particular note, this means that when REML is specified, one cannot use the change in the log likelihood statistic to test the difference between two models unless the predictor variables on the two MODEL statements (see below) are identical. For consistency, we use ML throughout this chapter.

7. Formally, this model states that the relationship between the residuals of any two reports obtained at times τ_t and $\tau_{t'}$ can be described by the equation $\varepsilon_{it} = \rho^{|\tau_t - \tau_{t'}|}\varepsilon_{it'} + \omega_{it}$, where each ω_{it} is assumed to be uncorrelated with all residuals prior to ε_{it}, to have a mean of zero, and to have a variance equal to $(1 - \rho^{2|\tau_t - \tau_{t'}|})\,\mathrm{Var}(\varepsilon_{it})$. Together, these assumptions imply that the $\mathrm{Var}(\varepsilon_{it})$ remains constant across time. For reports obtained 1 hour apart, $\tau_t - \tau_{t'} = 1$ and the correlation between the residuals is ρ; when 2 hours apart, the correlation is ρ^2, etc. Historically, this pattern of autocorrelated residuals was estimated on time series data where the interval between consecutive assessments was constant. Diggle (1988) extended this model to unevenly spaced assessments where the time interval between assessments was measured in continuous time (see Laird, Donnelly, & Ware, 1992).

8. SP(POW) stands for "spatial power." Although the SAS documentation describes an alternative "TYPE=" specification called AR(1), for first-order autoregressive, this specification treats the time variable as a categorical variable and assumes that assessments are made at fixed intervals. This specification is a special case of SP(POW), one that appears to offer no advantage and can sometimes be problematic.

9. This interpretation is consistent with the trait-state-error model proposed by Kenny and Zautra (1995), where δ_{0i}, μ_{it}, and ν_{it} correspond to the three sources of variance, assumed to be orthogonal. For those familiar with spectral analysis, an alternative interpretation of the ν_{it} is that they reflect a "high frequency" source of variance, one whose periodicity is substantially shorter than the typical interval between consecutive momentary assessments. In this case, the ν_{it} could reflect valid variance whose autocorrelation, if any, attenuates to zero as the interval between assessments increases. From a structural equation modeling perspective, the first-order autoregressive specification is closely related to Jöreskog's "simplex model," and the modified first-order auto-regressive specification parallels his "quasi-simplex" model (Jöreskog, 1970).

10. If each person had the exact same number of valid assessments and we ignored any autocorrelation of the within-person residuals, the two analytic methods would result in identical coefficient estimates and tests of the statistical significance, but differ in their estimates of total between-person variance and percent variance accounted for.

11. It is our impression that many published analyses that use multilevel modeling, including some of our own, have treated the primary moment-level predictors as fixed effects without adequately evaluating the validity of this assumption, thereby potentially exaggerating the statistical significance of the results.

12. If the mean of the predictor variable (pain) is substantially greater than zero, then there is a strong tendency for the intercepts and slopes to be negatively correlated; the

steeper the slope, the lower the intercept (predicted value of the outcome variable, frustration, when the predictor variable equals zero) is likely to be. Of note, subtraction of a constant from the pain variable implicitly redefines the intercept; as a result, the estimated variance of the intercept and the covariance and correlation of the intercept with the slope would change, but the variance of the slope would not be affected.

13. If the Proc MIXED statement includes the subcommand COVTEST, the software will provide a significance test of the null hypothesis that $\text{Var}(\delta_{1i}) = 0$. However, like many other global tests of significance, this is thought to be a low-power test.

14. It is possible that the use of lagged terms in the model would help to establish the causal direction of the relationship. However, this raises an issue concerning the correct lag period. Furthermore, while random timing of assessments is usually considered a strength in real-time data collection designs, analyses of lagged effects are greatly complicated when the time interval between assessments varies.

15. We note that had we obtained REML estimates instead of ML estimates, we could not have used the change in –2 LL and the chi-square distribution to test whether one model fit the data better than another (see footnote 6).

References

Bryk, A. S., & Raudenbush, S. W. (1992). *Hierarchical linear models: applications and data analysis methods.* Newbury Park, CA: Sage.

Bryk, A. S., Raudenbush, S. W., & Congdon, R. J. (1996). *HLM: Hierarchical linear and nonlinear modeling with the HLM/2L and HLM/3L programs.* Chicago: Scientific Software International.

Diggle, P. J. (1988). An approach to the analysis of repeated measurements. *Biometrics, 44,* 959–971.

Kenny, D. A., & Zautra, A. (1995). The trait-state-error model for multiwave data. *Journal of Consulting and Clinical Psychology, 63,* 52–59.

Jöreskog, K. G. (1970). Estimation and testing of simplex models. *British Journal of Mathematical and Statistical Psychology, 23,* 121–145.

Laird, N. M., & Ware, J. H. (1982). Random effects models for longitudinal data. *Biometrics, 38,* 963–974.

Laird, N. M., Donnelly, C., & Ware, J. H. (1992). Longitudinal studies with continuous responses. *Statistical Methods in Medical Research, 1,* 225–247.

Littell, R. C., Milliken, G. A., Stroup, W. W., & Wolfinger, R. D. (1996). *SAS system for mixed models.* Cary, NC: SAS Institute Inc.

Longford, N. T. (1993). *Random coefficient models.* Oxford: Clarendon Press.

Singer, J. D. (1998) Using SAS PROC MIXED to fit multilevel models, hierarchical models, and individual growth curve models. *Journal of Educational and Behavioral Statistics, 24,* 323–355.

Singer, J. D., & Willet, J. (2003). *Applied longitudinal data analysis.* Oxford: Oxford University Press.

Snijders, T. A. B., & Bosker, R. L. (1999). *Multilevel analysis: an introduction to basic and advanced multilevel modeling.* Thousand Oaks, CA: Sage.

Stone, A. A., Broderick, J. E., Schwartz, J. E., Shiffman, S. S., Litcher-Kelly, L., & Calvanese, P. (2003). Intensive momentary reporting of pain with an electronic diary: Reactivity, compliance, and patient satisfaction. *Pain, 104,* 343–351.

Stone, A. A., Broderick, J. E., Shiffman, S. S., & Schwartz, J. E. (2004). Understanding recall of weekly pain from a momentary assessment perspective: Absolute agreement, between- and within-person consistency, and judged change in weekly pain. *Pain, 107,* 61–69.

Walls, T. A., Jung, H., & Schwartz, J. E. (2006). Multilevel models for intensive longitudinal data. In T. A. Walls & J. L. Schafer (Eds.), *Models for intensive longitudinal data.* New York: Oxford University Press.

PART II

APPLICATION OF REAL-TIME DATA CAPTURE: EXEMPLARS OF REAL-TIME DATA RESEARCH

6

Real-Time Data Capture and Adolescent Cigarette Smoking: Moods and Smoking

Robin Mermelstein, Donald Hedeker,
Brian Flay, and Saul Shiffman

Cigarette smoking among adolescents remains a pressing public health challenge, considering the enormous toll smoking takes on health and health care resources. Most adolescents try smoking cigarettes. In 2003, almost 60 percent of twelfth-graders reported ever smoking (Johnston, O'Malley, & Bachman, 2003). However, not all of those who try smoking progress to regular use; 15.8 percent of twelfth-graders report daily smoking, and 8.4 percent report smoking half a pack or more a day (Johnston et al., 2003). Despite more than three decades of research on adolescent smoking, it is surprising how little is known about factors that predict the different trajectories or patterns of cigarette smoking beyond initial experimentation.

This chapter describes the use of Ecological Momentary Assessment (EMA) to help increase our understanding of how the immediate subjective and objective contexts of early trials of cigarette smoking may influence adolescents' patterns and progression of smoking. The objective contexts of smoking include the "who (with whom), what, and where" of smoking episodes. The subjective contexts include moods, perceived physiological sensations following smoking, and perceptions of the social environment, such as perceived peer pressure.

Numerous studies have identified individual difference variables (e.g., peer and parent smoking, temperament) and macro-contextual factors (e.g., tobacco advertising and marketing) as influencing adolescent smoking (e.g., see Conrad, Flay, & Hill, 1992; Turner, Mermelstein, & Flay, 2004, USHDDS, 1994). There are much fewer empirical data, though, about the immediate context in which early trials of smoking occur, and especially about adolescents' moods surrounding early experimentation with cigarettes. Until recently, attempts at investigating initial smoking episodes were limited to highly retrospective, anecdotal reports, gathered either through interviews or paper-and-pencil questionnaires. For example, Friedman and colleagues (1985) conducted structured interviews to explore the situational components of adolescents' first three smoking experiences and found that the vast majority (89%) of adolescents in their sample were with others during these times. Eissenberg and Balster (2000) reviewed research on initial tobacco use episodes and similarly concluded that most first smoking experiences occur in small, same-sex peer groups. Although the presence of peers and other smokers are likely common denominators running through the vast majority of first smoking experiences, what is still not known is why a particular context leads to smoking while at other times an apparently similar context does not result in smoking. Both objective situational factors and subjective moods may play a role in determining whether a given situation leads to smoking. Retrospective reports about such differences are likely to lead to a variety of attri-butional and recall biases. EMA provides a potentially less biased window into understanding differences between smoking and nonsmoking times.

Although social contexts may play a major role in understanding why adoles-cents initially try smoking, they may be less important in understanding why some adolescents progress beyond experimentation to more regular use. Recently, researchers have considered that adolescents' physiological responses to nicotine or smoking may be an important predictor of escalation (Eissenberg & Balster, 2000; Pomerleau, Collins, Shiffman, et al., 1993). Physical responses to early trials of smoking may be interpreted by youth as either pleasant or unpleasant sensa-tions, or these physical effects may also result in mood changes. Like adults, ado-lescent smokers report that they smoke to manage negative moods and stress (Mermelstein, 1999), and there is growing evidence that depression and adoles-cent smoking are linked (Brown, Lewinsohn, Seeley, et al., 1996; Choi, Patten, Gillin, et al., 1997; Patton, Hibbert, Rosier, et al., 1996). However, there is little direct evidence demonstrating the mood benefits of smoking among adoles-cents. It may be that adolescents who experience mood benefits from smoking are the ones most likely to escalate in their use.

Rationale for EMA Approach

EMA provides an excellent window into the lives of adolescents and a way to examine specific hypotheses about contextual influences on smoking. EMA cap-tures more accurately than other measurement modalities the frequency, inten-sity, and tone of social experiences as they occur, as well as the mood associated with those exchanges. Shiffman's work has amply demonstrated both the feasi-bility and utility of using EMA to study smoking, relapse, and temptations to smoke in adult smokers (e.g., Shiffman, Gnys, Richards, Paty, Hickcox, & Kassel, 1996; Shiffman, Paty, Gnys, Kassel, & Elash, 1995; Shiffman, Paty, Gnys, Kassel, & Hickcox, 1996), and the work of Jamner and colleagues has shown the feasibility of EMA with adolescents (e.g., Whalen, Jamner, Henker, et al., 2001). EMA is well suited for measuring internal, subjective states, intra-individual variability, and small shifts in mood that may play a role in cueing smoking (Shiffman, 1993). Finally, with the use of random assessments that are independent from the occurrence of specific behaviors and situations, EMA can provide useful comparison information about nontarget events. Thus, EMA can provide an ideal tool for studying the contextual micro-patterns of cigarette use, the micro-level antecedents of use, as well as the subjective experience of adolescent smoking.

A primary goal of the project reported here ("Context and Subjective Experience of Early Smoking" or "Early Smoking" study) was to increase our understanding of how adolescents' subjective experience and context of early trials of cigarette smoking affect their future smoking patterns. We focus here on addressing two questions: (1) *How do the subjective mood contexts of smoking episodes and nonsmoking decision times differ from random background times?* and (2) *Do moods prior to smoking differ by an adolescent's level of smoking experience?*

Method

Overview of Study

The data reported in this chapter come from a longitudinal study of the natural history of smoking among adolescents. The study used a multimethod approach to assess adolescents at four time points: baseline, 6 months, 12 months, and 18 months. The data collection modalities included a week-long time/event EMA sampling (through 12 months) via hand-held, palmtop computers (referred to as "ED" or Electronic Diary), self-report questionnaires, and in-depth interviews. We report here on the data from the baseline EMA collection.

The design of the "Early Smoking" study involved sampling eighth- and tenth-graders at baseline who fell into three early stages of cigarette use: (1) "susceptibles"—youth who had never smoked but who indicated high "suscepti-bility" to smoking based on questions about intentions; (2) "triers"—youth who had smoked within the past 90 days and who had no more than 20 cigarettes in their lifetimes; and (3) "experimenters"—youth who smoked in the past 30 days and smoked between 20 and 99 cigarettes in their lifetimes, and were not yet daily smokers. Our sampling rationale was based on our desire to follow youth who might have their first cigarette within the course of the study, as well as those who were still early in their smoking experiences. Adolescents were invited to participate in this longitudinal study based on their responses to a self-report screener. Across 11 middle schools and 7 high schools, 5,278 eighth- and tenth-graders completed the initial screening questionnaire, and 1,817 of those students fell into our three identified categories of eligible students. Of those eligible, a sample of 1,437 were invited to participate through a process of mailed recruitment letters to the adolescents' homes. Active parental consent was required for participation in the longitudinal study. Of those invited, 562 positively responded and completed the baseline measurement wave.

Sample Description

For the analyses reported here, we will focus on a subset of the 562 participants, including only those adolescents who event-reported either a smoking or nonsmoking decision episode (or both) on the ED during the baseline measurement wave. This analysis sample of 300 participants included 54.0 percent females ($n = 162$) and 48.3 percent eighth-graders ($n = 136$). Their ethnic distribution was 69.3 percent White ($n = 208$), 18.0 percent Hispanic ($n = 54$); 5.3 percent Black ($n = 16$); 4.0 percent Asian ($n = 12$); and 3.3 percent other ($n = 10$). Just prior to the ED data collection week, 18.3 percent ($n = 55$) reported never smoking, 15.3 percent ($n = 46$) reported having less than 6 cigarettes in their lifetimes, 51.0 percent ($n = 153$) reported having had between 6 and 99 lifetime cigarettes, and 15.3 percent ($n = 46$) reported having had 100 cigarettes or more. Considering that the baseline ED data collection occurred approximately 2 months after the screening for eligibility, some adolescents progressed in their smoking since screening, thus having had more than 100 cigarettes by the time of the baseline ED measurement.

Momentary Data Collection

TYPE OF SAMPLING

Data collection occurred via hand-held palmtop computers (ED), programmed specifically for our data collection needs, with all other residing programs disabled. Each data collection wave included 7 consecutive days of monitoring. The decision to monitor for 7 consecutive days involved a compromise among multiple factors: our desire to include both weekdays and weekends in order to obtain a more representative sample of the adolescents' daily lives than just weekends or weekdays, and the pragmatic factors of adolescent fatigue at monitoring as well as field issues of the hardware needing to be checked and batteries replaced after a longer time period. Three types of interviews were programmed onto the ED: random prompts, and smoke and "no smoke" events. Participants were trained to turn on the ED upon waking and to "put it to bed" upon going to sleep at night.

Random time prompts were initiated by the device on average five or six times per day. At these times, the ED would beep, signaling the participant to initiate an interview. The beeping noise would get increasingly louder until the participant responded. The participant needed to respond within 3 minutes of the prompt before the interview would be recorded as "missed." Each random prompt was date- and time-stamped and recorded whether the interview was completed, missed, or disbanded. The random interviews took 60 to 90 seconds to complete and asked about mood, activity (what the adolescent was doing), companionship (with whom or alone), presence of other smokers, where they were, and other behaviors (e.g., eating, drinking, substance use).

In addition to the random prompts, participants were trained to event-record both smoking and nonsmoking episodes. A smoking episode was defined as any time that a participant smoked, even a puff. Right after smoking, the participant would turn on the ED and initiate a "smoke" interview, which included the same questions as the random prompt, but in addition asked about specific smoking-related items (e.g., how much smoked, how the cigarette was obtained);

perceptions of the supportiveness, friendliness, or "pressuring" of others; and moods both right after smoking ("now") and then "just before" smoking.

A "no smoke" episode was defined as an occasion when the participant had the opportunity to smoke but made an active decision not to smoke. "No smoke" events were not times when the adolescent might have wanted to smoke but couldn't (e.g., in smoking-restricted areas or none available), but rather, active opportunity times. The "no smoke" interviews were similar to the smoke interviews but did not include the specific questions about cigarettes smoked.

Tailoring EMA to Adolescents

The ED had several features that made its use feasible for the adolescents. For example, the adolescents had the option to suspend the ED from randomly prompting them for up to 2 hours at a time. The suspension option was useful at times that were impractical for the adolescent to respond, such as during a school exam or while in an athletic event. The ED recorded all suspension times, along with the reason for the suspension. The suspension option did not interfere with the number of prompts answered overall. In addition, upon prompting, the adolescents could also initiate a "delay" option, allowing them to delay responding for up to 20 minutes (in 5-minute intervals) if they were not able to respond immediately. The brief interviews made it realistic for the adolescent to respond and complete the random prompts during the daily activities. The ED was programmed so that a response was required on each interview screen before the participant could move on to the next question. In addition, adolescents could not enter out-of-range values on an item. Thus, within an interview, there were no missing data.

Prior to finalizing all procedures with the ED, we conducted several focus groups of teens and piloted all procedures with teens in the field. Our focus groups covered topics such as what to call the device ("ED" was easiest for the teens), language/wording of questions and mood descriptors for items on the ED, anticipated problems with using the ED in real time and possible solutions, and also very pragmatic issues such as how the teens would actually carry around the ED (e.g., in a backpack, clipped to a belt), and whether they had concerns about their appearance in carrying and using the device. For example, we explored a variety of carrying case options with the teens, having the teens comment on their perceptions of the relative appeal of different options. To our surprise, the teens overwhelmingly preferred the use of seemingly less attractive, well-padded carrying cases, as opposed to the more sleek and aesthetically appealing leather cases. The teens were concerned more about not breaking the hardware and feeling responsible for it than they were about the appearance per se. To the teens, the sense of "coolness" came from being one of the relatively few in a school who were invited to participate in the study, rather than the looks of the devices.

There were also unique challenges to using the ED with adolescents. For example, during pilot work, we learned that we needed to password-protect the ED for initiating "smoke" or "no smoke" events as a way to prevent other adolescents from entering false data about a participant (as a prank). In addition, we programmed in a "demo" feature that included a very brief interview that allowed the adolescent to show friends, family, or teachers examples of what they were being asked to do. However, we also learned that we needed to limit the number of "demos" to prevent inappropriate overuse of this feature. In addition, following the pilot work, we decreased the number of random prompts per day from 7 to 9 to 5 or 6, after receiving feedback from the teens (and compliance data) about the perceived burden of the number of prompts.

Importantly, we also gained the cooperation and permission of the schools to allow the students to carry and use the ED while they were in school. We prepared the school administrators and teachers for the project through a series of in-person meetings (with administrators and teachers) and letters to teachers describing the study procedures, goals, and how the data collection and ED devices worked. We emphasized that the random prompts would be relatively rare in any one class and that the students had the option to suspend the program if requested. In any given school, data collection occurred during only 1 or 2 weeks in the school year. Students also received ID cards and letters (describing their study responsibilities and noting the permission of the school) to carry with them in case they were questioned about the devices. Data collection occurred throughout the full calendar year, including summer.

Procedures

TRAINING

At the beginning of each measurement wave, adolescents were individually trained on the use of the ED. Training took approximately 45 minutes and occurred either in a private location at the adolescent's school or a community location (e.g., library). Training was standardized with manuals for both the staff trainer and the participant. Training covered not only how to use and respond to the ED, but also role-playing how to deal with potentially awkward situations when the adolescent must either respond to a prompt or event record (e.g., smoking at a party). The trainer helped the adolescents to anticipate and problem-solve any difficulties or concerns they may have had about using the ED. Training reflected not only our suggested solutions to potentially awkward situations, but also suggestions by adolescents who participated in our pilot work and early waves of data collection. In addition, our staff trainers were selected based on their age, similarities to the adolescents, and ability to relate well to adolescents. The trainers underwent extensive training themselves in the use of the protocol, dealing with adolescents, and ways of enhancing compliance.

The trainers called each participant 1 day into the measurement week to check for potential problems and to reinforce compliance. Throughout the week, research staff were available via an 800 telephone number and pager to respond to any problems or issues (e.g., broken computers that needed to be replaced). At the end of each measurement week, the EDs were collected, and the trainer conducted an in-depth in-person interview with the participant.

During the interview, the trainer printed out a record of the adolescent's use of the ED, including details about compliance, and went over the printout with the adolescent, inquiring about any conflicting "problem reports" (times when the adolescent indicated a missed report). The printouts also served as additional training for subsequent waves, for the trainer to review compliance issues or difficulties with the adolescent. During the end-of-the-week interview, the trainer also inquired about potential reactivity, events that were not recorded, and the adolescent's impressions about the week.

MEASURES

To illustrate the use of EMA with one of its more unusual data collection options, we will focus here on the EMA measures of mood/affect. During the random prompt interviews, participants were asked, "Think about how you felt just before the signal." They were then shown a screen with the question stem, "Before signal, I felt . . ." One mood/affect adjective was presented per screen along with a 10-point visual analogue scale. The scale was anchored by "very" at the top, "somewhat" in the middle, and "not at all" at the bottom rung of the visual ladder. Participants used a stylus to point to the level on the scale that represented their response. A series of 12 adjectives (one per screen) was presented to the participants. The 12 adjectives factored into four scales: (a) positive mood scale (cheerful, happy, relaxed, coefficient alpha = .75); (b) negative mood scale (sad, embarrassed, angry, left out, lonely; coefficient alpha = .74); (c) stress/frustration scale (stressed, frustrated; coefficient alpha = .76); and (d) a tired/bored scale (tired, bored; coefficient alpha = .52).

During the "smoke" and "no smoke" event recorded interviews, participants were first asked, *"Think about how you feel right now." "Right now, I feel . . ."* They were then presented with the same set of adjectives as with the random prompt interview, with the addition of two other adjectives, sick and buzzed, to represent subjective physiological sensations that might be related to smoking. The ratings of feelings "right now" represented post-smoking or post-no smoking decision affect. After responding to the adjectives with the stem about how they felt right now, participants then were asked: *"Now think about the time just before you smoked/decided not to smoke." "Just before, I felt . . ."* and again, they rated each adjective. These ratings of just before the event represented pre-event affect/mood.

Assessing mood just prior to a smoke or no smoke event presented a measurement challenge. Unlike with adult smokers, who are more likely to be able to anticipate and plan when they smoke (or to add in a delay for recording just prior to the event), we expected that adolescents' decisions to smoke or not during the early stages of experimentation are likely to be far less routine than for adults. In addition, asking an adolescent to interrupt a stream of decisional and real-life situational complexities to complete an ED interview seemed unrealistic. Thus, we opted to have the "pre-event" mood assessment questions occur after the event. In addition, we decided to ask first about mood "now" right after smoking/not smoking, and then ask about mood "just before" smoking or the decision not to smoke, believing that we would be less likely to introduce any response biases about perceived changes in mood with both this question phrasing and ordering. As a result of our pilot work, we arrived at our final choice of question phrasing and ordering based on both methodological reasons and teens' perceptions of ease of answering specific questions.

DATA MANAGEMENT

The management of the EMA data involved several steps, including documentation, extraction, aggregation, and cleaning. At the subject debriefing at the end of the data collection week, a Microsoft Access database used by the EMA software to store data was uploaded onto a laptop and a report used to assist with debriefing was printed on site. The report contained a listing of random prompt, smoke, and no smoke interviews and a listing of events involving the subject's interaction with the ED during the week. The report was an important tool used by the trainer at debriefing to gauge compliance and to reinforce good efforts. The Microsoft Access database was split into four files: smoke interviews, no smoke interviews, random prompt interviews, and record events, which included data involving subject interaction and software operation (e.g., compliance record, number of suspends). All ASCII files of a single type of interview or event record were aggregated using MS-DOS batch commands, and the resulting aggregated ASCII was read into SAS and formatted. After cleaning, the four SAS files included all diary information for all subjects during the wave and were ready for analysis.

ANALYTIC APPROACH

The data were analyzed using mixed effects regression models for continuous outcomes (Verbeke & Molenberghs, 2000). These models are well suited for the EMA data since they can handle the repeated assessments within an individual over the measurement week, accounting for the data dependency of observations within an individual. In addition, they allow for the unequal number of observations across individuals. Thus, we did not exclude any subject or data due to level of "completeness," and neither did we aggregate data across days. Rather, all individual reports were included in the analysis. To address our questions about the effects of event type (random, smoke, or no smoke) and smoking level (<6 cigarettes/lifetime; 6–99 cigarettes; 100+ cigarettes), as well as their interactions, we ran separate mixed effects regression models for the EMA measures of positive and negative affect. Significant effects were followed up with a priori planned contrasts comparing random to smoke events and random to nonsmoking events. Significant interactions were followed up with a priori planned contrasts of random versus smoke events at each smoking level compared to the lowest (i.e., <6 cigarettes vs. 6–99; <6 cigarettes vs. 100+). Similar planned comparisons were made for the random versus nonsmoke events for the smoking level comparisons.

Results

Compliance

As one might expect with adolescents, there was some data loss due to damage to the equipment or to equipment loss. At our baseline wave, we had usable ED data from 516 of the 562 participants (92%). At the 6-month data collection, 15 adolescents declined to participate in the ED component of the study, and at 12 months, a total of 23 adolescents declined the ED component. For the most part, these adolescents found the ED component too difficult to complete given their other life commitments, or in a few cases, were not allowed to complete that component, given their multiple hardware losses. The level of useable data from the ED increased slightly at 6 and 12 months to 93.3 percent and 92.1 percent, respectively. Overall dropout from the study was relatively minimal; at 12 months, we retained 90.2 percent of the participants in the study.

Compliance with the ED among those with useable data ($n = 516$) was excellent. Table 6-1 shows various indices of compliance. As can be seen from the table, compliance remained relatively high and stable over time, with only very slight declines in the percent of random prompts answered. However, the total number of prompts answered remained the same, if not slightly higher, at 12 months. The number of times the participant "suspended" the ED is another measure of compliance. Overall, the amount of "suspension" time seemed reasonable within the context of adolescents' lives, averaging once per day for slightly over an hour.

We also examined compliance by calendar day (e.g., Monday–Sunday) and by study day (e.g., first day–seventh day of monitoring). As a note, the majority of initial training and study "first" days occurred on Tuesdays, Wednesdays, and Thursdays, with no study first days on Friday through Sunday. Table 6-2 presents compliance data (percentage of prompts answered, suspension data) by day of the week, and Table 6-3 presents these data by study day (monitoring day). As can be seen in Table 6-2, compliance was the best during the mid-week days (Tuesday through Thursday), which also were most frequently the first and second day of the monitoring period, and compliance with random prompts dropped off slightly over the weekend (Saturday and Sunday). Table 6-3 shows that there is an initial high level of responding to random prompts during the

Table 6-1. Compliance variables over time

	Baseline $n = 519$	6 Months $n = 487$	12 Months $n = 467$
Mean no. random prompts answered (SD)	33.8 (9.86)	33.8 (9.16)	36.0 (9.40)
Mean no. missed prompts (SD)	5.9 (6.01)	7.2 (6.39)	6.9 (6.40)
Mean % random prompts answered (SD)	85.0 (13.88)	82.5 (14.11)	83.9 (13.84)
Mean total no. suspends/week (SD)	9.5 (6.89)	7.6 (5.56)	7.1 (4.86)
Mean minutes per suspend (SD)	74.4 (19.80)	82.7 (20.88)	81.8 (19.27)

Table 6-2. Compliance by day of week at baseline

	% Prompts answered (SD)	Avg. # suspends (SD)	Avg. mins. suspend (SD)
Monday	85.1 (21.6)	1.4 (1.5)	73.9 (28.6)
Tuesday	86.4 (21.2)	1.3 (1.6)	75.2 (30.2)
Wednesday	88.8 (17.3)	1.5 (1.6)	69.4 (27.2)
Thursday	89.1 (17.7)	1.7 (1.7)	68.8 (26.8)
Friday	86.4 (21.2)	1.7 (1.7)	70.7 (25.8)
Saturday	81.8 (23.4)	1.1 (1.5)	87.6 (32.6)
Sunday	81.8 (24.3)	0.9 (1.2)	88.0 (31.3)

very first 2 days of the monitoring period at baseline, and then levels off to a narrower range after that. Over the subsequent measurement waves (6 and 12 months), the variability in compliance decreased and remained fairly stable across all days. For example, at the 6- and 12-month waves, the percentage of prompts answered ranged from approximately 82 to 86 percent regardless of whether one considers day of the week or day of the study.

Compliance with event-recording the "smoke" and "no smoke" interviews was assessed during the end-of-week in-person interviews, as well as with written responses to questionnaires. Although the adolescents acknowledged occasionally not recording an event, these omissions were relatively rare (accounting for approximately less than 3% of all events). Our end-of-the-week paper-and-pencil measure of smoking during the 7 days covering the ED monitoring period correlated highly (.75) with the number of smoke events recorded on the ED.

One potential validity check on adolescents' compliance with event-recording smoking events is to examine the frequency of these events by day of the week. Anecdotal and paper-and-pencil measures of adolescent smoking frequently note that adolescents smoke more on the weekends than during the week. Figure 6-1 plots the percentage of smoke reports on the ED by day of the week,

Table 6-3. Compliance by study day at baseline

	% Prompts answered (SD)	Avg. # suspends (SD)	Avg. mins. suspend (SD)
Day 1	90.8 (17.3)	1.0 (1.4)	69.6 (31.2)
Day 2	91.4 (14.5)	1.9 (1.9)	66.0 (25.2)
Day 3	85.9 (20.4)	1.6 (1.7)	72.9 (28.1)
Day 4	83.4 (22.2)	1.5 (1.6)	79.3 (30.6)
Day 5	83.4 (27.6)	1.2 (1.4)	79.9 (31.3)
Day 6	83.4 (22.9)	1.1 (1.4)	85.0 (31.0)
Day 7	82.4 (25.5)	1.2 (1.4)	77.7 (27.6)

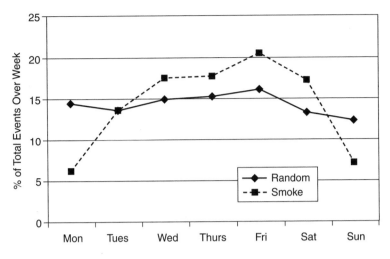

Figure 6-1. Frequency of event type by day of week.

along with the percentage of random events reports over the 7-day baseline period. We would expect that the percentage of random prompt responses should be relatively flat and stable over days of the week, given that the number of prompts does not vary by day, and indeed as can be seen in the figure, the percentage of random prompts responded to is relatively stable over the week. However, as can be seen in the figure, adolescents reported more smoking Wednesday through Saturday and a much lower percentage of smoking (of the total smoke reports) on Sunday or Monday.

Findings Related to Mood and Events

We were interested in the question of whether moods just prior to smoking or making a decision not to smoke differed from random times and also whether these differences varied by level of smoking experience. For the current analyses, we focused on the mood ratings just before the smoke or no smoke events compared to the random events. To be included in these analyses, adolescents needed to event-report either a smoking or a nonsmoking event ($n = 300$). Adolescents who responded only to random prompts and who did not report either smoking or making a nonsmoking decision were thus not included in these analyses.

Among the 300 participants for these analyses, there were three different possible patterns of data types: (1) random events and smoke events only ($n = 40$; 1,359 random events and 166 smoke events); (2) random events and no smoke events only ($n = 148$; 4,838 random events and 353 no smoke events); and (3) random events and both smoke and no smoke events ($n = 112$; 3,903 random events, 388 smoke events, and 331 no smoke events). To account for these different combinations of data, we controlled for data type in the analyses. Thus, for analyses comparing random to smoke events, data from 152 participants were used, which included comparisons of 5,262 random prompts and 554 smoke events. For comparisons of random to no smoke events, data from 188 participants were used, including 8,741 random prompts and 683 no smoke events.

Positive Mood

The random effects regression model with event type, smoking level, and the interactions of event type with smoking levels revealed a significant effect for event type (chi-square = 41.26, df = 2, p < 0.0001), and for the interaction of event type by smoking level (chi-square = 12.72, df = 4, p < 0.02). Overall, adolescents reported significantly higher positive moods during random times (M = 6.75, SD = 2.19) than just prior to smoking (M = 6.3, SD = 2.39). In addition, positive moods just prior to making a nonsmoking decision were significantly higher than moods at random times (M = 6.93, SD = 2.25 vs. M = 6.75, SD = 2.19). Examining the a priori planned contrasts for the interaction effect revealed that the difference in positive moods between random and smoke times was significantly greater for adolescents with the least smoking experience (<6 cigarettes) compared to those with either the middle level of experience (6–99 cigarettes in lifetime; estimate = –0.90, SE = 0.28, z = –3.24, p < 0.002) or to those with the most experience (100+ cigarettes in lifetime; estimate = –0.92, SE = 0.27, z = –3.41, p < 0.0001). These estimates mean that on average, the difference in positive moods between random and smoke times is .90 scale points greater for the lowest compared to the mid-level of smoking experience, and .92 scale points greater for the lowest compared to the highest level of smoking experience.

Figure 6-2 shows the mean values for the positive mood scale scores for the random and smoke events by smoking level. As can be seen, the difference between positive moods just prior to smoking and random times is greatest for the adolescents with the least smoking experience and is significantly different from the pattern for adolescents with more smoking experience. The adolescents with the least smoking experience feel significantly less positive just before smoking, compared to their random times. However, for adolescents with more smoking experience, there is not as great a difference in positive moods between random and smoke times; indeed, for the most experienced adolescents, positive moods before smoking are relatively high and equivalent to those of random times. There were no significant differences between positive mood prior to making a nonsmoking decision and random times by smoking level. The figure also shows the clear dose–response relationship between positive mood prior to smoking and smoking experience. As noted earlier, across all smoking levels, moods prior to deciding not to smoke were significantly higher at nonsmoking decision times than at random times.

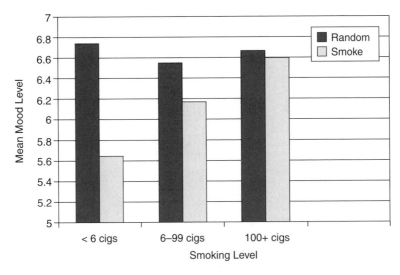

Figure 6-2. Mean positive mood just prior to smoking and at random times by smoking level.

Negative Mood

The random effects regression model for negative mood with event type, smoking level, and the interactions between event types and smoking level revealed significant effects for event type (chi square $= 44.86$, $df = 2$, $p < 0.0001$) and for the interaction between event type and smoking level (chi square $= 14.28$, $df = 4$, $p < 0.007$). Negative moods just prior to smoking were significantly higher (worse) than moods at random times (M $= 2.82$, SD $= 1.99$ vs. M $= 2.56$, SD $= 1.64$), and negative moods just prior to making a decision not to smoke were also significantly higher (worse) than negative moods at random times (M $= 2.73$, SD $= 1.72$ vs. M $= 2.46$, S $= 1.56$). Our a priori planned contrasts revealed that the significant interaction effect could be explained by differences in negative mood between random and smoking times for adolescents at the highest level of smoking compared to those at the two other levels of smoking. For adolescents at the highest level (100+ cigarettes in lifetime), the difference in negative mood between random and smoking times was significantly less than that for either the lowest smoking level (<6 cigarettes; estimate $= .63$, SE $= .19$, z $= 3.28$, $p < 0.002$) or for the middle level of smoking experience (6 to 99 cigarettes in lifetime; estimate $= .32$, SE $= .13$, z $= 2.46$, $p < 0.02$). In other words, the difference in negative mood scores between random and smoking times was approximately .63 points greater for adolescents in the lowest level of smoking compared to the highest level, and approximately .32 points greater for adolescents in the mid-level compared to the highest level of smoking.

Figure 6-3 shows the negative mood scores for both random and smoking times by smoking level. As can be seen, the difference in negative moods just

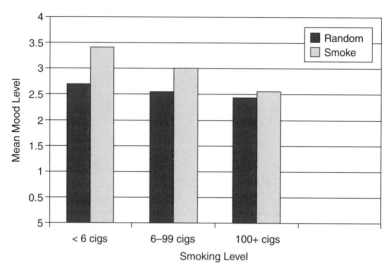

Figure 6-3. Mean negative mood just prior to smoking and at random times by smoking level.

prior to smoking and random times is greatest for the adolescents with the least smoking experience, and this difference between smoke and random times diminishes as smoking level increases, showing a clear dose–response relationship. Thus, adolescents with little smoking experience feel significantly worse just prior to smoking than they do at other times. For the most experienced smokers, there is no difference in negative moods between random times and presmoke times. There was no difference by smoking level between negative moods at random and nonsmoking decision times. For all smoking levels, negative moods were significantly higher (worse) at nonsmoking decision times than at random times.

Discussion

We addressed two primary questions with the EMA data: (1) Do moods just prior to smoking or prior to making a decision not to smoke differ from those of random, background times? and (2) Do the mood contexts of smoking and non-smoking decision times differ by level of smoking experience? We had hypothesized that, in general, moods prior to smoking would be less positive and more negative than those of random times. Our hypothesis was confirmed for the least experienced smokers; for adolescents who had smoked fewer than six cigarettes in their lifetimes, their moods just prior to smoking were significantly less positive and more negative than random times. However, for more experienced smokers, there was no difference in either positive or negative moods before smoking and at random times.

These findings suggest that for youth with little smoking experience, the subjective mood context of smoking events may be one of social discomfort—feeling lonely, sad, left out, and perhaps embarrassed. For these youth, smoking may be motivated by a desire to feel more positive about their immediate situation. Just prior to smoking, they also feel less happy, less cheerful, and less relaxed than they do at other times. However, for youth with substantially more smoking experience, smoking times are not less positive or more negative than other times. Indeed, there is no suggestion that adolescents with more smoking experience smoke at times that are affectively or subjectively different on a positive/negative dimension than other times. Importantly, the overall level of positive and negative moods at random times did not differ by smoking level.

Nonsmoking decision times for all of the adolescents were a curious combination of moods, somewhat more negative than random times, but also more positive than random times. Recall that the nonsmoking events reflected a time when adolescents actively considered smoking, had the opportunity to do so, but decided not to smoke. These may indeed be times when the adolescent's somewhat higher negative moods reflect a potentially awkward social situation. However, these times are different from smoking times in that the adolescent's overall positive mood is very high, more so than at random times. It may be that this overall positive affect in the moment buffers the adolescents against any perceived social pressures, allowing them to make a decision not to smoke.

Insights Gained from a Real-Time Approach

The real-time data collection allowed us to examine adolescents' moods immediately prior to smoking in a way that has not been captured before with more retrospective, paper-and-pencil or interview methods. In addition, because we were gathering adolescents' reports in real time, we were able to obtain more fine-grained subjective mood ratings along both a positive and negative affect dimension than is usually found with more retrospective methodologies. These data are unique, too, in that we captured nonsmoking decision times as well as smoking times. As difficult as it may be for adolescents to recall retrospectively months or years after an event how they felt in the early stages of smoking, it is even more difficult for them to recall moods surrounding specific cognitions or decisions that are not necessarily marked by overt behaviors. The EMA method allowed us to capture moods surrounding these more cognitive events.

Our data are provocative in that they point to the importance of examining moods surrounding smoking as a function of the level of experience that the adolescent has with smoking. Our findings also suggest that the emotional contexts surrounding smoking for novice smokers are very different from the emotional contexts of smoking for more experienced adolescent smokers. Contrary to expectations and more retrospective adolescent reports (e.g., Mermelstein, 1999), more experienced adolescent smokers are not smoking at times when they feel "down" or more negative than their norm.

Our analyses here focused on the mood experience of adolescents just prior to smoking or making a nonsmoking decision. We did not present adolescents' subjective mood responses following smoking or following a decision not to smoke. Thus, it is possible that adolescents who continue to experiment with smoking beyond the first few trials experience a mood boost following smoking even if their smoking was not initially preceded by subjectively negative mood states. It is also possible that adolescents who fail to experience mood relief following smoking are the ones who do not progress in their habit and stop "experimenting." Alternatively, one could also hypothesize that as adolescents progress in their smoking, they become more comfortable in what might otherwise be a socially difficult or awkward moment when they perceive a norm to smoke. Our sample of adolescents with little smoking experience is likely to be a heterogeneous one in that some of these youth will discontinue their smoking, while others will go on to become more regular smokers. The mood aftermath of smoking may be critical to predicting progression. Similarly, subjective affect following a decision not to smoke may also be important to understanding an adolescent's ability to continue to reject smoking or not. The data presented in this chapter are cross-sectional and as such do not allow us to make inferences yet about how moods both prior to and after smoking and not smoking relate to progression.

These data are invaluable in helping to start to understand why some situations lead to smoking and others do not. Our findings highlight the potential role of positive affect in tipping the balance toward not smoking in a given moment. Positive affect has been a relatively understudied dimension in smoking research, and these findings suggest a need to focus more efforts on both positive and negative emotional domains.

Success and Challenges

Our experience in using EMA with the adolescents to examine the contexts of smoking and nonsmoking has led us to conclude that the successes clearly outweighed the challenges. We have continued to be both surprised and pleased by the richness of the data. The methodology has allowed us to address questions about the immediate contexts surrounding smoking that have not been possible before. For example, by combining the objective data about the presence of other smokers and the subjective mood data, we can ask questions about how subjective moods differ when other smokers are present or not, and whether these differences in context are more likely to lead to a smoking or nonsmoking decision.

Our surprise has been how "well behaved" the data were. One of our concerns prior to initiating this study was that the adolescents would not take the task seriously or that they could not accommodate the demands of the data collection, potentially leading to careless or random responding, or a high rate of noncompliance. None of these have been our experience. We attribute much of this success to careful preparation of the participants in terms of training. From debriefing participants we also learned that participant payment was important, and because of the payment ($40 for the baseline EMA weeklong, with escalating payments over waves), participants reported treating the task as a "job" and one that they had to take seriously.

One might ask how representative our participants were of the pool of possible candidates. Adolescents who completed the baseline wave did not differ from the broader sample of adolescents who met inclusion criteria in terms of level of smoking experience, but males were slightly less likely than females to respond to our recruitment efforts and nonwhite youth were slightly less likely to respond than white youth (Diviak, Wahl, O'Keefe, et al., 2006). In addition, the more experienced smokers were somewhat less likely to drop out of the study. Anecdotally, the youth with more smoking experience were less busy with competing activities than were nonsmoking youth and had both the time and sense of commitment to the project to follow through (they reported feeling pleased to have been asked to participate). Clearly, not all adolescents can handle the requirements of this intensive data collection and navigate some of the social complexities of interacting with the ED. However, in each school, all students in the grade were aware of the study, and we engendered a sense of "specialness" among students for being invited to participate. It was rare for a student to report negative social reactions to carrying and responding to the ED.

There were additional ethical and pragmatic challenges in using EMA to study adolescent smoking. From an ethical perspective, we needed to include both smokers and nonsmokers in the study to avoid the possible implication that the adolescent participants were all "smokers." Given that smoking among adolescents is frequently a covert and punishable behavior, we were also concerned about participants' potential reluctance both to participate and to event record smoking episodes. Very explicit information to the adolescents, parents, and teachers explaining issues of confidentiality helped to assuage these concerns.

From a pragmatic standpoint, a major challenge was the enormous personnel time that was required to ensure participants' engagement and compliance. Developing a strong sense of a collaborative research relationship between our field staff and the participants, through one-on-one in-person training, personalized follow-up phone calls, and consistency in contact people, was important to the success of the data collection efforts. Anticipating hardware malfunctions and being prepared to respond quickly with replacements was also time-demanding. Finally, there was the occasional reminder that adolescents may indeed act out as adolescents at times and find ways to use the devices to annoy teachers, parents, and study staff.

Prospects for Application of EMA Methods

The EMA methods provide a wealth of opportunities for addressing important questions in the field of adolescent smoking. As noted earlier, the ability to examine concurrently both the objective and subjective components of the context of smoking or nonsmoking decision times allows researchers to answer questions about adolescent smoking in ways that will greatly increase our understanding of factors that may lead to the progression of smoking.

Longitudinal EMA data will be especially valuable in addressing questions about the development of dependence and changes that occur over time in subjective responses to smoking. For example, we might hypothesize that as an adolescent gains experience with smoking and starts to develop signs of dependence, we might see a decrease in certain subjective responses to smoking (c.f., Hedeker, Mermelstein & Flay, 2006). One might also see changes in situational antecedents over time as adolescents become more established smokers. For example, one might hypothesize that smoking alone, versus more social smoking, may be an early marker of dependence.

The EMA procedures also potentially produce enormous amounts of data, thus allowing researchers to address within-subject questions of interest that have been difficult to address with other methodologies. For example, one could examine the cross-situational variability (or consistency) in mood changes that might occur with smoking and start to address questions about how situational factors versus intraindividual factors contribute to emotional responses to smoking.

In sum, EMA methods provide a unique window into studying the contexts and subjective experiences of adolescents as they initially try, experiment, and become dependent on smoking. Our experience has demonstrated the feasibility and value of EMA data in gaining new insights into the antecedents and immediate consequences of both smoking and nonsmoking decisions among adolescents relatively early in their smoking "careers." Future work will need to focus on more established smokers as well.

ACKNOWLEDGMENTS

Work on this chapter was funded in part by grant CA80266 from the National Cancer Institute and by a grant from the Tobacco Etiology Network, Robert Wood Johnson Foundation.

References

Brown, R. A., Lewinsohn, P. M., Seeley, J. R., & Wagner, E. F. (1996). Cigarette smoking, major depression, and other psychiatric disorders among adolescents. *Journal of the American Academy of Child and Adolescent Psychiatry, 35,* 1602–1610.

Choi, W., Patten, C., Gillin, J., Kaplan, R., & Pierce, J. (1997). Cigarette smoking predicts development of depressive symptoms among U.S. adolescents. *Annals of Behavioral Medicine, 19,* 42–50.

Conrad, K., Flay, B. R., & Hill, D. (1992). Why children start smoking cigarettes: Predictors of onset. *British Journal of Addiction, 87,* 1711–1724.

Diviak, K., Wahl, S., O'Keefe, J., Mermelstein, R., & Flay, B. (2006). Recruitment and retention of adolescents in a smoking trajectory study: Who participates and lessons learned. *Substance Use and Misuse, 41,* 1–8.

Eissenberg, T., & Balster, R. (2000). Initial tobacco use episodes in children and adolescents: current knowledge and future directions. *Drug and Alcohol Dependence, 59,* S41–60.

Friedman, L., Lichtenstein, E., & Biglan, A. (1985). Smoking onset among teens: An empirical analysis of initial situations. *Addictive Behaviors, 10,* 1–13.

Hedeker, D., Mermelstein, R., & Flay, B. (2006). Application of item response theory models for intensive longitudinal data. In T. Walls & J. Schafer (Eds.), *Models for intensive longitudinal data* (pp. 84–108). Oxford University Press.

Johnston, L. D., O'Malley, P. M., & Bachman, J. C. (Dec.19, 2003). *Teen smoking continues to decline in 2003, but declines are slowing.* University of Michigan News and Information Services: Ann Arbor, MI. Available on-line at: www.monitoringthefuture.org.

Mermelstein, R. (1999). Explanations of ethnic and gender differences in youth smoking: A multi-site, qualitative investigation. *Nicotine and Tobacco Research, 1,* S91–S98.

Patton, G. C., Hibbert, M., Rosier, M. J., Carline, J. B., Caust, J., & Bowes, G. (1996). Is smoking associated with depression and anxiety in teenagers? *American Journal of Public Health, 86,* 225–230.

Pomerleau, O. F., Collins, A. C., Shiffman, S., & Pomerleau, C. (1993). Why some people smoke and others do not: New perspectives. *Journal of Consulting and Clinical Psychology, 61,* 723–731.

Shiffman, S. (1993). Assessing smoking patterns and motives. *Journal of Consulting and Clinical Psychology, 61,* 732–742.

Shiffman, S., Gnys, M., Richards, T. J., Paty, J. A., Hickcox, M., & Kassel, J. D. (1996). Temptations to smoke after quitting: A comparison of lapsers and maintainers. *Health Psychology, 15,* 455–461.

Shiffman, S., Paty, J. A., Gnys, M., Kassel, J. D., & Elash, C. (1995). Nicotine withdrawal in chippers and regular smokers: Subjective and cognitive effects. *Health Psychology, 14,* 301–309.

Shiffman, S., Paty, J. A., Gnys, M., Kassel, J. D., & Hickcox, M. (1996). First lapses of smoking: Within-subjects analysis of real-time reports. *Journal of Consulting and Clinical Psychology, 64,* 366–379.

Turner, L., Mermelstein, R., & Flay, B. (2004). Individual and contextual influences on adolescent smoking. *Annals of the New York Academy of Science, 1021,* 1–23.

U.S. Department of Health and Human Services. (1994). *Preventing tobacco use among young people: A report of the Surgeon General.* Atlanta, GA: U.S. Department of Health and Human Services. Public Health Service. Centers for Disease Control and Prevention. National Center for Chronic Disease Prevention and Health Promotion. Office on Smoking and Health.

Verbeke, G., & Molenberghs, G. (2000). *Linear mixed models for longitudinal data.* New York: Springer.

Whalen, C. K., Jamner, L. D., Henker, B., & Delfino, R. J. (2001). Smoking and moods in adolescents with depressive and aggressive dispositions. Evidence from surveys and electronic diaries. *Health Psychology, 20,* 99–111.

7

Ecological Momentary Assessment of Physical Activity in Hispanics/Latinos Using Pedometers and Diaries

Elva M. Arredondo, John P. Elder, Simon Marshall, and Barbara Baquero

Assessment of the overt performance of any behavior, including physical activity, is a distinguishing feature of both behavioral assessment and behavior analysis (Kazdin, 1981). Through direct assessment, minimal inference is needed about the relationship between the actual behavior and the subject's interpretation of that behavior. Ideal measures of physical activity are those that are objective, valid, and reliable. To meet the criterion of objectivity, observers must not allow their own feelings or interpretations to affect their recordings (Sulzer-Azaroff & Mayer, 1991). Ultimately, the utility of the assessment is judged with respect to how it contributes to interventions that increase the participant's adaptive behaviors (Hayes, Nelson, & Jarrett, 1987; Nelson, 1983; Sulzer-Azaroff & Mayer, 1991). Thus, it is important to collect as much information as possible about the behavior and the environment in which it occurs to better understand antecedents of behavior change.

Physical activity is defined as any bodily movement produced by skeletal muscles that results in an expenditure of energy. In this sense, physical activity itself does not require any subjective estimation as to whether the individual is active or not, as would be in the case when measuring feelings of stress or depression. Numerous objective methods have been designed and validated for measuring physical activity, including direct observation, heart rate monitors, accelerometers, and doubly labeled water (Montoye, Kemple, Saris, & Washburn, 1996). Direct observation is best for current, frequent, and regular (i.e., day-to-day) activity (Stone, McKenzie, Welk, & Booth, 1998). For example, McKenzie and colleagues have applied structured observations of physical activity to the physical education and open playground environments in both elementary and middle-school children (McKenzie, Marshall, Sallis, & Conway, 2000; McKenzie, Sallis, & Nader, 1991). However, direct observation methods are often not practical in larger studies because they are expensive, have the potential to create subject reactivity, may have findings limited in generalizability, and place a high burden on the observer

(McKenzie, 2002; Stone et al., 1998). This is one reason researchers often rely on self-reports of physical activity to determine whether specific interventions promoting physical activity have been effective.

Self-report and diaries are among the most common methods for assessing physical activity, primarily because of their low cost, ease of administration, and potential for nonreactivity. However, investigators have questioned the accuracy of self-report measures in the assessment of physical activity (Sallis & Saelens, 2000). They note that individuals tend to overreport their level of physical activity when assessed via paper and pencil (Duncan, Sydeman, Perri, et al., 2001; Montoye et al., 1996). One reason why individuals may not be accurate reporters of their physical activity is because of recall (Montoye et al., 1996).

The pedometer has recently been used as a cost-effective alternative to both objective and self-report methods of assessing physical activity (Tudor-Locke, Williams, Reis, & Pluto, 2002). There is a wide range of concordance between self-reported physical activities and pedometer-derived counts (median of reported correlations $r = 0.33$, range $= 0.02$ to 0.94). While pedometers cannot assess the intensity of physical activity, they appear to be a valid tool for assessing the total volume of ambulatory physical activity accrued over a specific period (Schneider, Crouter, & Bassett, 2004). It may be that pedometers offer an advantage over traditional self-report methods, particularly when the outcome of interest is ambulation-based physical activity or when a detailed assessment of intensity is unimportant.

One method of behavior assessment that is cheaper than direct observation and has the potential for minimizing recall bias is referred to as Ecological Momentary Assessment (EMA) (Stone & Shiffman, 2002). EMA requires that individuals provide a report (following an event or time-specific) of experiences (e.g., beliefs, emotions, cognitions) and behaviors (e.g., physical activity) in their natural environment. EMA refers to a collection of techniques based on principles of momentary time sampling, which can yield valid behavioral samples (Stone & Shiffman, 2002) and reduce the bias typically associated with recall. An important decision when conducting an EMA study is the selection of an appropriate sampling approach that ensures that the spectrum of behaviors or experiences is adequately represented (Stone & Shiffman, 2002). Sampling approaches include event contingent reporting (assessments are completed when a particular event occurs), interval contingent reporting (assessments are completed at regular intervals), and signal contingent reporting (assessments are completed when an external stimulus cues recording) (Wheeler & Reis, 1991).

The feasibility and validity of most of the aforementioned assessment methods have mostly been examined in White populations and not in ethnic minorities. Due to a variety of tangible (e.g., economic) and intangible (e.g., beliefs) barriers, Hispanic/Latino and other minority women get less physical activity than do White women (King, Castro, Wilcox, et al., 2000; Sternfeld, Ainsworth, & Quesenberry, 1999). Recent data suggest that 46 percent of Mexican-American women report no leisure time physical activity compared to 23 percent of White women (Kriska, 2000). However, these differences also may be attributable to ethnic-specific interpretations of "leisure," "physical activity," or "exercise" (Kriska, 2000). These factors highlight the difficulties of using self-report measures with certain populations and reinforce the need to develop viable alternatives that minimize factors known to bias study findings.

Rationale for a Momentary Approach to Data Collection

As discussed above, self-reported data gathered through paper-and-pencil diaries or questionnaires are subject to a variety of recall-related biases, including memory decay and the current salience of the phenomena during the time of report. Therefore, the primary purpose of the current pilot study was to evaluate the correspondence between self-reports of different levels of physical activity and pedometer-derived counts of physical activity. These data will allow us to examine the correspondence between pedometer counts and moderate, vigorous, and very vigorous reports of physical activity.

A secondary goal was to examine whether participants who were paged reported more accurate accounts of moderate, vigorous, and very vigorous physical activity compared to those who were not prompted. Studies show that individuals may overestimate the frequency of events when asked to recall over a long time frame (Bradburn, Rips, & Shevell, 1987). Thus, it was expected that individuals who recorded particular events of their activity levels at the time they were paged would be less susceptible to recall bias. A third aim was to examine the feasibility of using ecological momentary data among a Hispanic/Latino sample as, to our knowledge, no studies have examined the use of EMA with this community. The need to include such populations is important to better understand physical activity patterns and ways to improve accuracy in reporting physical activity.

Method

This was an experimental study in which the units of analyses were pedometer counts and self-report by Hispanics/Latinos of minutes of moderate, vigorous, and very vigorous physical activity. Participants were randomly assigned to either the control or experimental group. Pagers were chosen in order to page/prompt participants throughout each block of the day (e.g., morning, afternoon, and evening). We also wanted to avoid paging participants at the exact time each day in case they could not complete the diary when paged (e.g., during a class). Those in the experimental group were paged about every 4 hours (usually once in the morning, afternoon, and evening) and asked to record the type and intensity of activity and number of minutes of physical activity when paged (i.e., signal contingent). Participants in the control group were asked to record this information at their convenience, or by the end of the day.

Sample

Study participants were a convenience sample of Hispanics/Latinos recruited from the larger Secretos de la Buena Vida study that used random digit dialing to a tailored nutrition communication intervention. Detailed recruitment procedures are described elsewhere (Elder, Ayala, Campbell, et al., 2005). Female participants eligible for the study had to be between 18 and 65 years and Spanish-language dominant (i.e., able to read in Spanish). Participants were not eligible if they were pregnant, were on a strict diet for medical reasons, or intended to leave the study area within the subsequent 18 months. As part of the larger study, a bilingual, bicultural female research assistant (RA) scheduled home visits with the female head of the household to collect baseline data. During the home visits, the RA collected demographic, psychosocial, and anthropometric information such as height and weight using a portable scale and stadiometer.

For the current study, an RA called potential participants in sequential order within 6 months of their completion of the Secretos de la Buena Vida study to invite them to participate in the experimental study; the first 54 who agreed to participate were enrolled (none refused). All women who participated in the larger study gave prior approval to be called back for future studies. However, the three women who did not attend their first appointment were subsequently excluded from the study. A total of 51 women were included and randomly assigned to either the experimental or control condition. Instead of financial compensation, women were each given a pedometer to compensate for their time in the study.

Momentary Data Collection

We employed an interval contingent sampling approach because we expected the physical activity to vary and we wanted to attain an overall representative sample of the physical activity engaged throughout the day. Attaining a sample in the morning, afternoon, and evening (hence 4 to 5 hours) would give us the most representative sample of physical activity. At the end of the day, both groups were asked to record the number of steps displayed in their pedometer. Participants were asked to follow these procedures for 3 days. Because of staff and instrumentation availability, the procedure schedule was spread out for 5 weeks (e.g., 10 participants per week). There were no compliance checks, but participants were asked whether they followed protocol.

Measures

SELF-REPORT OF PHYSICAL ACTIVITY

The 3-day Physical Activity Record (3-day PAR) used in the current study is a modified version of the 7-day PAR (Sallis, Strikmiller, Harsha, et al., 1996), which has been validated with Hispanic/Latino populations (Sallis, Buono, Roby, et al., 1993), and of the Previous Day Physical Activity Recall (Weston, Petosa, & Pate, 1997).

The latter is a self-administered instrument that was used in minority populations (Trost, Pate, Dowda, et al., 2002) and is designed to assess weekday physical activity (e.g., kcals/kg/day). Participants were asked to report the type of activity and the number of hours and minutes of moderate, vigorous, and very vigorous physical activity during morning, afternoon, and evening.

To help participants select the correct intensity level, the instrument provides pictorial representations of three levels of physical activity. Moderate activity was defined as normal movement such as walking, cleaning the house, and gardening and was given the perceptual anchor of being "slightly out of breath, but still able to hold a conversation." Vigorous activity was defined as activity that requires more effort than walking (not as intense as running) such as swimming and dancing. The perceptual anchor for vigorous activity was "breathing rapidly and barely able to hold a conversation." Very vigorous activity was defined as fast movement such as running, cycling fast, and playing soccer. The perceptual anchor for very vigorous activity was "breathing rapidly and having difficulty holding a conversation." The number of minutes spent in each category of activity intensity was summed for each day.

STEPS

The Walk for Life digital walker (LS 2500) is an electronic pedometer that operates on a horizontal, spring-suspended level arm that moves up and down in response to vertical displacement. When a threshold of vertical displacement has been exceeded, the level arm completes an electrical circuit, and one step is recorded. The digital walker is mounted on the waistband over the midline of the dominant leg. One of the goals for using the pedometer is to provide construct validity of the self-report of physical activity.

BMI MEASUREMENT

Body mass index (BMI) is the ratio of weight in kilograms divided by the square of the height in meters. It is a reliable indicator of obesity (Garrow & Webster, 1985) and has a high correlation with body fatness (Bray & Gray, 1988; Manson, Colditz, Stampfer, et al., 1990; Simopoulos, 1985). BMI is related to mortality (Rockhill, Willett, Manson, et al., 2001), suggesting that it has construct validity when used as a health outcome. We included the measurement to ensure that there were no BMI differences between the experimental and control groups.

ACCULTURATION

The Acculturation Rating Scale for Mexican-Americans by Cuéllar et al. (Cuellar, Arnold, & Maldonado, 1995; ARSMA-II) assesses five elements of acculturation: (a) language familiarity and usage, (b) ethnic pride and identity, (c) ethnic interaction, (d) cultural heritage, and (e) generational proximity. We included acculturation in the analysis to better understand whether this variable did not account for physical activity differences between groups. Studies have shown that acculturation is associated with physical activity (Crespo, Smit, Carter-Pokras, & Andersen, 2001).

DEMOGRAPHIC

Participants were asked to provide information about their age, marital status, income, country of origin, years of residence in the United States, employment status, years of formal education, country of formal education, and number of adults and children under the age of 18 living in the household.

EXIT INTERVIEW

The RAs conducted a structured in-person interview asking participants whether they had changed their routine (activity level) or encountered special events during their participation in the study, the number of days they used the pedometer, pager (if applicable), whether they completed the 3-day PAR, whether they worked (the number of days/hours), whether they found the pager easy to use, whether there were special events in the past 3 days, whether they changed their routine, whether they encountered any challenges in participating (*"Tell us if you had problems filling out the survey"* [translated] and *"Tell us if you have other comments about participating in the study"* [translated]), and whether they planned to exercise following the program.

Procedures

Each participant was instructed to attach the pedometer to her clothing on the waist, over the dominant foot. She was also instructed to attach the pedometer upon waking and remove it just before going to bed. A bilingual/bicultural RA visited each participant's home to drop off a pedometer, the study survey (translated Spanish form of the 3-day PAR), and a pager (experimental group only) during the weekdays. The RA briefly trained each participant to complete the paper-and-pencil 3-day PAR and record the type and duration of physical activity for 3 days; it was estimated that the recordings would take approximately 1 to 3 minutes. Participants were shown how to operate and attach the pedometer. Those in the pager condition practiced turning off the pager following the auditory signal; each was asked to record the number of pedometer counts at the end of the day prior to bed and to reset it.

During data collection, all participants were asked to continue their usual routines and all were assessed during the weekday. The RA was available by telephone, during the day, all 3 days in case participants had difficulty completing the task or in case they had further questions. Participants were told to carry the diary with them so that an entry could be made. They were also told that completion of the assessment within 15 minutes of data entry was acceptable.

At the end of the third day, a bicultural/bilingual RA collected the research materials (pedometer, survey, and pager) and administered an exit interview that included a series of questions regarding any challenges participants encountered in adhering to the study protocol. The RA reviewed each sheet and checked for inconsistencies. The protocol of the current study was approved by the Institutional Review Board to ensure the protection of human participants.

Data Analysis

The total number of steps and the number of minutes spent at each level of physical activity intensity were averaged across 3 days of assessments. Prior to data analysis, the normality of the distributions for all variables was evaluated. Data revealed that reports of vigorous and very vigorous physical activity were negatively skewed and kurtotic because many women did not engage in physical activity at either of these intensity levels. Thus, it was decided to dichotomize these two variables (e.g., those who did not engage in any physical activity vs. those who engaged in vigorous activity level). The distribution of steps per day (from the pedometers) was also found to be non-normal, and so a square root transformation was applied to normalize these data.

A series of t-tests and chi-squares were conducted to examine whether there were a priori group differences in demographics. Pearson correlations were used to evaluate relations between self-reports of physical activity and pedometer counts. Descriptive analyses and chi-squares were conducted to evaluate whether group differences existed in terms of adherence to study protocol and change in routine. Subject and measure effects were considered random. Where intraclass correlations were less than .8, the Spearman-Brown prophecy formula was used to calculate the number of days of assessment needed to estimate stable (i.e., habitual) patterns. Finally, qualitative data were analyzed for content. All quantitative data analyses were conducted using SAS 6.12 and SPSS 11.01, with alpha set to .05 to determine statistical significance.

Results

Demographic

The mean age of the participants was 41 years; most were married (76%), had a low socioeconomic status (SES; 49% had a family income of $2,000 or less), and had a low level of education ($M_{education}$ = third grade). The majority of the participants were first-generation immigrants from Mexico (90%), most reported a homemaker status, and most received their education in Mexico (78%) (Table 7-1). Approximately 59 percent had two or fewer children under the age of 18 living in the household, and 67 percent had two or fewer adult members living in the household.

Table 7-1. Demographics

	Frequency (%)	Means (SD)
Age[1]		41 (9.5)
Marital status[1]		
Married/common law	38 (76)	
Divorced/widowed/separated/single	12 (16)	
Income[1]		
Less than $500	1 (2)	
$501–$1,000	4 (8)	
$1,001–$1,500	12 (24)	
$1,501–2,000	8 (15)	
Greater than $2,000	21 (41)	
Country of origin[1]		
Mexico	45 (90)	
Other	1 (2)	
Years in the United States[1]		15.4 (9.4)
Employment status[1]		
Full/part-time	16 (32)	
Homemaker	30 (60)	
Years of formal education		3 (1.1)
Country of formal education[1]		
Mexico	78 (85)	
United States	3 (6)	
Both	3 (6)	
Acculturation[2]		−2.10 (.86)

[1] Missing values
[2] Acculturation scores range from −4.00 (Very Mexican) to +4.00 (Very Anglo)

No demographic differences were evident between participants in the experimental (n = 24) and control (n = 26) groups: by age (t(44) = −.56, $p < 0.57$), marital status ($\chi^2(1, n = 46) = .26, p < 0.61$), employment status ($\chi^2(1, n = 46) = .19, p < 0.66$), country of origin ($\chi^2(1, n = 46) = 1.26, p < 0.27$), family income ($\chi^2(1, n = 46) = .21, p < 0.64$), years of formal education (t(44) = −.34, $p < 0.73$), years of living in the United States (t(44) = −.15, $p < 0.88$), acculturation (t(44) = 1.00, $p < 0.32$), and BMI (t(43) = 1.15, $p < 0.25$).

Validity/Manipulation Check

Approximately 67 percent of the participants correctly stated that they were paged three times a day, 6 percent indicated that they were paged more than three times, 12 percent indicated that they heard it twice a day, and 8 percent indicated that they did not hear it at all.

Question 1: *Is pedometer count related to self-report activity level?*

Results in Table 7-2 indicate that self-reported minutes of moderate physical activity were negatively correlated with steps per day ($r = −.10$, 95% CI = −.39 to .19).

Table 7-2. Means and standard deviations (kcals/kg/day)*

	Control group (n = 25)	Experimental group (pager) (n = 26)	p-value
Moderate units?	476 (223)	507 (219)	.63
Vigorous	73 (112)	30 (39)	.08
Very vigorous	15 (33)	51 (184)	.25
Pedometer counts	8,717 (10,360)	10,730 (10,324)	.49

* Average number of 3 days.

In comparison, self-reported minutes of vigorous physical activity were positively but not significantly related to steps per day ($r = .23$, 95% CI $= -.05$ to .48). Similarly, self-reports of very vigorous activity were significantly and positively associated with steps per day ($r = .36$, 95% CI $= .08$ to .58). Self-reports of very vigorous physical activity level were significantly associated with vigorous activity ($r = .30$, 95% CI $= .02$ to .53), but neither vigorous nor very vigorous activity was related to moderate activity ($r_{vig} = -.19$, 95% CI $= -.45$ to .11; $r_{very\ vig} = -.21$, 95% CI $= -.47$ to .09). To examine whether each of the associations differed from each other, Fisher's z transformations were computed and contrasted. Moderate physical activity was the only relation that significantly differed from very vigorous activity.

Question 2: *Is group status related to self-report of physical activity?*

Group status was not associated with any of the self-reports of physical activity ($r_{mod} = -.10$, 95% CI $= -.38$ to .19; $r_{vig} = .01$, 95% CI $= -.28$ to .30; $r_{very\ vig} = .05$, 95% CI $= -.24$ to .33). Consistent with these findings, group status was not significantly associated with pedometer counts (Table 7-3). When examining group means, no significant differences emerged between group status and moderate, vigorous, and very vigorous activity (see Table 7-2). Participants in the experimental (pager prompt) condition were more likely to report higher pedometer counts, but these differences were not statistically different (see Table 7-2).

Question 3: *Is EMA easy to use for Hispanics/Latinos?*

GROUP DIFFERENCES IN ADHERENCE TO STUDY PROTOCOL

Chi-square was used to evaluate whether differences between groups (experimental vs. control) existed in terms of adherence to the study protocol, change in activity level, and adherence of pedometers and pager use. All of the participants indicated that they used the pedometer during the 3 days of assessment, and 88 percent of the participants in the experimental group indicated that they used the pager for 3 days (12% indicated that they used it 2 days) and reported writing in the diaries within protocol (within 15 minutes of hearing the auditory signal). Participants who used the pager (88%)[1] indicated that it was easy to use. Twelve percent of pager users reported that they would not use it again.

Table 7-3. Pearson correlations between mean steps per day and minutes per day of self-reported moderate, vigorous, and very vigorous activity, and group level

Number of steps as measured by the pedometer	r	95% CI
Moderate	−.10	−.39 to .19
Vigorous	.23	−.05 to −.48
Very vigorous	.36	.08 to −.58
Group level*	.21	−.12 −.42

* "0" = control and "1" = experimental

Compared to women in the control group, women in the experimental group were no more likely to have been employed in the last 3 days ($\chi^2(1, n = 50) = .0007, p < 1.00$), to change their routine due to their participation in the study ($\chi^2(1, n = 50) = .66, p < 0.68$), to report special events (i.e., pregnancy, illness, accident, other) occurring in the past 3 days ($\chi^2(1, n = 50) = .29, p < 0.58$), and to change their activity ($\chi^2(1, n = 46) = 1.38, p < 0.23$). Because all ($n = 51$) women reported that they did not have difficulty using the pedometer and almost all ($n = 49$) stated that it was very easy to record it, chi-squares examining group differences were not performed. Of the women who were in the experimental group, 32 percent ($n = 16$) reported that they planned to exercise "more than usual" as a result of participation in the program. However, 26 percent ($n = 13$) of women in the control group also reported that they planned to exercise "more than usual" as a result of participation.

QUALITATIVE RESULTS

Women were asked in an open-ended format whether they had difficulty completing the survey (*"Tell us if you had problems filling out the survey"* [translated]). Several of the participants, particularly those with low levels of literacy, indicated that they found the 3-day PAR difficult to use. More specifically, they indicated that the forms requested too much information in each time period, namely the time of activity, minutes spent on it, and the type of activity; several women noted that they would like a simpler form. Other women indicated that some of the pictures in the survey (e.g., running, bicycling, playing soccer), particularly those depicting very vigorous activity levels, did not accurately reflect the daily activities of the participants, and they were therefore less likely to report very vigorous activity.

Participants were also asked in an open-ended format about their experience participating in the current study (*"Tell us if you have other comments about participating in the study"* [translated]). Several Hispanics/Latinos noted that they found the study interesting and that they would not change any aspect. Many Hispanics/Latinos indicated that participating in the current study increased their awareness of their physical activity. One 34-year-old participant noted, *"The experience was good because I had no idea I was as physically active"* [translated]. Other women explained that participation in the pilot study motivated them to be physically active. For instance, one said, *"The pedometer is good; it wasn't difficult. I noticed the total number of steps and it was increasing every day and I wanted to have this number increase the other day"* [translated]. Another participant said, *"I found it interesting. I don't see where it* [the program] *needs to change but to continue with these programs for us. The pedometer motivates one to increase physical activity and to keep in mind that one can exercise instead of watching television"* [translated].

Most women were interested in receiving some type of feedback regarding their physical activity because they said it would help them understand whether they need to increase their daily physical activity. Only one participant commented on her form that she found the pager helpful in reminding her to record the level and duration of physical activity engaged in over a period of 3 to 4 hours.

Discussion

Study findings highlight some of the challenges of assessing physical activity behavior using pedometers and paper-and-pencil self-report of physical activity. The current study evaluates the construct validity of self-reported physical activity at different levels of intensity by comparing the data to the number of steps taken by study participants. Pedometer correlations with self-reported moderate, vigorous, and very vigorous activity were $-.10$, $.23$, and $.36$. These findings indicate that steps per day correspond more closely to those who reported very vigorous physical activity and, to a lesser extent, vigorous activity. In contrast, self-report of moderate physical activity was inversely related to steps per day.

One possible explanation for the current findings may be that adults, particularly those who lead sedentary lifestyles, tend to overestimate the intensity of their moderate level activity (Duncan et al., 2001). Further, the reverse association between steps per day and moderate activity may be due to considerable error in these measures or the instruments may be assessing different constructs. Because pedometers account only for movement requiring vertical displacement of the hips, they cannot accurately assess activity that occurs predominantly at the upper extremities of the body (Tudor-Locke et al., 2002). Therefore, women in the current study may also have engaged in moderate-intensity physical activity that did not require much vertical hip displacement.

Measurement error in self-report of moderate levels of physical activity can also be influenced by cultural factors documented in health behavior research among Hispanics/Latinos (Marin & Triandis, 1985). Participants may have provided socially desirable answers in order to portray behavior in the best possible light, and this factor may have contributed to the high report of moderate activity level (Marin & Triandis, 1985). Another possible explanation for the poor correspondence between moderate intensity in physical activity and steps per day is that moderate-intensity physical activity is notoriously difficult to recall for many adults (Sallis & Saelens, 2000; Taylor, Coffey, Berra, et al., 1984), largely because these behaviors are more likely to be intermittent and unstructured and involve a perception of effort that may not be easily recalled by memory.

Our data also indicate that participants in the pager condition were no more accurate reporters of physical activity than those who were not paged. We expected the self-report of physical activity among prompted participants to closely correspond to the number of steps assessed by the pedometer because we believed that delay in recording physical activity would be subject to recall bias. However, it is unclear whether participants in the experimental condition completed an entry following a prompt. In the absence of objective data about recording latency (from initial prompt), it is not possible to estimate the effects of recall bias on the self-report data. Moreover, our qualitative data suggest that participants, particularly those in the experimental condition, encountered many challenges in using EMA via pagers. In addition to having less-than-ideal compliance,[2] 12 percent of those in the pager condition indicated that they would not use the pager again.

Insights Gained from a Real-Time Approach

Although more studies with larger samples are needed to confirm findings from the current study, it appears that prompting participants via a pager to record their physical activity may not be an effective strategy to increase accuracy of self-report. In a recent study, Broderick and colleagues (2003) examined compliance with a paper diary protocol using auditory signaling among adults with chronic pain. The authors found that although signaling (via a watch) produced a significant increment in verified compliance when compared with an identical trial without signaling, compliance of self-report diary entries was unsatisfactory. Taken together, signaling without verification of entry makes it difficult to know whether participants behaved according to protocol. It may be that participants had difficulty completing EMA via the pager because they found it cumbersome to wear a pager and a pedometer while carrying the pencil-and-paper forms. Moreover, if given a choice, participants may not consider using the pager as beneficial and therefore may have opted to wear only the pedometer.

Successes and Challenges

Given the challenges and lessons noted above, we would use different measurement instruments in future studies. Because it is uncertain whether prompting individuals with a pager creates questionnaire compliance, other types of EMAs such as the electronic diaries may be appropriate to use. Such instrumentation enables more objective assessment of compliance because each diary entry is electronically and independently "stamped" with the date and time of the recording. Electronic diaries also allow participants to suspend and "delay" their responses for up to 20 minutes (in case they are driving). Electronic diaries can reduce data entry errors as well, by eliminating missed questions or out-of-range responses.[3] Given our experience, this is a particularly important consideration when working with less acculturated and low-literacy populations.

Another benefit of using the electronic diaries is that the data can be downloaded and the quick receipt of data allows for the possibility of providing timely feedback to participants about their patterns of responding. Taken together, electronic diaries are the type of measurement that will help investigators better understand whether prompting does indeed increase accuracy in reporting.[4]

We would also conduct the study differently by including more participants in our experimental trial. A larger sample size would reduce the standard deviation in the mean number of steps per day, giving more power to detect true differences between groups. The small sample sizes in each group may have precluded the ability to detect differences in physical activity.[5] Given that the current pilot study was exploratory in nature, only a few participants were recruited.

Prospects for Applications of EMA Methods

There are a number of prospects for applications for EMA methods. Researchers could use EMA to link specific tangible (e.g., economic) and intangible barriers (e.g., mood) and facilitators (e.g., social support) to their physical activity. The results of studies that assess barriers and facilitators to physical activity before and after participation in an intervention may be confounded by participants' recall bias of their physical activity. Future studies could assess via electronic diaries the types of activities women engage in throughout the day, as well as the barriers and facilitators to engaging in physical activity. Assessing the barriers and facilitators through electronic diaries would further our understanding of mediators or moderators for the low physical activity evident in Hispanics/Latinos. Prior to conducting such studies, research is needed to examine how electronic diaries would be received by them and the training needed to ensure the technology is used correctly and that good adherence is achieved.

Notes

1. The intraclass correlation for 3 days of assessment was 0.33 (95% CI = 0.15 to 0.51). This suggests that the number of steps per day was highly variable within participants. At these levels of variability, approximately 25 days of assessment would be needed to achieve a reliability of .8. This length of assessment would place considerable burden on the participant, and so further research should examine factors that contribute to the day-to-day variability of stepping behavior in Hispanics/Latinos.

2. Eighty-eight percent of the participants indicated that they used the pager all 3 days.

3. The RAs indicated that the forms of almost all of the participants needed clarification and completion.

4. Interestingly, a trend was evident in that the group who received prompted recall accrued approximately 2,000 more steps per day than the unprompted group. This may have clinical importance, because 2,000 steps per day has been offered as a public health recommendation to help prevent weight gain (Hill, Wyatt, Reed, & Peters, 2003). Indeed, some participants in the current study commented that the pager prompt made them think more consciously about their physical activity.

5. Post hoc power analysis using .5 effect size (n = 25) with a $p < 0.05$ indicates a power of .41.

References

Bradburn, N. M., Rips, L. J., & Shevell, S. K. (1987). Answering autobiographical questions: the impact of memory and inference on surveys. *Science, 236*(4798), 157–161.

Bray, G. A., & Gray, D. S. (1988). Obesity. Part I—Pathogenesis. *Western Journal of Medicine, 149*(4), 429–441.

Broderick, J. E., Schwartz, J. E., Shiffman, S., Hufford, M. R., & Stone, A. A. (2003). Signaling does not adequately improve diary compliance. *Annals of Behavioral Medicine, 26*(2), 139, 148.

Crespo, C. J., Smit, E., Carter-Pokras, O., & Andersen, R. (2001). Acculturation and leisure-time physical inactivity in Mexican American adults: Results from NHANES III, 1988-1994. *American Journal of Public Health, 91*(8), 1254–1257.

Cuellar, I., Arnold, B., & Maldonado, R. (1995). Acculturation Rating Scale for Mexican Americans-II: A revision of the original ARSMA Scale. *Hispanic Journal of Behavioral Sciences, 17*(3), 275–304.

Duncan, G. E., Sydeman, S. J., Perri, M. G., Limacher, M. C., & Martin, A. D. (2001). Can sedentary adults accurately recall the intensity of their physical activity? *Preventive Medicine, 33*(1), 18–26.

Elder, J.P., Ayala, G.X., Campbell, N.R., Slymen, D., Lopez-Madurga, E.T., Engelberg, M. & Baquero, B. (2005). Interpersonal and print nutrition communication for a Spanish dominant Latino population. *Health Psychology*, 24(1), 49–57.

Garrow, J. S., & Webster, J. (1985). Quetelet's index (W/H2) as a measure of fatness. *International Journal of Obesity, 9*(2), 147–153.

Hayes, S. C., Nelson, R. O., & Jarrett, R. B. (1987). The treatment utility of assessment: A functional approach to evaluating assessment quality. *American Psychologist, 42*(11), 963–974.

Hill, J. O., Wyatt, H. R., Reed, G. W., & Peters, J. G. (2003). Obesity and the environment: Understanding where we go from here. *Science, 299*, 853–855.

Kazdin, A. E. (1981). Behavioral observation. In M. Hersen & A. S. Blerack (Eds.), *Behavioral assessment: A practical handbook* (2nd edition). New York: Kragrmin Press.

King, A. C., Castro, C., Wilcox, S., Eyler, A. A., Sallis, J. F., & Brownson, R. C. (2000). Personal and environmental factors associated with physical inactivity among different racial-ethnic groups of U.S. middle-aged and older-aged women. *Health Psychology, 19*(4), 354–364.

Kriska, A. (2000). Ethnic and cultural issues in assessing physical activity. *Research Quarterly for Exercise and Sport, 71*(2 Suppl), S47–53.

Manson, J. E., Colditz, G. A., Stampfer, M. J., Willett, W. C., Rosner, B., Monson, R. R., Speizer, F. E., & Hennekens, C. H. (1990). A prospective study of obesity and risk of coronary heart disease in women. *New England Journal of Medicine, 322*(13), 882–889.

Marin, G., & Triandis, H. C. (1985). Allocentrism as an important characteristic of the behavior of Latin Americans and Hispanics. In R. Diaz-Guerro (Ed.), *Cross-cultural and national studies.* Amsterdam: Elsevier.

McKenzie, T. L. (2002). Use of direct observation to assess physical activity. In G. J. Welk (Ed.), *Physical activity assessments for health-related research* (pp. 179, 195). Champaign, IL: Human Kinetics.

McKenzie, T. L., Marshall, S. J., Sallis, J. F., & Conway, T. L. (2000). Student activity levels, lesson context, and teacher behavior during middle school physical education. *Research Quarterly for Exercise and Sport, 71*(3), 249–259.

McKenzie, T. L., Sallis, J. F., & Nader, P. R. (1991). SOFIT: System for observing fitness instruction time. *Journal of Teaching in Physical Education, 11*, 195, 205.

Montoye, H. J., Kemple, H. C. G., Saris, W. H. M., & Washburn, R. A. (1996). *Measuring physical activity and energy expenditure.* Champaign, IL: Human Kinetics.

Nelson, R. O. (1983). Behavioral assessment: Past, present, and future. *Behavioral Assessment, 5,* 195, 206.

Rockhill, B., Willett, W. C., Manson, J. E., Leitzmann, M. F., Stampfer, M. J., Hunter, D. J., & Colditz, G. A. (2001). Physical activity and mortality: A prospective study among women. *American Journal of Public Health, 91*(4), 578–583.

Sallis, J. F., Buono, M. J., Roby, J. J., Micale, F. G., & Nelson, J. A. (1993). Seven-day recall and other physical activity self-reports in children and adolescents. *Medicine and Science in Sports and Exercise, 25*(1), 99–108.

Sallis, J. F., & Saelens, B. E. (2000). Assessment of physical activity by self-report: Status, limitations, and future directions. [erratum appears in *Res Q Exerc Sport* 2000 Dec; 71(4):409]. *Research Quarterly for Exercise and Sport, 71*(2 Suppl), S1–14.

Sallis, J. F., Strikmiller, P. K., Harsha, D. W., Feldman, H. A., Ehlinger, S., Williston, J., Woods, S., & Stone, E. J. (1996). Validation of interviewer- and self-administered physical activity checklists for fifth grade students. *Medicine and Science in Sports and Exercise, 28*(7), 840–851.

Schneider, P. L., Crouter, S. E., & Bassett, D. R. (2004). Pedometer measures of free-living physical activity: Comparison of 13 models. *Medicine and Science in Sports and Exercise, 36*(2), 331–335.

Simopoulos, A. P. (1985). The health implications of overweight and obesity. *Nutrition Reviews, 43*(2), 33–40.

Sternfeld, B., Ainsworth, B. E., & Quesenberry, C. P. (1999). Physical activity patterns in a diverse population of women. *Preventive Medicine, 28*(3), 313–323.

Stone, A. A., & Shiffman, S. (2002). Capturing momentary, self-report data: A proposal for reporting guidelines. *Annals of Behavioral Medicine, 24*(3), 236–243.

Stone, E. J., McKenzie, T. L., Welk, G. J., & Booth, M. L. (1998). Effects of physical activity interventions in youth. Review and synthesis. *American Journal of Preventive Medicine, 15*(4), 298–315.

Sulzer-Azaroff, B., & Mayer, G. (1991). *Behavior analysis for lasting change.* Fort Worth, TX: Harcourt Brace College Publisher.

Taylor, C. B., Coffey, T., Berra, K., Iaffaldano, R., Casey, K., & Haskell, W. L. (1984). Seven-day activity and self-report compared to a direct measure of physical activity. *American Journal of Epidemiology, 120*(6), 818–824.

Trost, S. G., Pate, R. R., Dowda, M., Ward, D. S., Felton, G., & Saunders, R. (2002). Psychosocial correlates of physical activity in white and African-American girls. *Journal of Adolescent Health, 31*(3), 226–233.

Tudor-Locke, C., Williams, J. E., Reis, J. P., & Pluto, D. (2002). Utility of pedometers for assessing physical activity: Convergent validity. *Sports Medicine, 32*(12), 795–808.

Weston, A. T., Petosa, R., & Pate, R. R. (1997). Validation of an instrument for measurement of physical activity in youth. *Medicine and Science in Sports and Exercise, 29*(1), 138–143.

Wheeler, L., & Reis, H. T. (1991). Self-recording of events in everyday life: Origins, types, and uses. *Journal of Personality, 59*(3), 339, 354.

8

Dietary Assessment and Monitoring in Real Time

Karen Glanz and Suzanne Murphy

Nutrition plays an important role in the risk of chronic diseases that are major causes of illness and death in America today. Good nutrition, often in combination with physical activity and maintenance of a healthy weight, can help prevent heart disease, stroke, hypertension, diabetes, and some types of cancer (DHHS, 1998; Norris, Harnack, Carmichael, et al., 1997; World Cancer Research Fund, 1997). About half of all U.S. adults are overweight (DHHS, 1998), and the mean percentage of daily total food intake from dietary fat is at 34 percent, well above the health recommendations of 30 percent energy from fat (Norris et al., 1997). Consumption of fruits and vegetables is essential to healthy nutrition and weight; it can help control weight and may also lead to eating fewer high-fat foods (USDA/DHHS, 2000). However, many people do not consume enough fruits and vegetables (Norris et al., 1997; World Cancer Research Fund, 1997), and there is a great public health need for prevention strategies to promote healthy nutrition among Americans.

Nutrition education and promotion have the potential to encourage people to eat more healthfully. The most successful nutrition promotion strategies are rooted in theory and research. They should also be systematically evaluated so that the most efficacious approaches can be widely adopted and sustained. Research on nutrition behavior depends on accurate, reliable, and unbiased assessment of what people eat, and clinical interventions also depend on accurate monitoring information.

Dietary behavior that contributes to increasing (or decreasing) the risk of chronic disease is habitual and practiced over time. It is also most often measured by asking study participants what they have eaten (i.e., by self-report). The potential of collecting dietary data in real time to improve dietary assessment and monitoring is an exciting development that is increasingly possible with new information technologies.

This chapter describes the rationale for considering a momentary, or real-time, approach to dietary data collection; reviews a range of nutrition assessment methodologies that provide a foundation for real-time data collection; and describes a pilot study that involved developing, implementing, and evaluating a hand-held computer-based system for diet self-monitoring in the Women's Health Initiative (WHI) Diet Modification Trial.

Rationale for a Momentary Approach to Data Collection

There are many challenges to collecting accurate and detailed self-reports of dietary behaviors. For dietary intake, issues include the following:

- Accuracy of recall
- Timeliness of recording
- Time sampling frame—most health risks/effects/associations are based on long-term dietary intake, not a single day
- Subject sampling frame—for population estimates of dietary intake, 1-day measures can be aggregated to get a good group assessment (but not an individual one); for individual assessment, a series of days over time can be used. Thus, nutrition data may or may not be easily interpreted for individuals, groups, or defined populations, depending on the purpose of the study (e.g., epidemiology, intervention, clinical).
- Portion size information/estimation
- Knowledge of the components of mixed dishes and prepared foods
- Possible systematic under- or overreporting (including the often-cited underreporting by overweight persons)

In the dietary change arena, as distinct from research that merely describes people's eating behaviors/patterns, there are good reasons to consider a momentary approach to data collection. In these situations, however, real-time data collection is not simply for the purpose of measurement. Self-monitoring has long been found to be associated with better adherence (Glanz, 1985), though we cannot separate cause and effect or the possible driving role of a third factor (i.e., motivation to comply). Self-monitoring is often cumbersome and time-consuming, so making it easier and more convenient might increase compliance with recording. Finally, feedback can improve adherence (Brug, Campbell, & van Assema, 1999; Brug, Glanz, van Assema, et al., 1998; DeVries & Brug, 1999; Skinner, Campbell, Rimer, et al., 1999), and real-time feedback and more accurate feedback seem likely to be most useful. Further, and importantly, in nutrition assessment, some commonly available data collection approaches may be considered (or strive to be) real-time or "momentary."

The focus of this chapter is primarily on momentary self-report information—with some limited coverage of momentary studies that do not rely on self-report—observations, other sources of data, unobtrusive assessments (e.g., cameras), and so forth.

Dietary Assessment Methods: Real-Time, Over Time, and Emerging Technologies

To understand why a real-time, or momentary, approach to collecting dietary data has important potential in health and health behavior research, it is useful to examine a range of traditional diet assessment methods; the extent to which they do (or do not) assess eating behavior in real time; and the advantages and limitations of various approaches. These methods are summarized in Table 8-1.

It is possible to record dietary intakes in real time using traditional self-reported assessment methods, although some methods lend themselves to real-time recording more than others. Food frequency questionnaires (FFQs) cannot be considered real-time assessment methods, as they collect summary information on intakes across time. A typical frame of reference is the past month or past year, and a respondent reports the frequency of consumption of a list of foods during the time period of interest. Thus, the consumer must remember both the types of foods and the average amounts of these foods that were eaten during the reference period. Although FFQs theoretically offer many advantages in measuring usual intakes across time, the errors incurred are often large (Subar, Kipnis, Troiano, et al., 2003). Dietary histories, like FFQs, are used to measure usual intakes over several days or months and thus cannot be considered real-time assessment methods. Dietary history methods usually include a FFQ as well as information about typical intakes at meals. As with FFQ's, there is ample opportunity for reporting errors (Thompson, Byers, & Kohlmeier, 1994).

Dietary recalls are typically used to collect information, either by self-report or by an interviewer, about foods consumed during the previous 24-hour period. Thus, the recall method captures intakes close to the time the foods were consumed, although not truly in real time.

Diet diaries and records, if used correctly, are a true real-time method of recording intakes. The consumer writes down (or enters into a computer) all foods consumed as they are consumed. Portion sizes can be estimated, measured using measuring cups, spoons, and so forth, or weighed using a scale. Because theoretically no foods are left out of the data collection, diet diaries should be a more accurate reflection of true intake during a given time period. Unfortunately, consumers often do not record their intakes in a true real-time mode, but wait until the end of the day to write down what they have eaten. If this occurs, diaries can sometimes resemble recalls more than actual records of intake collected at the time of consumption. Because diaries are collected in real time, they are the only assessment method that offers the potential to provide feedback that could influence the types and amounts of food chosen during the rest of the day.

Technology-Assisted Approaches

Technology can assist in collecting real-time reports of food consumption. Several tools have been developed as alternatives to the traditional paper-and-pencil methods of recording intakes. Because these tools simplify the task for

Table 8-1. Dietary assessment methods: Relevance to real-time measures, advantages, and limitations

Method	Key features	Advantages and limitations
Food frequency questionnaire (FFQ)	Collects summary dietary information over past month or year Not a real-time assessment method	*Advantage*: Evaluate average intake over time *Limitation*: Consumer must remember types and amounts of foods; measurement error
Dietary history	Usually includes FFQ plus questions about typical intakes at meals Not a real-time assessment method	*Advantage*: More depth than an FFQ alone *Limitation*: Reporting errors common
Dietary recall	Collects detailed data about foods consumed, usually past 24 hours Captures intakes close to the time of eating, though not not truly in real time	*Advantage*: Better recall, time close to behaviour *Limitation*: Expensive to code and analyze data
Diet diaries and records	Person records (write/computer) all foods eaten, as they are consumed When used as intended, a true real-time method of recording food intake	*Advantage*: Can include all food, portion sizes *Limitation*: Consumers often wait until the end of the day to write down what they ate
Tape recordings	Person carries small tape recorder and voice records all foods consumed Real-time method if used as directed	*Advantage*: Simplifies respondent burden *Limitation*: Need to retrieve tapes and convert them into food lists and amounts
Desktop or laptop computers	User enters information on foods eaten, ideally at the time of consumption If user eats when not near the computer, food not captured in real-time	*Advantage*: Can automate data analysis, potential prompting for completeness/detail *Limitation*: Hard to carry computer throughout the day
Hand-held computer or personal digital assistant (PDA)	Portable device used to record foods eaten at the time of consumption Ideal technology for capturing real time dietary choices	*Advantage*: Portable, automated, potential for prompting and recording time of entry *Limitation*: Screen size may be small, requires manual dexterity, database size may be limited
Observational methods—video, photography, direct observation	User or observer records food types and amounts on camera, video, or recording sheet Real-time data (but not self-report)	*Advantage*: Verifiable, can be reviewed later; may supplement other self-report method(s) *Limitation*: May provide incomplete information on food type/preparation; may be limited to aggregate assessment in some settings; could be reactive and may invade privacy

the consumer, there is likely to be greater compliance with the protocols. Tape recordings were one of the earliest tools to be used to assist consumers in keeping track of their intakes (see, for example, Todd, Hudes, & Calloway, 1983). The consumer carries a small tape recorder throughout the day, and records voice messages describing all foods consumed. The tapes are returned to the project staff at the end of the recording period. It is then necessary for a member of the staff to retrieve these messages and convert them to a list of foods and portion sizes.

A more modern alternative is to ask consumers to record their intakes on either a desktop or a laptop computer. Numerous interactive dietary data entry programs (e.g., the Interactive Healthy Eating Index from the Center for Nutrition Policy and Promotion (CNPP) [2004]) may be used for this purpose. The use of computers has many advantages as well, particularly if the data entry software is user-friendly. One innovative method combines an electronic food balance and bar code reader with a portable computer to more accurately capture portion sizes (Kretsch & Fong, 1990). However, use of computers for real-time collection has an obvious disadvantage because they are difficult to carry throughout the day. Thus, food consumed away from home or office may not be captured in real time but instead entered into the computer at a later time.

Hand-Held Computers or Personal Digital Assistants (PDAs)

PDAs provide the ideal technology for capturing real-time dietary choices. As capacity increases and costs decrease, they can provide essentially all of the advantages of larger computers but are lightweight enough to be carried by the consumer in much the same way as a tape recorder. Although screen size and quality may be limiting for some applications, these features are steadily improving as well.

Observational Methods

The most accurate method of recording dietary data in real time is through direct observation of food choices and the amounts consumed. Although this is usually expensive in terms of staff time required, the results can be considered a true gold standard measure of intake. However, to truly reflect usual intake, the observers must be unobtrusive so that consumers do not change their dietary choices. Because of the staff and equipment required, direct observation is often used for only a portion of the day—usually at congregate meal sites such as school and worksite cafeterias.

Video or photographic records can be used to capture both food choices and amounts consumed. One recently reported study used a PDA with a camera and mobile telephone card, and 20 college students took photos and recorded their food intake at the same time. The diet record and camera/PDA method yielded comparable data regarding dietary intake (Wang, Kogashiwa, Ohta, & Kira, 2002).

Direct observation of cafeteria lines and other central food service facilities by research project staff has been used successfully to record foods selected and to allow calculation of food consumption by subtracting leftovers remaining at the end of the meal (see, for example, Eck, Klesges, & Hanson, 1989; Shatenstein, Claveau, & Ferland, 2002). With the advent of itemized receipts, it is possible to simply collect the cafeteria or restaurant receipts for the consumers being tracked. The use of electronic itemized receipts from grocery stores can yield a real-time measure of food purchases, though it may be difficult to determine when, by whom, and how much of the food bought is consumed from these sources.

Real-Time Dietary Assessment with Feedback on Diet Quality

A unique opportunity for health behavior change that flows from real-time dietary assessment is real-time feedback on the quality of the diet at a given point in time. Feedback might evaluate intakes over the past meal, the past day, or some other time such as the past week or month. This type of evaluation is both feasible and practical using information technology tools such as PDAs.

Feedback to the consumer/user can take many forms. The most common are evaluations of nutrient adequacy and of compliance with recommendations such as the Dietary Guidelines (USDA/USDHHS, 2000) or Dietary Reference Intakes (DRIs) published by the Institute of Medicine (2000). Comparisons of nutrient intake to recommendations are possible using food composition tables based on the Standard Reference Database developed by the U.S. Department of Agriculture (Nutrient Data Laboratory, 2004).

Other options include evaluating food intake by comparing the number of servings of foods to the Food Guide Pyramid recommendations (USDA, 1992). Composite indexes of dietary quality can also be useful in tracking food intakes; one such index is the Healthy Eating Index (HEI) developed by the USDA (CNPP, 1998). An extensive set of consumer-friendly evaluation tools is included at the website for the Interactive Healthy Eating Index (CNPP, 2004).

Method and Context

A pilot study of momentary diet assessment and dietary adherence improvement was conducted in cooperation with Women's Health Hawaii, the Hawaii clinical site of the Women's Health Initiative (WHI). The aims of the pilot study were to (a) assess the feasibility of collecting real-time dietary data with a PDA and (b) to evaluate the use of real-time feedback for increasing the women's diet self-monitoring, reducing the burden and inconvenience of monitoring food intake, and increasing adherence to WHI dietary goals.

The federally funded WHI is designed to test whether long-term preventive measures will decrease the incidence of certain cancers, cardiovascular disease, and fractures (Roussow, Finnegan, Harlan, et al., 1995). It is the largest multicenter trial to date of dietary means for prevention, with more than 40,000 women in the Diet Modification Trial within WHI. In the Diet Modification Intervention arm of the trial, participants are taught and advised to follow a diet for up to 10 years that is low in fat and high in fruits, vegetables, and grains. Adherence is a critical concern in WHI: *"If we do not achieve reasonable adherence and high retention, we cannot test the intervention and we will have wasted millions of dollars, our time, and the participants' time, and have no unequivocal answers for women about these critical health issues"* (WHI, 1998). For this reason, it is important to continually try to identify new and potentially efficacious adherence-improving strategies as well as improved monitoring techniques. Therefore, we conducted a pilot study to evaluate the feasibility, acceptability, and short-term impact of a real-time diet monitoring and tailored feedback system on self-monitoring and adherence to WHI diet goals among the WHI participants.

Sample

Eligible participants were women in the Diet Modification Intervention arm of the trial who had completed their first year of group dietary change sessions. They were recruited by mail invitations. For the pilot study, efforts were made to secure at least one volunteer per WHI education group. The pilot study goal was 36 subjects in three cohorts. About half of the participants were expected to be women with access to a home computer and modem to allow for testing the system under different conditions.

Momentary Data Collection

The pilot study began with formative research to determine the features of computerized dietary monitoring and tailored feedback that would be acceptable, interesting, and motivating to WHI Diet Modification participants. This was accomplished by conducting focus groups with 29 women from the WHI Diet Modification group. We used input from the focus groups and consultation with study nutritionists to develop the diet monitoring method using hand-held computer technology. The platform for the diet monitoring system was a Palm Pilot V hand-held computer, custom-programmed using Puma Satellite Form and Pendragon software. These applications allow for storage of data in relational database tables, interface between the palmtop computer and a centralized database, and interactive feedback loops. Participants were not required to have access to a desktop computer to use the system.

Table 8-2 summarizes design issues and how they were addressed in this study, using the guidelines proposed by Stone and Shiffman (2002).

The system was initialized with personal data about participants, included a time-date stamp, and had cumulative memory for up to 1 week. The food list was taken from existing WHI food booklets (e.g., the Fat Scan food reference guide) and included local (Hawaii) foods, customized foods, and favorite recipes. Three components of each food item were entered into the foods database on the PDA: grams of fat, servings of fruits and vegetables, and servings of grains per serving of the food. These values were obtained from WHI food booklets and from the Cancer Research Center of Hawaii's food composition database.

Table 8-2. Summary of how design issues were addressed in WHI real-time diet assessment and feedback pilot study

Design issue	How issue was addressed
Sampling	**Rationale:** collect data on all foods consumed depending on participants' willingness to record foods **Sampling density and schedule:** event-based sampling encouraged, ≥ 3 days/week **Implications for bias and validity:** event-based sampling maximizes accuracy of recall of foods. Completeness of data depends on whether recording occurs. Awarness increased by recording might influence eating behavior.
Monetary procedures	**Prompting and recording methods:** records were entered into PDA/Palm Pilot. Event-based sampling, so only self-prompting was used. **Description and definition of participant-initiated event entries:** any eating occasion; entries were foods, including preparation information (as applicable) and portion sizes **How nonresponse was handled:** as a feasibility study, the aim was simply to observe response **Were response-delaying procedures available?** Yes, it was possible to enter a food later but only on the same day before midnight **Definition of immediate and timely response:** food entries throughout the day rather than all entries in the evening
Data acquisition interface	**Description of physical characteristics of diary or palmtop computer:** Palm Pilot V hand-held computer; charger base and modem also provided **Mode of item presentation:** drop-down menus using main categories of foods based on food guide booklets already in use for WHI **Important algorithm features:** fat grams, fruit/vegetables servings, grain servings; based in personal fat goals. Custom foods/meals could be added **Text of items and response options and how they were derived or modified:** (1) food, (2) preparation, (3) serving size and number of servings, based on WHI food lists plus individuals' custom recipes or food combinations

158

Compliance	**Rationale for compliance decisions:** for recording, based on feasibility in consultation with study nutritionist; for diet intake, comparison to WHI/individual goals for fat, fruit and vegetable, and grain serving intake
	Presentation of systematic compliance rates: evaluated based on data downloaded from PDAs, at the end of individuals' study periods
	Demonstration that compliance was accurately and objectively assessed: time-date stamp in the PDA revealed when data entries were made
Participant training and monitoring	**Description of training procedures:** orientation, demonstration, instruction manual, and completion of a sample assessment with study coordinator's help
	Use of run-in or training periods: orientation completed only when participant demonstrated adequate mastery of the PDA-based recording system
	Procedures to enhance compliance: telephone and e-mail helplines available for troubleshooting and questions; weekly telephone reminder to submit data via modem
Data management procedures	**Data management decisions that affects data analyses:** preprogrammed PDAs to download to an Excel spreadsheet, which could be imported into SAS for analysis
	Define missing data criteria and actions: as a feasibility/exploratory study, missing data provided important information
Data analysis	**Rationale for aggregated or disaggregated approach:** both approaches were used to "mine" the data for maximum possible interpretation
	Clearly specified model used in analysis: described in narrative (see text)
	Details of procedures: described in narrative (see text); supplemented PDA data with surveys and qualitative debriefing information from participants

159

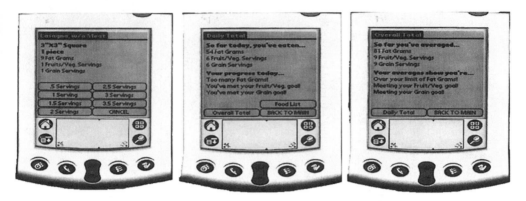

Figure 8-1. Sample PDA screens. (Reprinted with permission of the *American Journal of Health Promotion.*)

The touch-screens used a drop-down menu format with foods grouped as they were in the WHI food reference guides. Users would enter their food choices as well as the number of servings, with the screen providing information about portion sizes. Additional features included the option of creating "custom foods" or meals that were often consumed by individual women. Recipe analysis by study nutritionists was used to determine nutritional values of favorite recipes submitted by the participants.

Women used the system to record and monitor their food intake throughout the day, using an event-based sampling scheme. They received immediate on-screen feedback giving current progress toward attainment of their goals (Figure 8-1) and transmitted the accumulated data once a week via telephone modem. A 1-week interval for submitting data was used because of the electronic program's capacity, the practical feasibility of requesting weekly data transmission, and the WHI Diet Modification Program guidelines to achieve weekly dietary goals. Mailed feedback each week provided motivational messages to assist the women in reaching their daily and weekly dietary goals for fat, fruits and vegetables, and grain servings. Two feedback formats were used for maximum usefulness (Figure 8-2).

Procedures

RECRUITMENT AND ORIENTATION

Thirty-six women were recruited for the pilot test, in three 1-month cohorts of 12 participants each. To participate in the pilot test, women were asked for a 1-month commitment to use the system at least 3 days per week. At an enrollment visit, each woman received an orientation including an instruction manual, watched a demonstration of the PDA diet monitoring system, and completed a sample assessment with the study coordinator's help.

Palm Pilot Project

Dear Diane,

Thank you so much for participating in our Pilot study using the Palm Pilot. This report is generated from the data you entered on the Palm Pilot and sent to us over the telephone lines for the week of November 12 to November 18. Any data sent to us that is incomplete for a specific day will not be included in this report.

Your average dietary intake per day for this period was:

		Goals
Fat Grams	22.5	25
Fruit/Vegetable	6.6	5
Grain Servings	7.9	6

Your cumulative dietary intake was:

		Goals
Fat Grams	24.0	25
Fruit/Vegetable	7.3	5
Grain Servings	7.0	6

Summary

Fat Grams

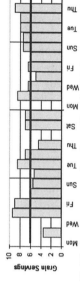

Yea!! Over the past month, you have met your fat gram goal each period. You have done an excellent job meeting your goal.

Fruit and Vegetable Servings

Hurray!! Each week you were over your vegetable/fruit servings goal. Fabulous!

Grain Servings

Wow!! You have been over your grain servings goal for each period. Over the past month you have done an outstanding job. Keep it up!

Figure 8-2. Sample feedback letters: preintervention (left) and postintervention (right). (Reprinted with permission of the *American Journal of Health Promotion*.)

SAMPLE CHARACTERISTICS

Thirty-six women enrolled in the pilot study. They ranged in age from 54 to 82 years old, with a mean of 64.4 years ($\pm$ 7.6), and were 50 percent Asian or Pacific Islander and 50 percent White. A portion of 81.8 percent had been in the WHI study for 3 years or more. Only 30.3 percent reported "a fair amount" or "a lot" of experience with computers at baseline, and 23.2 percent said they were uncomfortable with computers at baseline. Three participants did not complete the study because of personal or family illness.

INTERVENTION AND DATA TRANSMISSION PROCEDURES

After becoming familiar with the system, the participants received ongoing, daily, and weekly on-screen feedback. Telephone and e-mail helplines were available for troubleshooting and questions. The women submitted weekly data by telephone modem or by e-mail (if they had a desktop computer) and received weekly feedback by mail.

DATA COLLECTION

The results of each woman's use of the system and her food choices, as submitted by modem each week, were recorded on a relational database, using an Excel spreadsheet that showed the day and time of recording, food choices, portion sizes, and nutrient values. Participants also completed a WHI food frequency questionnaire (FFQ) (Patterson, Kristal, Carter, et al., 1999) before and after the pilot study period, to see whether their adherence, as measured independently by an FFQ, had changed. The time frame for the follow-up FFQ was modified from 3 months to 1 month to match the study period.

Participants completed a short baseline survey before the orientation and an end-of-study survey when they returned their PDAs. A debriefing session was held for each group, and an end-of-study party was held to thank those who completed the study. All women who completed the pilot study were part of a lottery to win one of two Palm Pilots with the monitoring system, as well as other door prizes.

STATISTICAL METHODS

The study sample included 36 women at baseline and 33 women at follow-up. For the main analyses, we included only the 33 respondents who completed the entire 1-month study period and usable surveys at both baseline and follow-up.

The FFQs were analyzed at the WHI Coordinating Center (Patterson et al., 1999). Statistical analysis was completed using SAS statistical software. Several summary variables were created from weekly PDA-entered data submitted by the participants, including the number of days foods were recorded; timing of food entry; attainment of dietary goals for fat, fruit and vegetables, and grain servings; and changes across the 4 study weeks. Paired t-tests were used to compare baseline and end-of-month dietary intakes based on the FFQs. Descriptive statistics were used to analyze the baseline and end-of-study interviews.

Results

As reported in the previous section, the aims of the pilot study were to evaluate the feasibility, acceptability, and short-term impact of a real-time diet monitoring and tailored feedback system on self-monitoring and adherence to WHI diet goals. Here we report the findings for each of these aims.

Feasibility, Acceptability, and Self-Reported Adherence to Self-Monitoring

Baseline and end-of-study surveys provided data regarding the use of the PDA for real-time dietary self-monitoring. The survey responses supported the feasibility and acceptability of the PDA-based method for diet assessment. The women's attitudes toward monitoring their food intake improved across the period of study. At baseline, 61.3 percent considered recording their food intake to be a burden, but only 13 percent reported this view at follow-up. The proportion who rated recording their foods as very easy nearly doubled during the study period, from 31.0 percent to 60.6 percent, and ratings of convenience more than tripled, from 20.7 percent to 76.6 percent. On the follow-up survey, 63 percent reported that they used food recording to help meet their dietary goals often, usually, or always. More than 90 percent of the participants said they would continue to use the Palm Pilot over the long term if they had one.

In debriefing interviews, women who participated in the pilot study expanded on their survey responses and offered comments and suggestions for the future use of similar innovations. Most importantly, they reported on how easy, convenient, informative, and reinforcing the PDA was for diet self-monitoring and adherence. The calculation of running daily and weekly totals was an often-mentioned popular feature. They suggested adding more foods to the database, having most-often-consumed foods come up first on the screens, and including more "local" Hawaii foods.

Participant self-reports of adherence and self-monitoring before and after the pilot study period indicated significant increases in both monitoring and adherence. At followup, two thirds of the women said they recorded their food either 3 or 4 days per week (45.5%) or at least 5 days per week (21.2%). This level of monitoring was a substantial increase from baseline monitoring, when a large majority of the women (78.1%) said they usually recorded their food intake less than once a week. Few of the women (18.2%) said they recorded their food when they ate it prior to the beginning of the study, but this increased to 54.6 percent at followup ($p < 0.001$). In addition, only 39.4 percent of participants rated their adherence to the dietary plan as high or very high ("4" or "5" on a scale of 1 to 5) at baseline, while 65.6 percent reported high levels of adherence at followup ($p < 0.001$).

MOMENTARY DATA CAPTURE: FREQUENCY OF MONITORING AND GOAL ATTAINMENT

Weekly food record data, based on momentary data captured on the PDAs, were obtained from the transmissions sent by modem to the study center. Across all weeks and participants, food choices were entered on an average of 5.0 days per week. Approximately half of the women entered their food data 6 or 7 days per week. There were no trends of increasing or decreasing food entry across the month of participation and no significant differences between the three 1-month cohorts of women. Analysis of the time-date stamps on submitted food data revealed that on 62 percent of all days, foods were entered at least three distinct times each day (at least 2 hours between entries).

Daily dietary goals for fat and fruit and vegetable intake were met on about 60 percent of days, and grain intake goals were met on 40 percent of the days. Average weekly goals were met most often for fat intake (55 to 68 percent of the time), followed by fruit and vegetable consumption goals (48 to 59 percent), and grain intake goals (24 to 32 percent). The only change in weekly goal attainment was an increase in meeting grain serving goals in the last 2 weeks of the month.

ADHERENCE TO DIETARY GOALS

As described in the procedures section above, we used FFQs to evaluate change in adherence to dietary goals before and after the real-time data collection system (i.e., self-monitoring) was in place. Comparisons of baseline and follow-up FFQ data showed a significant decrease in total daily fat grams (42.2 to 36.3, $p < 0.05$) and percent energy from fat (25.7 to 23.7 percent, $p < 0.05$), and a trend toward lower mean caloric intake (1,477 to 1,359 kcal; $p < 0.10$). There were no significant changes in daily fruit and vegetable consumption (5.5 to 5.4 servings), daily grain intake (5.1 to 4.9 servings), dietary fiber intake (20.4 to 19.1 g), or fiber density (13.8 to 14.1 g/1,000 kcal).

Discussion

The aims of this pilot study were achieved, with positive findings. The participants found the system easy, convenient, informative, and reinforcing and significantly increased the frequency of their self-monitoring. The women were also able to reduce their total daily fat intake, energy intake, and energy from fat, as shown by the follow-up FFQ results. Despite the possibility that using repeated FFQs just 1 month apart might be insensitive to change, the FFQ findings were consistent with more frequent attainment of dietary fat goals revealed by the PDA data received from the participants. Thus, using this conservative measure, the PDA system for self-monitoring and feedback appears to have helped participants to achieve better adherence to several key dietary goals.

The fact that there were no significant reported changes in fruit, vegetable, and grain consumption from the FFQ data may be because most people can easily identify what constitutes a fruit, vegetable, or grain serving, whereas identifying the fat content of different foods and sources of fat is more challenging. This finding is also consistent with previous experimental research on tailored communications where fat intake was reduced but little or no change in fruit and vegetable intake was found (Brug et al., 1998).

Insights Gained from a Real-Time Approach

Our experience and findings support the utility of momentary assessment methods for dietary assessment. The real-time approach was well received and was useful for self-monitoring, for reporting to the research center, and for increasing adherence to dietary goals. The portability of the PDA-based system was shown to be important for real-time recording of food consumption. This study also confirmed the feasibility of using real-time diet assessment and feedback among adults who had limited computer experience, without requiring them to own a desktop or laptop computer. We determined that we could use the Ecological Momentary Assessment (EMA) methods in a study with older women, and that it was preferred to a pencil-and-paper approach to recording food intake.

Successes and Challenges

To our knowledge, this is the first report of behavioral results using a PDA-based dietary monitoring and feedback intervention. While there are several commercially available portable diet self-monitoring tools, there are no professional or scientific reports about how they are designed, how they are used, or whether they are accurate or efficacious.

Strengths of the pilot study include the high rate of compliance with study procedures; the availability of objectively provided "real-time" food intake data in addition to food habits information; the ease of data transmission for use in central monitoring and evaluation of dietary compliance; and the potential for both hand-held and central feedback. The system we developed had an easily adaptable database and almost limitless potential for individual tailoring of feedback. We added some "local" ethnic foods to the database, and the participants expressed a desire for even more of these foods; such additions to the PDA database could be made with relative ease. Despite the upfront cost of hardware and systems design, this is likely to be more cost-effective and practical than other intensive interpersonal or counseling adherence-improving programs. It takes advantage of the increasing computer literacy of the population, and yet the pilot demonstrates that the benefits are not limited to those who are already computer literate.

Limitations of the study include its short time frame, small sample size, and pre/post test design without a control group. Another limitation is the use of volunteer participants; however, this pilot study was greatly over-subscribed and could not accommodate as many women as were interested in participating.

Prospects for Application of Real-Time Data Collection (EMA) Methods

Preventive dietary practices offer the potential to help reduce morbidity and mortality from a number of chronic diseases. However, our ability to achieve lasting long-term dietary changes is limited and rarely attained outside of research settings. New methods for aiding individuals to make such changes, and for evaluating the impacts, are needed.

The hand-held computer-based system described in this chapter offers the potential for improving scientists' ability to monitor the success of dietary interventions and provides a tool that individuals can use to enhance their ability to make and maintain long-term dietary changes. This innovative method combines the features of storing real-time dietary data and providing more immediate feedback on diet than is possible using paper-based home monitoring systems.

This method can also be used for planning food intake—the system used in this study had a "back" button for correcting entry errors, which could also be used if a planned meal seemed too high in fat, too low in fruits and vegetables, or the like. Such a system could also be used to collect real-time data without providing feedback, although compliance with recording food consumption might be lower than in our study, because there would be no feedback. PDA technology is readily accessible and was easy to use for the older women in the WHI, even those who do not regularly use computers.

Future research should examine the utility of PDAs to monitor dietary behavior without a feedback intervention and to test the impact of this PDA intervention on diet over longer periods, in large samples, in men, and among other age and ethnic groups. Strategies for diffusion of successful program models will also need to be developed. The findings reported here provide initial insight into the use of this potentially powerful new tool to improve dietary patterns and promote adherence to clinical trial protocols. This type of intervention, if feasible and efficacious over the longer term, can produce a significant improvement in healthful eating behaviors.

Note

Portions of this chapter appeared in Glanz, K., Murphy, S., Moylan, J., Evensen, D. & Curb, J. (2006). "Improving dietary self-monitoring and adherence with hand-held computers: A pilot study." *American Journal of Health Promotion, 20*: 165–170. Used with permission.

References

Brug, J., Campbell, M., & van Assema, P. (1999). The application and impact of computer-generated personalized nutrition education. *Patient Education and Counseling, 36*, 145–156.

Brug, J., Glanz, K., van Assema, P., Kok, G., & van Breukelen, G. (1998). The impact of computer-tailored feedback and iterative feedback on fat, fruit and vegetable intake. *Health Education and Behavior, 25*, 517–531.

Center for Nutrition Policy and Promotion, U.S. Department of Agriculture. (2004). *The Interactive Healthy Eating Index.* Accessed at www.usda.gov/cnpp on March 18, 2004.

Center for Nutrition Policy and Promotion, U.S. Department of Agriculture. (1998). *The Healthy Eating Index, 1994-96.* CNPP-5. CNPP, Washington, DC.

Department of Health and Human Services. (1998). National Health and Nutrition *Examination Survey (NHANES).* U.S. Centers for Disease Control and Prevention, and National Center for Health Statistics. Washington, DC: U.S. Government Printing Office.

De Vries, H., & Brug, J. (1999). Computer-tailored interventions motivating people to adopt health promoting behaviors. *Patient Education and Counseling, 36,* 99–105.

Eck, L. H., Klesges, R. C., & Hanson, C. L. (1989). Recall of a child's intake from one meal: are parents accurate? *Journal of the American Dietetic Association, 89,* 784–789.

Glanz, K. (1985). Nutrition education for risk factor reduction and patient education: A review. *Preventive Medicine, 14,* 721–752.

Institute of Medicine. (2000). *Dietary Reference Intakes, Applications in Dietary Assessment.* National Academy Press, Washington, DC.

Kretsch, M. J., & Fong, A. K. H. (1990). Validation of a new computerized technique for quantitating individual dietary intake: The Nutrition Evaluation Scale System (NESSy) vs. the weighed food record. *American Journal of Clinical Nutrition, 51,* 477–484.

Norris, J., Harnack, L., Carmichael, S., Pouan, T., Wakmoto, P., & Block, G. (1997). U.S. trends in nutrient intake: The 1987 and 1992 National Health Interview Surveys. *American Journal of Public Health, 87,* 740–746.

Nutrient Data Laboratory, U.S. Department of Agriculture. (2004). *USDA National Nutrient Database for Standard Reference, Release 16-1.* Accessed at www.nal.usda.gov/fnic/foodcomp on March 19, 2004.

Patterson, R. E., Kristal, A., Carter, R. A., Fels-Tinker, L., Bolton, M. P., & Agurs-Collins, T. (1999). Measurement characteristics of the Women's Health Initiative Food Frequency Questionnaire. *Annals of Epidemiology, 9,* 178–187.

Roussow, J. E., Finnegan, L. P., Harlan, W. R., Pinn, V. W., Clifford, C., & McGowan, J. A. (1995). The evolution of the Women's Health Initiative: Perspectives from the NIH. *Journal of the American Medical Women's Association, 50,* 50–55.

Shatenstein, B., Claveau, D., & Ferland, G. (2002). Visual observation is a valid means of assessing dietary consumption among older adults with cognitive deficits in long-term care settings. *Journal of the American Dietetic Association, 102,* 250–252.

Skinner, C. S., Campbell, M. K., Rimer, B. K., Curry, S., & Prochaska, J. O. (1999). How effective is tailored print communication? *Annals of Behavioral Medicine, 21,* 290–298.

Stone, A. A., & Shiffman, S. (2002). Capturing momentary, self-report data: A proposal for reporting guidelines. *Annals of Behavioral Medicine, 24,* 236–243.

Subar, A. F., Kipnis, V., Troiano, R. P., Midthune, D., Schoeller, D. A., Bingham, S., Sharbaugh, C. O., Trabulsi, J., Runswick, S., Ballard-Barbash, R., Sunshine, J., & Schatzkin, A. (2003). Using intake biomarkers to evaluate the extent of dietary misreporting in a large sample of adults: the OPEN study. *American Journal of Epidemiology, 158,* 1–13.

Todd, K. S., Hudes, M., & Calloway, D. H. (1983). Food intake measurement: Problems and approaches. *American Journal of Clinical Nutrition, 37,* 139–146.

Thompson, F. E., Byers, T., & Kohlmeier, L. (1994). Dietary Assessment Resource Manual. *Journal of Nutrition, 124,* 2245S–2317S.

U.S. Department of Agriculture, U.S. Department of Health and Human Services. (2000). *Nutrition and Your Health: Dietary Guidelines for Americans* (5th ed.). U.S. Government Printing Office, Washington, DC.

U.S. Department of Agriculture. (1992). *The Food Guide Pyramid.* Home and Garden Bulletin No. 252. USDA, Hyattsville, MD.

Wang, D. H., Kogashiwa, M., Ohta, S., & Kira, S. (2002). Validity and reliability of a dietary assessment method: The application of a digital camera with a mobile phone card attachment. *Journal of Nutrition Science and Vitaminology, 48,* 498–504.

Women's Health Initiative. (April 1998). WHI *Adherence and Retention Workshop Materials.*

World Cancer Research Fund, American Institute for Cancer Research. (1997). *Food, Nutrition and the Prevention of Cancer: A Global Perspective.* Washington, DC: American Institute for Cancer Research.

9

Real-Time Data Capture: Ecological Momentary Assessment of Behavioral Symptoms Associated with Eating Disorders

Karen Farchaus Stein and Pamela E. Paulson

The eating disorders of anorexia nervosa (AN) and bulimia nervosa (BN) are serious health problems that affect as many as 5 million American adolescent and young adult women each year and cause life-threatening physical complications and compromised states of emotional health. Although a number of approaches to treatment of the eating disorders have been developed, their effectiveness in producing long- and short-term recovery is alarmingly low (Keel & Mitchell, 1997; Walsh & Devlin, 1998). These disappointing outcomes have led to renewed calls for the development of new, theoretically based approaches to the treatment of eating disorders (Walsh & Devlin, 1998; Walsh & Kahn, 1997).

Our program of research focuses on the role of self-cognitions in the etiology of AN and BN and the development of an approach to intervention that focuses on self-cognitions as a means to promote recovery from these disorders. Currently, we are conducting a randomized clinical trial of cognitive-behavioral psychotherapy that focuses on self-cognitions as a means to promote recovery from eating disorders. It is within this clinical trial that Ecological Momentary Assessment (EMA) is being used to measure change in the eating disorder behavioral outcomes (Shiffman & Stone, 1998; Stone & Shiffman, 1994).

AN and BN are conceptualized as behavioral and psychological syndromes (American Psychiatric Association, 2000). BN is characterized by a behavioral pattern that consists of a binge eating episode followed by compensatory behaviors to lose weight or prevent weight gain. Compensatory behavior falls into one of two types: purging type, which includes self-induced vomiting or laxative or diuretic use to avoid weight gain, and nonpurging type, consisting of excessive exercise, food restricting, and fasting to control weight. The defining symptoms of AN focus on physical symptoms (e.g., body weight and menstrual status) and attitudes toward weight/shape.

Although the BN and AN diagnostic categories are theoretically discrete, clinically there is considerable overlap in behavioral symptomatology. Women within a single diagnostic category (either AN or BN) engage in diverse sets of behaviors, and even within an individual woman, the behavioral pattern frequently shifts and changes over time (Agras, Brandt, Bulik, et al., 2004). Yet the most commonly used outcome measures focus on select subsets of behaviors. While these measures typically address absolute change in the number of targeted behaviors, they fail to provide a comprehensive overview of the eating disorder behavioral symptomatology over time.

There are two important consequences of this limited focus of study. First, very little is known about individual differences in eating disorder behavioral patterns, and the consequences of this variability in the etiology and treatment of the disorders have yet to be explored. Furthermore, existing measures that focus narrowly on a subset of behaviors limit the ability to fully understand the consequences of the intervention and to distinguish interventions that lead to full remission of eating disorder behaviors from those that simply promote shifts or substitutions of alternative behavioral patterns. For example, an intervention may reduce the number of vomiting and laxative episodes but fail to change underlying feelings of fatness and fears related to weight gain. Consequently, nonpurging behaviors such as excessive exercise and calorie restriction may be used as a substitute to the purging behaviors to cope with the persisting fears regarding body weight.

In this chapter, we argue that Ecological Momentary Assessment (EMA) is a feasible and reliable methodology that can be used to gain a comprehensive understanding of the profile of eating-disordered behaviors over time. We begin by discussing the limitations of retrospective methodology often used to measure eating disorder behavioral patterns and provide a rationale for the use of EMA in this area of research. Next, we address specific features of implementing EMA methodology in an eating disorders treatment randomized clinical trial and report preliminary findings that demonstrate that EMA methodology can be profitably used to capture important therapeutic change in eating disorder behaviors.

Rationale for a Momentary Approach to Data Collection

The majority of randomized clinical trials of interventions for AN and BN have used retrospective measures to examine change in frequency of eating disorder behaviors, the most common being the Eating Disorder Examination (EDE) (Fairburn & Cooper, 1993). The EDE is a standardized semi-structured clinical interview designed to measure frequency of eating disorder behaviors over the previous 4 weeks. This measure is administered by a clinically experienced interviewer who elicits detailed descriptions of target behaviors and judges their presence based on the *Diagnostic and Statistical Manual* (*DSM-IV*) definitions (American Psychiatric Association, 2000).

Although use of an expert interviewer reduces reporting errors from question interpretations and definitions of the target behaviors, potential threats to the accuracy of the data remain. The most obvious threat to accurate reporting of eating disorder behaviors in clinical trial research stems from participants' purposeful editing of responses due to issues of social desirability and self-presentation. Since eating disorder behaviors are undesirable and embarrassing, the respondent may alter her response, an effect that may be heightened by the face-to-face format of the EDE interview (DeMaio, 1984). Perceptions of interviewer expectancies may also contribute to edited responses (Smyth, Wonderlich, Crosby, et al., 2001). This effect may be particularly powerful in eating disorder intervention studies due to (1) the insecure and compliant personality style associated with AN and BN (Perry, Silvera, & Rosenvinge, 2002) and (2) a sense of obligation to report levels of eating disorder behavior that conform to perceived expectancies of the research team after participation in an intensive intervention protocol.

The second threat to reliable retrospective reporting has to do with the nature of eating disorder behaviors and their recall. The diagnostic criteria for BN specify a minimum of two binge eating and compensatory behavior cycles per week on average over a period of at least 3 months (American Psychiatric Association, 2000). Diagnostic criteria for AN do not address specific behavioral parameters. Within these relatively broad diagnostic parameters, marked variability exists in the pattern of behaviors over time, characterized by (1) frequency (number of times within a day, across a week and month); (2) regularity (day of week and time of day); and (3) similarity (number and type of behaviors used and contexts within which they occur).

Studies have shown that these three dimensions of the target behaviors influence both encoding and retrieval processes and, therefore, the reliability of self-report data (Brown, 1995; Menon, 1993). For example, behaviors that are infrequent and dissimilar tend to be encoded in autobiographical memory as discrete events, and frequency estimates are reached by a scanning and counting process. In contrast, behaviors that are frequent, regular, and similar are less likely to be encoded as individual episodes but rather stored in summary form as higher-level semantic knowledge that is retrieved and used as the foundation for computation of a response. While both of these retrieval strategies are associated with significant recall error, estimation errors tend to be unsystematic and, therefore, introduce less bias into the results than the counting process (Sudman, Bradburn, & Schwarz, 1996).

Given that little is currently known about patterns of eating disorder behaviors in clinical and subclinical populations, the nature and significance of the biases associated with retrospective measurement of the behaviors remain unknown. Furthermore, studies that have compared retrospective and real-time data measurement of eating disorder behaviors have shown that concordance is low (for review, see Stein & Corte, 2003). The use of EMA to measure the frequency of eating disorder behaviors should reduce or eliminate the effects of social desirability and recall error that are associated with the standard retrospective measures.

Another important advantage of the EMA methodology is that it provides detailed information about the structure and pattern of eating disorder behavior over time. Although considerable research has focused on variability in experiences of hunger, appetite, and satiety in women with eating disorders (see Hetherington & Rolls, 2001, for a review), very little is known about variability in eating disorder behavioral patterns and the importance of this variability in understanding etiology and treatment outcomes (Walsh & Kahn, 1997). We anticipated that EMA would enable us to explore whether common patterns of these behaviors can be reliably identified and, if so, to examine their relationship to participant attrition and responsiveness to therapy.

Method

An experimental pretest/posttest design was used with three posttest data collection points occurring immediately, 6, and 12 months after intervention. The experimental condition was a 20-week manual-based psychotherapy program that focused on identifying and building new domains of self-definition and consisted of weekly individual and group sessions. The control condition was a manual-based supportive psychotherapy for eating disorders developed by Walsh and Wilson (1997). Participants in both conditions also received standardized manual-based nutritional counseling and medical monitoring. The effects of the intervention on self-cognitions, eating disorder attitudes and behaviors, and nutritional, psychological and functional health, were measured before and after the intervention. The EMA methodology was used to measure change in eight eating disorder behaviors: six active behaviors (binge eating, self-induced vomiting, laxative use, diuretic use, diet pill use, and excessive exercise) and two passive behaviors (calorie restricting and fasting).

Participants

The participants were nonpregnant women with a DSM-IV threshold or subthreshold diagnosis of AN or BN. Participants also had to meet the following eligibility criteria: (1) no other concurrent threshold level Axis I DSM-IV diagnosis, (2) no concurrent psychotropic medications or psychotherapy, and (3) no indications for inpatient treatment. Currently, data are available on a total of 34 women with a diagnosed eating disorder. The average age of our participants was 24.4 ± 0.1 years. Participants were 70 percent White, 10 percent Black/African-American, 15 percent Asian, and 5 percent Hispanic/Latino. The majority of participants had some college education (58%), 19 percent had a college degree, and the remaining 23 percent had a postgraduate degree. Our participants reported engaging in eating disorder behaviors for an average of 8.6 years.

Participants were recruited through advertisements and referrals from local health care providers. The Structured Clinical Interview (SCID) (First, Spitzer, Gibbon, & Williams, 1997) was used to establish the AN or BN diagnosis and the absence of all other Axis I disorders. An experienced clinician who was trained in the administration of the SCID completed all interviews.

Momentary Data Collection

A combined event-based and time-based, single end-of-the-day recording approach was used to measure the eating disorder behaviors. Event-based sampling is most commonly used for low-frequency events and was selected for this study for several reasons. First, even at full threshold level of the disorders, eating disorder behaviors may occur no more frequently than twice a week. To signal participants repeatedly throughout the day would be highly burdensome and likely to undermine recording compliance. Furthermore, results of a previous study using time-based approach showed that eating disorder behaviors were difficult to capture (Corte & Stein, in press). Use of less frequent signals with instructions to report all behaviors that occurred in the interval since the last signal would increase the risk of significant delays between the event and the recording and potentially undermine the basic logic of the EMA approach. The use of either the time- or signal-based approach might also result in recordings occurring while the participant was in social contexts in which completion of this sensitive questionnaire would be difficult, and therefore compliance with the measure could be compromised.

The final reason why an event-based recording approach was selected for this study has to do with the cognitive consequences of the signal itself. The basic logic of the identity intervention psychotherapy is to decrease the accessibility of weight- and food-related self-cognitions by promoting the development of new domains of self-definition. Several studies have shown that the duration and frequency of activation of a cognitive structure influence both the levels of elaboration of the structure and its influence on behavior (Davachi, Maril, & Wagner, 2001; Dijksterhuis, Aarts, Bargh, & van Knippenberg, 2000; Macrae, Stangor, & Milne, 1994). Thus, we reasoned that a time- or signal-based recording approach could actually contribute to further activation and elaboration of the dysfunctional self-cognitions and thereby attenuate the effects of the intervention.

A time-based single end-of-day recording of two eating disorder behaviors— food restricting and fasting—was included in our protocol for two reasons. First, food restricting and fasting are passive behaviors that occur over an extended period of time that is not clearly demarcated. Therefore, selection of the point in time to record the behavior would be unclear. Second, while there are no objective means of verifying the occurrence and recording of the eating disorder behaviors, bedtime recordings of these passive behaviors provide one means of evaluating participant compliance with the recording instructions and the EMA protocol.

A 22-day interval was selected for the study to ensure adequate sampling of intermittent eating disorder behaviors, to provide time for habituation to the measurement approach so that reactivity effects would not compromise the quality of the data, and, finally, because this interval is generally comparable to the time frame used for retrospective measures. A menu-driven computerized questionnaire was developed and programmed for use on a hand-held computer. A hand-held computer (Palm, Inc., Santa Clara, CA) was chosen as the recording device based on population characteristics, features of the behaviors of interest, and goals of the study.

We anticipated that our sample would comprise highly educated young adult women who would be familiar, comfortable, and even enthusiastic about using hand-held computer technology. In addition, use of password-protected access to the questionnaire decreases the risk of participants' family members or friends inadvertently seeing the highly personal and sensitive recordings that might occur with recordings using paper-and-pencil diaries. Finally, the date and time signature feature of the device enabled us to investigate issues such as data hoarding related to the reliability of the data and, potentially, to examine more subtle structural properties of eating disorder behaviors over time.

Items were derived from commonly used eating disorder questionnaires, including the EDE (Fairburn & Cooper, 1993) and the Questionnaire on Eating and Weight Patterns-Revised (Spitzer, Yanovski, & Marcus, 1994). Items were rewritten to focus on the single episode of the behavior that had just occurred. For simple eating disorder behaviors such as vomiting, laxative and diuretic use, diet pill use, food restricting, and fasting, definitions were included as a part of the items. For example, as shown in Figure 9-1, vomiting was measured with one item that captured the definition of the behavior.

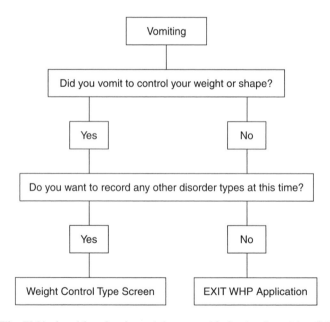

Figure 9-1. The EMA algorithm for the weight control behavior "vomiting." After a participant endorses vomiting on the initial Palm Pilot screen, she is then asked the two additional questions shown in this figure, each question displayed on a new screen. Depending on the answers, the participant may either record another behavior or exit the Palm Pilot application. The vomiting algorithm is the simples in the application.

The definitions of other eating disorder behaviors, including a binge eating and excessive exercise episodes, were more complex and dependent on several subjective and objective indicators. For example, a binge eating episode was defined based on three criteria: (1) eating an objectively large quantity of food, (2) within a 2-hour period, and (3) accompanied by a sense of being out of control (American Psychiatric Association, 2000). Similarly, an excessive exercise episode was defined as engaging in physical activity for 1 hour or more, primarily to control weight or shape or to burn calories. For these behaviors, algorithms were designed to enable querying of specific characteristics of the behaviors so that true episodes of the behaviors could be distinguished.

As shown in Figure 9-2, the binge eating algorithm consisted of seven questions that reflected specific defining properties of the behavior. The last three questions

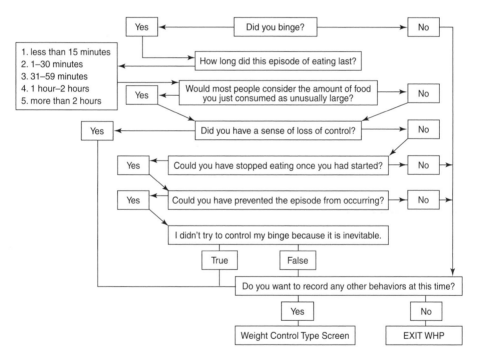

Figure 9-2. The EMA algorithm for the weight control behavior "binge eating." The binge eating algorithm is the most complex in the Palm Pilot application. Endorsement of a binge can lead the participant through a series of as few as two to as many as nine screens, with one new question displayed on each screen. The series of questions the participant answers allows us to determine whether the binge the participant is reporting meets *DSM-IV* criteria as a binge episode. For a binge to be counted as a binge episode, the participant must report that she consumed what other people would consider to be a large amount of food in a short period of time, experienced a loss of control, and could not have prevented the episode.

were alternative ways that a sense of loss of control could be expressed and were displayed only if the characteristic was not endorsed on the previous question.

Procedures

An overview of the study design is provided in Figure 9-3. For four 22-day intervals (before the intervention and immediately, 6 months, and 12 months after the intervention), participants carried a Palm Pilot and recorded all eating disorder behaviors at the time they occurred. They were also asked to record each day at bedtime food-restricting and fasting behaviors that occurred over the last 24 hours. Instruction on use of the Palm Pilot and procedures for recording eating disorder behaviors were provided in an individual 45-minute orientation session. A written manual with step-by-step descriptions of the recording procedure, along with an error log, were provided. Participants were asked to use the error log in the event they forgot or could not record behaviors on the Palm Pilot immediately after the behavior occurred. They were seen weekly over the 3-week period for Palm Pilot data downloads.

This clinical trial was complex and followed participants through an intense 18-month protocol. EMA was used to capture eating disorder behaviors four times in the protocol (before the intervention and immediately, 6 months, and 12 months after the intervention), providing a baseline from which we could measure remission (immediate) and recovery (6 and 12 months) from eating disorder behaviors. The EMA in this study was only one of a variety of outcome measures; we also administered 12 paper-and-pencil measures, collected menstrual status with a 6-week diary, collected food diaries, and collected blood/urine samples to provide indicators of nutritional health.

Data Management

The data from each of the 34 participants were saved in Excel, corrected with error log entries, and imported into a SPSS file. The most common error log

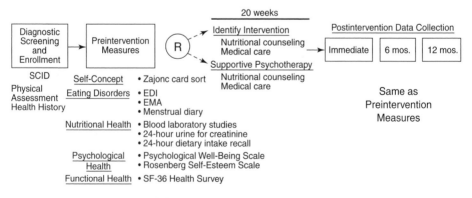

Figure 9-3. A schematic of the study protocol.

entry was an omission of recording a behavior—particularly, the failure to record end-of-day behaviors. The second most common error was documentation of a discrepancy between the time of occurrence of the behavior and its recording. Multiple error log entries indicated that a behavior had actually occurred hours, sometimes days, prior to when the behavior was recorded, as indicated by the time and date stamp of the Palm Pilot. The third type of error log entry occurred when a participant falsely endorsed a behavior; for example, the participant recorded diuretic use when she intended to endorse the use of a laxative. The occurrence of this type of error was very low, resulting in the modification of only five entries.

Hierarchical Linear Modeling

When every person is observed at the same fixed number of time points, it is conventional to view the design as occasions crossed by persons. However, when the number and spacing of time points vary from person to person, we may view occasions as nested within persons. Hierarchical linear models (HLMs) (Raudenbush & Bryk, 2002) use the latter approach to analyze data, allowing us to model the within-person variation, as well as between-persons variation, and to study the structure and predictors of individual change.

To examine overall pre- to postintervention differences in the trajectory of total number of active eating disorder behaviors, a two-level HLM was performed using HLM 5.62 (Raudenbush, Bryk, Cheong, & Congdon 2001). Since the initial data structure had separate instances of eating disorder behavioral episodes nested within day and individual, data were transformed to compute daily totals of active behaviors and a person-period data set was created. Level 1, or within-subject analysis, assumed a Poisson distribution to model the daily number of active behaviors an individual engaged in at a specific time. Within-subject correlations were accounted for with the estimation of a dispersion parameter. Both pre- and postintervention trajectories were modeled as a linear function of time. At the between-subject level (level 2), the four parameters from the level 1 model (average number of active behaviors pre- and postintervention and expected daily changes in active behaviors pre- and postintervention) were allowed to vary randomly. At level 2, individual covariates (e.g., treatment group) could be added to explain the variations in individual trajectories. However, for simplicity, no such covariates were included in this model.

Eating Disorder Behavioral Pattern Changes

To begin to develop a more complex characterization of the structure of eating disorder behaviors, we identified a number of properties that address regularity and similarity of behaviors over time using Menon's (1993) definitions of behavioral regularity and similarity. "Regularity" refers to the periodicity of the eating disorder behavioral episodes or the distribution of behaviors across the total time. We characterized individual differences in regularity of eating disorder behaviors with three variables: (1) the number of "no behavior" days across the 22-day EMA interval, (2) the mean number of "no behavior" days between behavioral episodes, and (3) the standard deviation or average variability in "no behavior" days between behavioral episodes. "Similarity" refers to the specific behaviors enacted in an episode or the extent to which the same or different behaviors are used. We characterized individual differences in behavioral similarity by two properties: (1) the total number of different eating disorder behaviors engaged in over the 22-day interval and (2) the number of unique behavioral combinations engaged in over the 22-day period.

Results

The 5-year clinical trial addressed in this chapter is approximately 2 years into data collection. Consequently, preliminary analyses are based on the small sample with preintervention and immediate postintervention data currently available ($n = 34$). This chapter addresses fundamental questions about whether eating disorder behaviors are altered by the psychotherapies.

Participant Compliance/Dropout

The end-of-day report was used to assess participant compliance; a compliant participant should record 22 end-of-day entries. For the preintervention data EMA period, the average number of end-of-day reports completed was 16.65 (SE = 0.29) days, or 77.17 percent. Comparison of participant compliance between those who completed both the pre- and immediate postintervention EMA data collection (completers, $n = 17$) and those who completed only the preintervention phase (noncompleters, $n = 17$) revealed that the completers had a significantly higher preintervention compliance rate ($p = 0.01$) than the noncompleters. The completer group had 18 end-of-day reports (85 percent compliance) during the preintervention EMA compared to 15 end-of-day reports (69 percent compliance) from the noncompleter group. No other significant differences in mean number of active and passive eating disorder behaviors per day were found between the completer and noncompleter groups.

Eating Disorder Behaviors

The mean number of eating disorder behaviors expressed per day during the 22-day period pre- and postintervention phases is shown in Figure 9-4. As can be seen, vomiting was the most frequently occurring active behavior. Consistent with the findings of previous studies, daily rates of laxative, diuretic, and diet pill use were low (Stein & Corte, 2003). In addition, restricting food intake was reported more frequently than was fasting, accounting for the majority of passive behaviors reported.

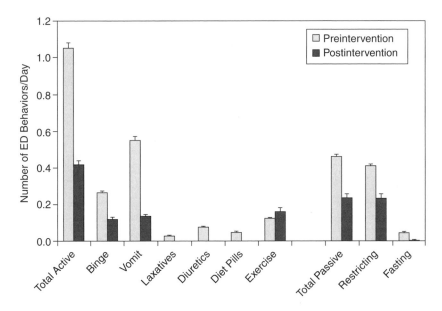

Figure 9-4. Mean number of eating disorder behaviors per day recorded with EMA.

The bar graph shows the mean ($\pm$ SD) number of eating disorder behaviors that participants engaged in daily during the pre- and immediate postintervention EMA periods. Participants reported more active behaviors than passive behaviors; the incidence of vomiting was the most prevalent, with binge and exercise also frequently reported. As in previous studies, laxative, diuretic, and diet pills were used frequently as a means to control weight or shape. The passive eating disorder behavior most frequently reported was restricting food/calorie intake.

The population-average model estimates based on the HLM analysis are shown in Table 9-1. There was a nonsignificant decrease in the log of the active behaviors over the pre- and postintervention 22-day EMA period (Figure 9-5), reflected by the negative slopes of the trajectories (–0.01 and –0.02, respectively). In addition, the slopes of the average daily changes in active eating disorder behaviors were not significantly different between the pre- and postintervention

Table 1-1. Population-average model: Estimation of fixed effects

Fixed effect	Coefficient	Standard error	T ratio	p value
Preintervention intercept	0.46	0.13	3.42	0.002
Preintervention slope	−0.01	0.01	−1.73	0.091
Postintervention intercept	−0.91	0.30	−3.01	0.005
Postintervention slope	−0.02	0.02	−1.18	0.248

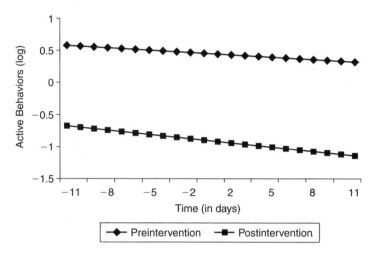

Figure 9-5. The log of active eating disorder behaviors reported over the 22-day EMA period during pre- and postintervention.

EMA periods [$\chi^2(df=1) = 0.25$, $p > 0.50$]. The downward trend of the slopes indicates that participants reported fewer behaviors at the end of the 22-day EMA period compared to the beginning.

The line graph depicts the log of active eating disorder behaviors over the 22-day EMA recording period before the intervention (diamonds) and immediately after the intervention (squares). Time 0 is the midpoint of EMA data collection.

The log of the expected average number of active behaviors the participants reported during both the pre- and postintervention EMA periods was significantly different from zero (see Table 9-1; $p = 0.002$ and 0.005, respectively), indicating that the participants were engaging in more eating disorder behaviors than would be expected based on the null hypothesis. However, although participants continued to report more eating disorder behaviors than expected based on the null hypothesis in the postintervention EMA period, there was a significant decrease in level of active behaviors after treatment. Results showed that the log of the expected average number of active behaviors in the middle of the postintervention period (intercept) was significantly lower than that of the preintervention period, [$\chi^2(df = 1) = 19.12$, $p < 0.001$], showing a significant effect of the overall intervention. Individual level covariates (e.g., age, treatment, group) can be added to this model at level 2 to explain individual variations in trajectories.

The EMA technology allowed us to examine individual eating disorder behavioral patterns, revealing distinctly different profiles among participants. Preliminary characterizations of two types of eating disorder behavioral profiles are presented below.

PARTICIPANT 1

This participant met SCID diagnostic criteria for BN and reported experiencing eating disorder behaviors for 8 years. The profile of eating disorder behaviors reported by the participant before the intervention and immediately after the intervention is shown in Figure 9-6. The eating disorder behavioral episodes were irregular in the preintervention phase, with 15 of the 22 days with no episodes, a mean number of 1.9 days between episodes, and considerable variability in the number of days between episodes (SD = 2.36 days); they were more irregular

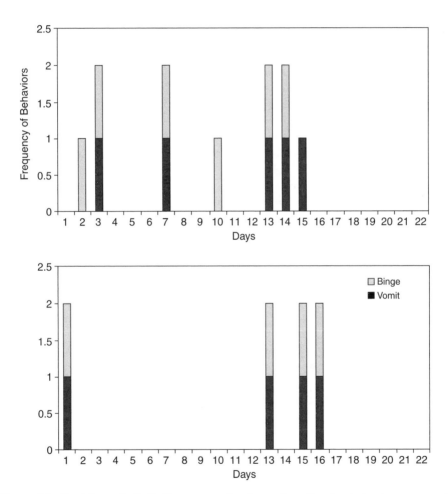

Figure 9-6. Participant 1: Daily frequency of active eating disorder behaviors, pre- and postintervention. The bar graph shows the mean daily pattern of eating disorder behaviors reported by a single participant. This participant engaged in only two eating disorder behaviors: binge and vomit. Note that the participant showed a decreased frequency of behaviors in the postintervention period.

after the intervention (number of "no behavior" days = 18; mean number of days between episodes = 3.6, SD = 4.8). For this participant, behavioral episodes were very similar before and after the intervention. She engaged in two types of behaviors at both time points. At preintervention she engaged in three unique combinations of eating disorder behaviors: binging alone, binging and vomiting, and vomiting alone. At postintervention, all episodes consisted of binge and vomit behaviors.

Participant 2

This participant met SCID diagnostic criteria for BN and reported engaging in eating disorder behaviors for over 17 years. This participant had a distinctly different eating disorder behavioral structure from the previous case (Figure 9-7), with behaviors highly regular and dissimilar in the preintervention phase, changing to a more irregular and similar pattern in the postintervention phase. Before the intervention the participant reported zero "no behavior" days, with a 0 mean and standard deviation for days between episodes. Over the preintervention phase, the participant engaged in four different eating disorder behaviors and reported a total of eight unique combinations of behaviors over the 22-day EMA period. In sharp contrast, the profile of eating disorder behaviors at the immediate postintervention phase (panel B) showed a dramatic change compared to preintervention. After the intervention she reported a total of 13 "no behavior" days, with a mean of 1.3 days between episodes and a standard deviation of 2.1 days. Behavioral episodes also became more similar, reflecting a total of two different behaviors and three unique combinations over the EMA period.

Discussion

Because the results reported in this chapter are preliminary and are based on a small sample, conclusions drawn from these findings should be viewed with caution. Overall, the preliminary findings provide evidence to suggest that participants in both treatment conditions experienced a significant decrease in their eating disorder behaviors. Furthermore, examination of individual case profiles provides some very early evidence to suggest that although the interventions do not lead to a total elimination of the active eating disorder behaviors, important changes in the behavioral regularity and similarity do occur.

One interesting and unexpected finding was the tendency to decrease the frequency of the active eating disorder behaviors during the 22-day EMA recording period. Although a recent collection of studies failed to find evidence of reactivity to the EMA methodology in measurement of eating disorder (Corte & Stein, in press) and other health risk behaviors (Hufford, Shields, Shiffman, et al., 2002), this finding raises an important question about whether the process of recording behaviors and/or the contact with the research team related to the EMA methodology may itself alter the pattern of behaviors.

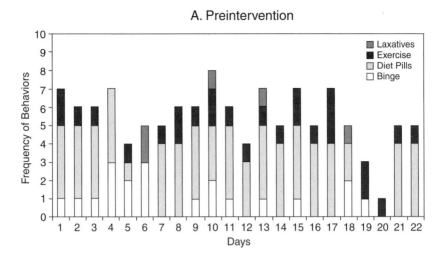

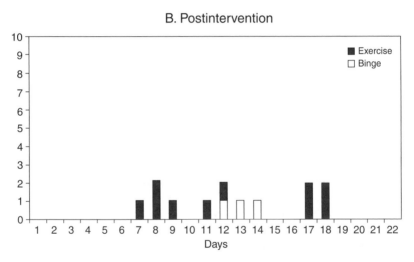

Figure 9-7. Participant 2: Daily frequency of active eating disorder behaviors, pre- and postintervention. The bar graph shows the mean daily pattern of eating disorder behaviors reported by a single participant. This participant engaged in a wide variety of eating disorder behaviors in the preintervention period and reported multiple behaviors on a daily basis. Note that the participant showed not only a decreased frequency of behaviors in the postintervention period but also reduced the variety of eating disorder behaviors to only binge and exercise.

One possible explanation for the inconsistency in the reactivity study findings is that change in the rate of behavior is gradual and occurs after monitoring one's own behaviors after a period of several weeks. In this study, self-monitoring of eating disorder behaviors extended over a 3-week period, which may provide sufficient time for a participant to recognize the high rate of behaviors and initiate a gradual decrease in behavioral frequency (for similar findings using EMA to record drinking behaviors, see Collins, Morsheimer, Shiffman, et al., 1998). Many previous studies that examined reactivity used shorter recording periods and therefore may not have captured the reactivity process (Cruise, Broderick, Porter, et al., 1996; LeGrange, Gorin, Dymek, & Stone, 2002). Our findings, although tentative, raise the possibility that EMA periods of 2 weeks or less may provide the most reliable, nonreactive measurement of eating disorder behaviors.

Insights Gained

To the best of our knowledge, this study is the first attempt to use EMA to measure an outcome variable in randomized clinical trials with persons with a major mental disorder. Characteristics of this type of study pose unique challenges for effective use of EMA methodology, including participant burden, diverse and high level of research staff responsibilities, and characteristics of the population.

First and foremost, the complexity and duration of the study protocol greatly increased participant burden, issues, and problems. Before beginning this clinical trial, a pilot study was completed in which 16 women with a clinically diagnosed eating disorder of AN or BN recorded eating disorder behaviors using event-triggered EMA methodology (Stein & Corte, 2003). The protocol for that study included diagnostic screening, a 28-day EMA behavioral recording period, and completion of a retrospective measure of eating disorder behaviors at the end of the EMA period. Since it was the primary focus of the study, participant investment in recording was high, and energy and commitment were singularly focused on this aspect of the study. The attrition rate for the pilot study was 11 percent. Although we received negative feedback regarding the EMA only from participants in the full trial, the attrition rate during the preintervention data collection phase was 21 percent. The high attrition rate was not likely to stem solely from the 22-day EMA. However, the combined effects of EMA, along with other labor-intensive outcome measurement activities (e.g., six weekly blood draws, collection of a 24-hour urine sample, and four 24-hour food recalls), is most likely a factor in the participants' decision to discontinue participation.

In addition to the burden associated with the recording of behaviors, the time interval between initial contact and start of the intervention is increased by the EMA data collection. We used a 22-day EMA period to increase the reliability of our behavioral frequency estimates. However, the length of time associated with EMA data collection may be of particularly high importance in participant retention, given that those who initiate contact are often experiencing high levels of distress stemming from their symptoms and have decided to seek treatment. Within this context, a several-week-long period from initial contact to the start of intervention may be frustrating and may contribute to increased levels of attrition during this period.

The complexity of the protocol also had implications for research staff and their focus on the EMA dimensions of the study. Even with extensive pilot testing, which included a study focused solely on the EMA of eating disorder behaviors and a second pilot study of the full protocol, once the full trial started, an additional challenging period of adjustment occurred. The consequences of the greater study complexity on research staff were most pronounced during the start-up phase of the clinical trial, while they were learning to manage a larger and more complicated array of issues and problems. Project changes, including an increase in the number of research staff members handling the personal digital assistants (PDAs) and the data, a much longer participant enrollment period so that hardware and software replacements were essential, and the addition of treatment and follow-up components of the study that required intense levels of attention, resulted in EMA problems stemming from small issues that were not recognized and handled in a timely manner. Issues such as seasonal time changes (e.g., Eastern and Standard time shifts), battery difficulties, and hardware and software changes affected the structure of the data in the earliest stages of the trial.

Successes and Challenges

In hindsight, it is clear that we made two key mistakes that reflected our novice status with the methodology. First, we hired a single independent computer programmer to develop our PDA interview and laptop interface software. Access to this programmer was limited and channels of communication were not well developed. Many of the problems that we experienced could have been avoided by hiring an experienced electronic provider company and working closely with it, particularly around issues of data structure. Second, the success of our small pilot study left us with a false sense of competency, and therefore we did not immediately begin to merge individual data files to construct a large data file. While we had well-developed procedures for downloading, backing up, checking, and storing individual data files, we did not attempt to merge files into a large data file for several months into the study. Consequently, data structure problems stemming from hardware and software changes were not immediately detected and became larger over time. Given our limited experience with EMA methodology and related technologies, a collaborative partnership with an experienced electronic diary provider company would have facilitated a smoother transition between the pilot and full trial phases of the project.

Prospects for Application of EMA Methods

Despite the many challenges encountered, our work suggests that EMA is a feasible and reliable approach to measuring eating disorder behaviors. Based on our preliminary exploratory analysis, we believe that the EMA approach will improve the reliability of the measurement of eating disorder behaviors as an outcome variable. In addition, it will enable a more detailed description of individual differences in patterns of eating disorder behaviors and, in doing so, may contribute to a more refined understanding of the disorders, their etiologies, and responses to treatment.

The EMA may also be used to examine antecedents or proximal triggers of eating disorder behavioral episodes. Wegner and colleagues effectively used EMA methodology to measure mood immediately before and just after binge episodes. In this study, signal and event-based recording methods were used to examine the association between negative mood and binge eating episodes in a sample of college women with subthreshold levels of binge eating disorder (Wegner, Smyth, Crosby, et al., 2002). Greeno used the methodology to examine mood, appetite, and setting as triggers in a similar sample (Greeno, Wing, & Shiffman, 2000). Other studies that have investigated social stressors, dietary restraint, social context, and mood as antecedents to eating disorder behaviors have relied on paper-and-pencil diaries for data collection (Davis, Freeman, & Garner, 1988; Johnson & Larson, 1982; Johnson, Schlundt, Barclay, et al., 1995; Larson & Johnson, 1985; Steiger, Gauvin, Jabalpurwala, et al., 1999; Steiger, Lehoux, & Gauvin, 1999) and could profitably use EMA methodology to improve the validity of the results.

Another potentially important application of EMA methodology is exploration of the development of disorders and identification of factors that distinguish those who experiment with the behaviors from those who move into full threshold disorders and their chronic variants. Little is currently known about the developmental trajectories of the disorders. While many women experiment with eating disorder behaviors, only a small subset progresses to manifest a diagnosable eating disorder. Whether specific entry-level behaviors are predictive of the development of a diagnosable disorder and whether specific profiles can distinguish subthreshold, threshold, and chronic variants of the disorders are unknown. Using methodology similar to that described by Mermelstein (chapter 6, this volume) in which multiple periods of EMA data collection take place over an extended period of months or years may enable identification of discrete developmental trajectories of eating disorder behaviors, and the psychological and social risk factors that are predictive of these trajectories.

Summary

The EMA is a costly, resource- and energy-intensive methodology. However, given the limited methodologies available to measure highly personal and complex health-related behaviors such as binge eating, self-induced vomiting, and laxative use and the rich array of information that can be collected regarding these behaviors from even the most simple set of questions, the EMA approach holds great potential for both reliable and in-depth measurement of these phenomena.

References

Agras, W., Brandt, H., Bulik, C., Dolan-Sewell, R., Fairburn, C., Halmi, K., Herzog, D., Jimerson, D., Kaplan, A., Kaye, W., le Grange, D., Lock, J., Mitchell, J., Rudorfer, M., Street, L., Striegel-Moore, R., Vitousek, K., Walsh, B., & Wilfley, D. (2004). Report of the National Institutes of Health Workshop on Overcoming Barriers to Treatment Research in Anorexia Nervosa. *International Journal of Eating Disorders, 35*, 509–521.

American Psychiatric Association. (2000). *Diagnostic and Statistical Manual of Mental Disorders, 4th Ed., Text Revision.* Washington, DC: American Psychiatric Association.

Brown, N. (1995). Estimation strategies and the judgment of event frequency. *Journal of Experimental Psychology, 21,* 1539–1553.

Collins, R. L., Morsheimer, E., Shiffman, S., Paty, J., Gnys, M., & Papandonatos, G. (1998). Ecological momentary assessment in a behavioral drinking modification training program. *Experimental and Clinical Psychopharmacology, 6,* 306–315.

Corte, C., & Stein, K. F. (in press). Body-weight self-schema: Determinant of mood and behavior in women with an eating disorder. *Journal of Applied Social Psychology.*

Cruise, C., Broderick, J., Porter, L., Kaell, A., & Stone, A. (1996). Reactive effects of diary self-assessment in chronic pain patients. *Pain, 67,* 253–258.

Davachi, L., Maril, A., & Wagner, A. (2001). When keeping in mind supports later bringing to mind: Neural markers of phonological rehearsal predict subsequent remembering. *Journal of Cognitive Neuroscience, 13,* 1059–1070.

Davis, R., Freeman, R., & Garner, D. (1988). A naturalistic investigation of eating behavior in bulimia nervosa. *Journal of Consulting and Clinical Psychology, 56,* 273–279.

DeMaio, T.J. (1984). Social desirability and survey measurement: A review. In C. F. Turner and E. Martin, *Eating disorders: Surveying subjective phenomena* (Vol. 2, pp. 257–281). New York: Russell Sage.

Dijksterhuis, A., Aarts, H., Bargh, J., & van Knippenberg, A. (2000). On the relation between associative strength and automatic behavior. *Journal of Experimental Social Psychology, 36,* 531–544.

Fairburn, C. G., & Cooper, Z. (1993). The eating disorder examination. In C. G. Fairburn & T. G. Wilson, *Eating disorders: Binge eating: Nature, assessment and treatment* (12th ed., pp. 317–360). New York: Guilford Press.

First, M. B., Spitzer, R. L., Gibbon, M., & Williams, J. (1997). *User's guide for the Structured Clinical Interview for DSM-IV Axis I Disorders.* Washington, DC: American Psychiatric Press Inc.

Greeno, C., Wing, R., & Shiffman, S. (2000). Binge antecedents in obese women with and without binge eating disorder. *Journal of Consulting and Clinical Psychology, 68,* 95–102.

Hetherington, M. & Rolls, B. (2001). Dysfunctional eating in the eating disorders. *The Psychiatric Clinics of North America, 24,* 235–248.

Hufford, M., Shields, A., Shiffman, S., Paty, J., & Balabanis, M. (2002). Reactivity to ecological momentary assessment: An example using undergraduate problem drinkers. *Psychology of Addictive Behaviors, 16,* 205–211.

Johnson, C., & Larson, R. (1982). Bulimia: An analysis of mood and behavior. *Psychosomatic Medicine, 44,* 341–351.

Johnson, W., Schlundt, D., Barclay, D., Carr-Nangle, R., & Engler, L. (1995). A naturalistic functional analysis of binge eating. *Behavior Therapy, 26,* 101–118.

Keel, P. K., & Mitchell, J. E. (1997). Outcome in bulimia nervosa. *American Journal of Psychiatry, 154,* 313–321.

Larson, R., & Johnson, C. (1985). Bulimia: Disturbed patterns of solitude. *Addictive Behaviors, 10,* 281–290.

Le Grange, D., Gorin, A., Dymek, M., & Stone, A. (2002). Does ecological momentary assessment improve cognitive behavioral therapy for binge eating disorder? A pilot study. *European Eating Disorder Review, 10,* 316–328.

Macrae, C., Stangor, C., & Milne, A. (1994). Activating social stereotypes: A functional analysis. *Journal of Experimental Social Psychology, 30,* 370–389.

Menon, G. (1993). The effects of accessibility of information in memory on judgments of behavioral frequencies. *Journal of Consumer Research, 20,* 431–440.

Perry, J., Silvera, D., & Rosenvinge, J. (2002). Are oral, obsessive and hysterical personality traits related to disturbed eating patterns? A general population study of 6,313 men and women. *Journal of Personality Assessment, 78,* 405–416.

Raudenbush, S. W., & Bryk, A. S. (2002). *Hierarchical linear models: Applications and data analysis methods* (2nd ed). Thousand Oaks, CA: Sage.

Raudenbush, S. W., Bryk, A. S., Cheong, Y. F., & Congdon, R. T. (2001). *HLM 5: Hierarchical linear and nonlinear modeling*. Chicago: Scientific Software International.

Shiffman, S., & Stone, A. (1998). Ecological momentary assessment in health psychology. *Health Psychology, 17,* 3–5.

Smyth, J., Wonderlich, S., Crosby, R., Miltenberger, R., Mitchell, J., & Rorty, M. (2001). The use of ecological momentary assessment approaches in eating disorder research. *International Journal of Eating Disorders, 30,* 83–95.

Spitzer, R., Yanovski, & Marcus, S. (1994). *Questionnaire on Eating and Weight Patterns-Revised (QEWP-R)*. Pittsburgh, PA: Behavioral Measurement Database Services.

Steiger, H., Gauvin, L., Jabalpurwala, S., Seguin, J., & Stotl, S. (1999). Hypersensitivity to social interactions in bulimic syndromes relationship to binge eating. *Journal of Consulting and Clinical Psychology, 67,* 765–775.

Steiger, H., Lehoux, P. M., & Gauvin, L. (1999). Impulsivity, dieting control and the urge to binge in bulimic syndromes. *International Journal of Eating Disorders, 26,* 261–274.

Stein, K. F., & Corte, C. (2003). Ecologic momentary assessment of eating-disordered behaviors. *International Journal of Eating Disorders, 34,* 1–12.

Stone, A., & Shiffman, S. (1994). Ecological momentary assessment: Measuring real world processes in behavioral medicine. *Annals of Behavioral Medicine, 16,* 199–202.

Sudman, S., Bradburn, N., & Schwarz, N. (1996). *Thinking about answers: The application of cognitive processes to survey methodology*. San Francisco: Jossey-Bass.

Walsh, B. T., & Devlin, M. J. (1998). Eating disorders: Progress and problems. *Science, 280,* 1387–1390.

Walsh, T., & Kahn, C. (1997). Diagnostic criteria for eating disorders: Current concerns and future directions. *Psychopharmacology Bulletin, 33,* 369–372.

Walsh, B. T., & Wilson, G. T. (1997). *Supportive Psychotherapy Manual*.

Wegner, K., Smyth, J., Crosby, R., Wittrock, D., Wonderlich, S., & Mitchell, J. (2002). An evaluation of the relationship between mood and binge eating in the natural environment using ecological momentary assessment. *International Journal of Eating Disorders, 32,* 352–361.

10

Ecological Momentary Assessment of Alcohol Consumption

R. Lorraine Collins and Mark Muraven

Drinking Restraint and the Regulation of Alcohol Intake

The drinking restraint model suggests that excessive/binge drinking occurs in a cognitive context in which the individual alternates between being attracted to alcohol and being concerned about the need to restrict/regulate alcohol intake (Bensley, 1991; Collins, 1993). Some "restrained drinkers" may be so preoccupied with the need to lessen or control their alcohol intake that they invoke rules and set limits on alcohol use (Collins, 1993; Ruderman & McKirnan, 1984). Paradoxically, the thinking about the need to limit/regulate alcohol intake, while not being successful at such regulation, can precipitate excessive drinking (Collins & Lapp, 1991; Marlatt, 1985). In this way, drinking restraint may be a risk factor for excessive drinking and alcohol-related problems (Bensley, Kuna, & Steele, 1990; Collins, 1993; Connor, Young, Williams, & Ricciardelli, 2000; Connors, Collins, Dermen, & Koutsky, 1998; Curry, Southwick, & Steele, 1987).

Drinking Restraint, the Limit Violation Effect, and Excessive Drinking

We propose that the Limit Violation Effect (LVE) describes the process that moves restrained drinkers to engage in excessive drinking (Collins & Lapp, 1991, 1992; Collins, Lapp, & Izzo, 1994). The LVE, which is based on Marlatt and Gordon's (Marlatt, 1985; Marlatt & Gordon, 1980) Abstinence Violation Effect, involves a cycle of limit setting, limit violation, self-blame, negative affective reactions, and excessive drinking. It provides the conceptual framework for our use of Ecological Momentary Assessment (EMA) to examine social drinkers' risk for excessive drinking and alcohol-related problems. We proposed that restrained social drinkers regard consuming more than a predetermined amount of alcohol as a personal failure. If they violate their limits on drinking and then blame themselves for the violations, they subsequently experience negative affective reactions such as guilt, anger, and sadness. They continue to drink (i.e., excessively) to alleviate the negative emotions they feel as a result of this self-blame.

Equivocal Evidence of the Occurrence of the LVE

Although the LVE was conceptually compelling, evidence regarding its occurrence in alcohol use has not been conclusive. In a cross-sectional questionnaire study, Collins and Lapp (1991) found that perceived difficulty in controlling drinking (one aspect of drinking restraint) and self-blame for negative drinking-related outcomes predicted alcohol problems in a sample of social drinkers. However, the cross-sectional data meant that the causal linkages in the LVE model could not be directly tested.

Laboratory experiments offered a better opportunity to test the LVE but still had limitations. In the earliest such experiments, participants were given a preload of wine (to precipitate a violation) and then were offered the opportunity to drink more during a subsequent taste-rating task (Bensley et al., 1990; Ruderman & McKirnan, 1984). These experiments generally failed to produce the LVE, possibly because the experimental designs ignored the participants' need to take responsibility for the violation (Collins & Lapp, 1991) and because of the relatively short duration of time. To address the first limitation, Collins and Lapp (1991) conducted an experiment in which they maintained the possibility that participants could blame themselves for violating their drinking limits. Their procedures produced limit violations to which participants reacted with negative affect, particularly anger. However, the participants did not continue to drink, thereby showing the excessive drinking predicted by the LVE. This possibly was because they could attribute their alcohol intake to the experimental situation rather than to themselves and the relatively short (30 minutes) drinking period. These inconsistent findings about the occurrence of the LVE made it impossible to draw any firm conclusions. However, the LVE's potential importance as an explanatory model of excessive drinking provided the impetus to find new methods that could better capture its components.

Rationale for a Real-Time Momentary Approach to Data Collection

EMA Provides a Valid Method for Field Testing the LVE

To provide valid tests of predictions derived from the LVE, we needed a methodology with which to self-monitor drinking behavior and ever-changing subjective experiences (e.g., moods) in real time within and across episodes of drinking. The resulting data could be used to examine the complex relationships among subjective reactions and drinking. Traditionally, self-monitoring of alcohol use has relied on paper-and-pencil reports (e.g., daily diaries, calendars; Samo, Tucker, & Vuchinich, 1989; Sobell, Bogardis, Schuller, et al., 1989; Vuchinich, Tucker, & Harllee, 1988). Although these self-reports allowed researchers to capture subjective states and ongoing behavior, paper-and-pencil methods had limitations that were not easily addressed. These included poor or faked compliance and deficient data (e.g., missing data, ambiguous responses; Broderick, Schwartz, Shiffman, et al., 2003; Litt, Cooney, & Morse, 1998; Stone, Shiffman, Schwartz, et al., 2002).

EMA provided the methodology of choice for examining the occurrence of the LVE. It allowed us to assess the subjective precursors of drinking (e.g., mood), alcohol intake (e.g., number of drinks), reactions to drinking (e.g., mood, self-blame), as well as subsequent drinking either proximal to (next drinking episode) and/or distal to (over days or weeks) a specific episode of drinking and limit violation. We also could collect base rate data (e.g., on mood) as a context for understanding assessments linked to specific drinking episodes. Using EMA also enhanced the validity of self-reports of subjective states and drinking behavior (Stone & Shiffman, 1994). This enhanced validity is related to the advantages of EMA. They include (1) compliance with self-monitoring cannot be faked because each entry is tagged with a time and date; (2) compliance can be tracked because failures to respond to prompts are tagged and stored; and (3) once initiated, participants must complete a standard interview, thereby providing quality control of data (Shiffman, 2000). Finally, collecting EMA data on alcohol use generated little reactivity, even among alcoholics (Litt et al., 1998).

Method

In this chapter we describe three studies in which we have used EMA methods to collect data (see Collins, Morsheimer, Shiffman, et al., 1998; Muraven, Collins, Morsheimer, et al., 2005 a, b; Muraven, Collins, Shiffman, & Paty, 2005). Each study focused on social drinkers who used electronic diaries (EDs) to self-monitor drinking behavior and its antecedents and consequences, as well as their activities, locations, and social contexts. The studies typically involved a session in which participants completed questionnaires, followed by a training session in which they learned how to use the ED. These two sessions were followed by weekly individual sessions to download data, receive feedback on the use of the ED, and change batteries. Our screening procedures helped to ensure that participants were willing and able to use the ED. Thus, we were able to achieve relatively good compliance with ED procedures. Table 10-1 gives information on demographics and the EMA study characteristics.

Samples

Our research focused on the LVE as a risk factor for excessive drinking and alcohol problems. We used newspaper advertisements and flyers to recruit participants from the broader community and from colleges. Typically, participants had to meet

Table 10-1. Demographic and EMA study characteristics

| | Collins et al., 1998 | Muraven et al., 2005 | Muraven et al., 2005a | | Muraven et al., 2005b |
			Study 1	Study 2	
SAMPLE (*n*)	37	106	106	38	38
Men	22	49	49	20	20
Women	15	57	57	18	18
ETHNICITY (%)					
European American	89	86	86	82	82
Minority	11	14	14	18	18
MARITAL STATUS (%)					
Single	35	100	100	73.7	73.7
Other	65	0	0	26.3	26.3
Mean age (years)	35.9	19.3	19.3	26.9	26.9
Mean no. drinks/week	22	18.6	18.6	15.8	15.8
EMA platform	Psion	Palm Pilot	Palm Pilot	Psion	Psion
No. weeks of EMA	8	3	2	2	2
Intervention	Yes	No	No	No	No
Type of intervention	Behavioral				

eligibility criteria such as a willingness to drink a minimum of four drinks per week; no previous medical diagnosis or treatment for abuse of alcohol or other drugs; and no psychological, physical, medical, or legal contraindications to drinking alcohol. Table 10-1 contains information on the participants' demographic characteristics.

Momentary Data Collection

We applied EMA methods to collecting data relevant to testing the LVE, our conceptual model of risk for alcohol abuse. In our earliest studies, the ED hardware consisted of a Psion business organizer (Psion, Ltd., London, England). In later studies participants carried a Palm Pilot Professional (Palm, Inc., Milpitas, CA, USA). Each platform used software specifically developed for our projects. In each of our studies (see "Results" section), participants both initiated entries related to each episode of drinking and responded to audible random prompts to provide base rate information on the occurrence of subjective phenomena (e.g., moods) that were central to our conceptual model. Research participants were trained to interact with the ED during all of their waking hours. At night, they put the ED to sleep when they went to sleep and in the morning they used the ED as their alarm clock to wake up.

The ED had a main menu from which participants could choose one of five different interviews, report a problem, suspend random prompting, and so on. The ED interviews were as follows: (1) participants initiated a morning interview when they awoke; (2) they responded to an audible random prompt (four or five times/day); (3) they initiated a "begin drinking" interview just before they started each episode of drinking; and (4) they initiated an "end drinking" interview just after they stopped drinking. In some of our more recent studies, we added a fifth daily interview called an evening report, which was scheduled to be prompted in the early evening (6 to 8 p.m.). Examples of some of the varied topics assessed in each type of interview are as follows: (1) the morning interview included the likelihood of drinking during different periods of the coming day/week; (2) the random prompt interview included positive and negative mood (to provide information on base rates); (3) the "begin drinking" interview included mood and time since drinking started (to assess compliance); (4) the "end drinking" interview included mood and the number of drinks consumed during the episode; (5) the evening report included intention to drink and plans to limit alcohol intake.

The ED software was designed to prevent missing data, out-of-range responses, and the option of abandoning (i.e., failure to complete) an interview. Response formats varied based on the type of question. Participants could use an 11-point sliding scale to make ratings, check one of many choice boxes, or select a specific number (e.g., number of drinks). To facilitate integration of the ED into everyday life and increase compliance with responding to random prompts, the software included *delay*, *suspend*, and *nap* functions. Participants could delay completing (for up to 20 minutes) a randomly prompted interview, if the prompt occurred at an inauspicious time. They could suspend (i.e., turn off) random prompting for up to 2 hours, but they were asked to indicate a reason for suspending (e.g., driving a car). They could use the *nap* function if they slept during the day (length of time unspecified).

Procedures

Eligible participants first completed a series of individual-difference measures in small groups. At the end of that session, we invited interested individuals to return to the research site for 1.5 to 2 hours of individualized training in the procedures for using the ED. In the training session, research staff used a manual to explain concepts and participants practiced with an ED until they were comfortable with the procedures. We then instructed them to use the ED to self-monitor ongoing behavior 24 hours per day for the duration of the study. An initial ED-feedback appointment took place 2 to 3 days after training. In this way, our staff could catch errors and troubleshoot problems before participants had been in the field for a long time. Feedback usually focused on problems related to compliance with the protocol or using the different features of the ED. A staff person was "on call" 24 hours each day, so participants could contact staff if they experienced an ED emergency (e.g., dead battery, software malfunction). In this way, participants who ran into trouble either could be talked through a solution or were scheduled for an immediate appointment, at which the malfunctioning ED was replaced.

The raw data from the ED were compiled and concatenated using a database program (Microsoft Access). Initially, we examined these tables to extract participants' compliance with the protocols and the descriptive information from the various assessments. From there, we used multilevel regression (e.g., Schwartz & Stone, 1998) to examine our hypotheses and to test our model. We focused on both the antecedents and the consequences of excessive drinking. In particular, we specified a priori relationships between excessive drinking and mood. These relationships, as fixed in our model, guided the statistical equations we tested.

In the multilevel models, we person-centered all independent variables (Kreft, de Leeuw, & Aiken, 1995; Schwartz & Stone, 1998) because our conceptual focus was on how intraindividual changes (i.e., the individual's mood at one moment compared to his or her average mood) were related to outcomes such as alcohol intake. We used hierarchical linear modeling (HLM) software (Bryk, Raudenbush, & Congdon, 2000) and we examined the residuals using numerical outputs and graphs to determine whether there were any significant outliers or influential cases. We also tested whether the data violated assumptions of the analyses (Singer & Willett, 2003).

Results

Our hypotheses were well suited to EMA because they focused on how behaviors unfold over time. Rather than just examining behavior at static intervals, our primary interest was how negative affective states were dynamically related to subsequent alcohol intake. Indeed, the richness of the data allowed us to test hypotheses in several different and distinct ways and to help rule out alternative explanations. In the studies to be described, we treated alcohol intake as a continuous variable, and we define heavier and lighter drinkers with reference to the mean number of drinks the sample reported consuming during a typical week (see Table 10-1).

Mood Immediately after Drinking

In our first test of the LVE model, we related alcohol consumption during a drinking episode to mood after consumption (Muraven et al., 2005b). As outlined above, restrained social drinkers who blame themselves for drinking to excess should experience regret over their alcohol intake. We measured mood in real time, at the start and end of a drinking episode, and related the change in mood over the course of the drinking episode to the amount consumed and attributions made immediately after drinking. From these within-person analyses, we found that mood declined after episodes in which individuals consumed more alcohol than their personal average and engaged in more than average self-blame, compared to episodes in which they consumed less alcohol than average and engaged in less self-blame. Moreover, consistent with the LVE model, this effect was stronger for heavier drinkers than for lighter drinkers, suggesting that heavier drinkers were more sensitive to self-blame.

In the same study, we found that participants' mood after drinking was a predictor of how much alcohol they consumed in their next drinking episode. Consistent with the LVE, following drinking episodes in which participants felt worse than average, they returned to drinking sooner and they consumed more alcohol in their subsequent episode. This was true even after controlling for mood at the start of the next episode, time between episodes, and day of the week. Likewise, participants' self-blame for excessive drinking at the end of one episode was related to how much they consumed in the next episode. Our examination of individual differences further reinforced the predictions of the LVE model. Heavier drinkers drank more in their subsequent episode as compared to lighter drinkers, even when both groups felt equally bad after drinking. This is consistent with the theoretical prediction that negative affect should be more dysregulating to individuals who consume larger amounts of alcohol as compared to lighter drinkers (cf. Cunningham, Sobell, Sobell, et al., 1995; Greeley & Oei, 1999).

Morning after Drinking

Our finding that negative affect influences drinking during an episode was replicated for daily drinking. We examined how feelings and thoughts about drinking one day were related to actual alcohol intake the next day (Muraven et al., 2005a). Across two samples, our within-person analyses indicated that when participants felt that they violated their personal limits (measured just after the drinking episode) by drinking more than average, they experienced greater guilt the next day, even after controlling for hangover symptoms and actual amount consumed. Replicating the episode-level data, we found that the effects of limit violations on mood were stronger for heavier drinkers than for lighter drinkers in each of the two studies.

Reciprocally, guilt led to poorer self-regulation of alcohol intake; greater distress than average over alcohol consumption in the morning was linked to greater alcohol intake, higher levels of intoxication, and more limit violations later that day. Consistent with the LVE model, regret over alcohol intake on the previous day paradoxically led to more alcohol consumption that day. Finally, like the results seen when examining drinking at the episode level, these effects were stronger for individuals who drank more alcohol on average. When heavier drinkers felt guiltier than average in the morning, they consumed more alcohol that day compared to equally guilty lighter drinkers, suggesting that negative affect is more dysregulating for heavier drinkers.

Discussion

Across several levels of analyses and different samples, our use of EMA methods avoided the difficulties found in cross-sectional and laboratory studies and provided strong support for the LVE model. As theorized in the model, we found that negative mood due to excessive drinking was associated with poorer self-regulation of subsequent alcohol intake. We examined the relationship between mood and drinking at both the day level (how drinking one day affected drinking the next day) and episode level (how mood at the end of a drinking episode was related to subsequent drinking). Individuals who drank more than they wanted, and who blamed themselves for that excessive drinking, experienced more negative affect immediately after drinking and the morning after drinking. Consistent with our model of restrained drinking and the LVE, experiencing negative affective states after drinking was dysregulating and was related to greater subsequent alcohol intake, especially for heavier drinkers.

Insights from the Real-Time Approach

To test the LVE model, it was necessary to study the unfolding of processes related to alcohol use in the real world over time. A laboratory study (Collins, Lapp, & Izzo, 1994) had provided a useful first step. However, such studies were limited because of the difficulty of evoking strong emotions in an experiment, the passage of time that is needed for the LVE processes to evolve, and the changes that occur when participants drink in experimental settings (cf. George, Phillips, & Skinner, 1988). The real-time EMA approach allowed us to examine the self-regulation of alcohol intake in a prospective and conceptually meaningful way. Participants regularly interacted with their EDs, thereby providing a steady flow of complex data. Indeed, we could investigate the antecedents of behavior (i.e., excessive drinking) that participants had no idea they were about to engage in and, in fact, wished to avoid. Real-time data capture and the associated data analysis techniques helped to reduce the influence of extraneous variables and allowed for tight control over data collection. As a result, we were able to test our hypotheses in a dynamic manner that would be difficult or impossible using other data collection methods.

Another benefit of EMA data is its ideographic nature. We used a within-subject approach to analyze the antecedents and consequences of alcohol consumption. This approach helped to reduce alternative explanations for the results and permitted a strong statement on how processes occurred within a person. At the same time, the between-subjects analyses provided insight into how these processes differed between people. For example, by collecting many instances of drinking for each participant and comparing the relationship between mood and subsequent consumption across drinkers, we were able to show that negative affect is more dysregulating for heavier drinkers than for lighter drinkers. Obviously, testing such a model in a laboratory setting would be difficult, as it would require recruiting a large number of drinkers.

We had strong conceptual reasons for examining the antecedents and consequences of excessive drinking. These conceptual rationales guided our data analyses as well as the overall methodology, including how the data were collected, when participants were signaled or told to initiate assessments, and the contents of the different interviews. EMA data collection minimized biases, such as memory distortions or concerns about self-presentation, while permitting tight control over data collection. The data helped us to test and develop our model and provided us with opportunities to consider and rule out alternative explanations. For example, all the analyses controlled for day of the week, to help eliminate weekly patterns of drinking such as binge drinking on the weekends. Similarly, when we examined the relationship between reporting a limit violation immediately after drinking and remorse the next morning, we controlled for previous days' alcohol intake and hangover symptoms to get a sense of the effects of limit violation on guilt, beyond the effects of acute physical symptoms or amount consumed.

Successes and Challenges

In this chapter we have described many benefits of the real-time EMA approach, most notably the success of model testing in an ecologically valid manner. In particular, the LVE model posited mechanisms that developed and changed over time and hence required testing in real-world settings. The benefits of EMA methods came with some costs and challenges, which we outline below. Although these challenges are offset by EMA's benefits, they can serve as threats to the external validity of EMA data and can create certain practical problems.

MONITORING BURDEN AND THE GENERALIZABILITY OF RESEARCH FINDINGS

An issue faced by all users of EMA is the potential burden of the frequent and intense monitoring of behavior. As a result of either self-selection related to burden or other criteria, EMA studies may be populated by unique participants who are willing to undergo the training and self-monitoring and therefore are not representative of the populations to which the researcher wishes to generalize. In our studies, some potential participants refused to interact with an ED for 24 hours each day for weeks at a time. On the other hand, many participants enjoyed interacting with their EDs and reported that it helped them to understand their behaviors and feelings and/or that it was fun and interesting.

RELIANCE ON SELF-REPORT

Despite all the strengths of EMA data, ultimately it relies on each participant's self-report. There is evidence that data collected on the computer are more valid than data collected in other ways (Corkrey & Parkinson, 2002). Yet it still would be useful to augment EMA data by collecting behavioral data, collateral reports, or biological data where possible. Although EMA's collection of prospective data enhanced our ability to make causal statements (Shiffman & Stone, 1998), our research relies on correlational analyses and lacks the control conditions that would allow for stronger statements of causality. Advances in hand-held computing may eventually allow for even more dynamic and multifaceted data collection, which could address some of these limitations.

DATA MANAGEMENT AND ANALYSES

The large amount of data generated in our EMA studies presented a challenge, and our examination of how behaviors change over time compounded that problem. In particular, separate databases containing the different assessments (i.e., morning, evening, random prompt, and before and after drinking) needed to be combined. Matching assessments required skillful manipulation of the databases. For example, selecting the random prompt closest to the beginning of a multidrinking episode was a complex, multistep process. Over time, as more sophisticated data analytic approaches (e.g., HLM) become more readily available, they will enhance researchers' abilities to handle the complex data generated using the EMA real-time approach.

PDA HARDWARE AND SOFTWARE

Our use of EMA included some practical challenges, beginning with the personal digital assistant's (PDA) hardware. In the beginning, there were frustrating losses of data because of battery failure or other malfunctions. The relatively low volume of the PDA alarm meant that we could not accommodate participants who worked in noisy environments and reported that they could not hear the random prompts. Random prompting also meant that we had to screen out participants who presented other constraints for using our software. For example, some employees had bosses who would not allow them to respond to the random prompts while at work.

We also experienced challenges specific to assessing drinking behavior. They included (1) how to define a drinking episode, (2) the pharmacological effects of alcohol on cognitive and motor performance, and (3) the drinking and sleeping patterns of our samples of young adults.

DEFINING DRINKING EPISODES

Compliance with entry of each specific drink might be burdensome, might lead to reactivity, and was not necessary to provide data for the model being tested. Therefore, we sought to facilitate self-monitoring by defining an episode of drinking as "the period of time during which you consume alcohol." We then trained participants to self-define when an episode of drinking began and ended by using criteria such as change in their physical surroundings (e.g., going from drinking at home to drinking at a bar), change in activities (drinking while watching TV to drinking while eating), and the passage of time (drinking at lunch vs. dinner). This led to very large ranges in the time between episodes (e.g., 2 minutes to 1 week; Collins et al., 1998) and very large ranges in the number of episodes per participant (e.g., 5 to 58 during 8 weeks; Collins et al., 1998). Although this did not create problems for analyzing our data, it contrasted with other approaches for assessing alcohol intake. For example, Swendsen and colleagues programmed their EMA software to collect drinking data using two different formats

(Swendsen, Tennen, Carney, et al., 2000): participants either could record each drink as it was being consumed or could initiate a program that prompted them once each hour to assess their consumption since the previous prompt 1 hour earlier. At this time, there is no standard way of defining a drinking episode or assessing alcohol intake using EMA. Current approaches need to be evaluated and new approaches need to be developed.

ALCOHOL'S EFFECTS ON COGNITIVE AND MOTOR PERFORMANCE

Imbibing large amounts of alcohol can affect cognitive and motor performance (Fillmore & Vogel Sprott, 1998). Thus, the reliability and validity of EMA data could deteriorate as a function of heavier drinking by research participants. Litt and colleagues (1998) reported that about half of their treated alcoholic sample stopped EMA recording during and after drinking. Our experience with heavier drinkers (e.g., average intake of 22 drinks/week) has not shown the same level of disruption. Collins and colleagues (1998) reported that compliance with initiating the "begin drinking" interview was somewhat better (87% within 1 minute) than compliance with initiating the "end drinking" interview (48% within 1 minute). However, some of this delay may be a function of deciding whether an episode of drinking had truly ended rather than a reflection of the slowing of cognitive and motor functions as a result of high blood-alcohol levels. Even so, researchers should continue to examine the role of the pharmacological effects of alcohol, particularly when blood-alcohol levels are very high.

IRREGULAR DRINKING AND SLEEPING PATTERNS

Many of our samples consisted of young adults whose weekend drinking episodes began around 11 p.m. and ended when the bars closed at 4 a.m. They then went to sleep at around 8 a.m. and woke up around 4 p.m. These wake and sleep patterns created problems for defining a "morning" assessment and for defining and programming a period of sleep for our software. Although we were able to address these problems, particularly during our weekly review of each participant's data printout, they clearly presented some training and interpretational challenges. These challenges may not be unique to assessing drinking, but rather may reflect issues that arise with young adult populations.

Prospects for Application of EMA Methods

We believe that EMA methods represent an important step forward in testing and building a model of alcohol use and abuse. The ability to assess internal and external phenomena as they occur over time, in an ecologically valid manner, presents researchers with the opportunity to study alcohol-related phenomena in much greater detail and to examine hypotheses that heretofore have been difficult or nearly impossible to investigate. Indeed, EMA approaches already have been applied to the examination of other complex and dynamic models of alcohol use and abuse. For example, EMA methods have been successfully applied to testing the self-control strength model (Muraven, Collins, Shiffman, & Paty, 2005) and the self-medication hypothesis (Swendsen et al., 2000) as they pertain to alcohol use.

Muraven, Collins, Shiffman, and Paty (2005) used EMA data to examine whether naturally occurring self-control demands were associated with drinking behavior. The assumption was that the exertion of self-control in daily life may undermine an individual's subsequent ability to use self-control to regulate alcohol intake (cf. Muraven, Collins, & Nienhaus, 2002). Consistent with self-control strength theory (Muraven & Baumeister, 2000; Muraven, Tice, & Baumeister, 1998), they found that participants who experienced greater self-control demands during the day were more likely to drink to excess that night. In addition, experiencing greater than average self-control demands led to more drinking on occasions when the individual planned to limit alcohol intake.

The self-medication hypothesis states that alcohol is used to medicate/relieve negative affective symptoms such as anxiety and depression. The experience of this relief positively reinforces further drinking. Over time, regular intake of large amounts of alcohol in response to negative affective states could explain the comorbidity of alcoholism with mood and anxiety disorders. Consistent with this hypothesis, Swendsen and colleagues (2000) found that negative affect (particularly nervousness) earlier in the evening was associated with drinking later in the night. After drinking, participants reported experiencing less nervousness/negative affect.

The successful use of EMA data to test different conceptual models of alcohol use is only the beginning. The EMA method could easily be applied to clinical contexts to monitor alcohol use and related symptoms during different phases of treatment (cf. Collins et al., 1998). This ongoing self-monitoring could be useful for many different alcohol treatments, including pharmaceutical and/or behavioral interventions. Real-time EMA methods could be applied to assessing changes in symptoms as well as physical and psychological side effects of treatment. In the case of cognitive-behavioral treatment, the flexibility of EMA software makes it possible to develop interactive programs that include suggestions for using specific strategies and/or reminders of goals/outcomes that the individual wants to achieve. The only limits are those imposed by the imagination of the researcher/clinician as well as the hardware and software.

In the future, the platform on which EMA data is collected will likely expand beyond PDAs. Although we pioneered the use of hand-held computers to collect EMA data on drinking and related phenomena (Collins et al., 1998), and saw many benefits to using PDAs, we also became aware of limitations related to storing data and incorporating the technology into the participants' daily lives. Thus, we explored the use of cellular telephones and interactive voice response (IVR) technology as an alternative, more convenient and cost-effective method for collecting EMA data from social drinkers (Collins, Kashdan, & Gollnisch, 2003). For this cellular monitoring, we used a data collection format similar to what we had used with PDAs. Using IVR, we verbally presented our interviews and used a multiple-choice response format, to which the participant responded by pressing a number on the telephone keypad. Participants carried the cellular telephones at all times and when appropriate (either in response to a random prompt or to initiate an interview) used them to call the IVR software on a central computer. The combination of IVR and cellular phones provided participants with the mobility and flexibility to self-monitor in almost any context. Participants were compliant in their use of cellular monitoring, and we found few differences in consumer satisfaction as compared to traditional paper-and-pencil monitoring.

Relative to data collection on PDAs, the benefits of using cellular telephones included the following: (1) pervasive knowledge and use of cellular telephones that lessened the amount of training needed and made it easier to integrate data collection into the participant's daily life; (2) instantaneous entry of data into a central database, thereby limiting data loss and enhancing data storage; (3) the possibility of ongoing monitoring of compliance with the research protocol so as to provide participants with more immediate feedback; and (4) lower software, hardware, and data management costs. These features and benefits provided an alternative to PDAs and expanded upon previous use of IVR and home telephones to collect daily reports of drinking (cf. Searles, Helzer, Rose, & Badger, 2002; Searles, Helzer, & Walter, 2000).

Changes in PDAs and cellular telephones promise many exciting possibilities for the future hardware used to collect EMA data. Recent advances in memory technology (e.g., flash memory) may help forestall data losses from PDAs. It now is possible to present cellular monitoring in text as well as audio formats. Participants can use picture telephones to provide detailed information on their location and/or social context. Who knows what will be possible in a few years? These and other technological advancements will enhance the ability to use EMA methods to reach target populations in real-world contexts and to examine dynamic process related to alcohol use and related behaviors over time.

ACKNOWLEDGMENTS

Our research on the LVE model was supported by Grant AA07595 from the National Institute on Alcohol Abuse and Alcoholism of the National Institutes of Health awarded to R. Lorraine Collins. Our research on the self-control strength model also was supported by Grant AA12770 from the National Institute on Alcohol Abuse and Alcoholism of the National Institutes of Health awarded to Mark Muraven.

References

Bensley, L. S. (1991). Construct validity evidence for the interpretation of drinking restraint as a response conflict. *Addictive Behaviors, 16*, 139–150.

Bensley, L. S., Kuna, P. H., & Steele, C. (1990). The role of drinking restraint success in subsequent alcohol consumption. *Addictive Behaviors, 15*, 491–496.

Broderick, J. E., Schwartz, J. E., Shiffman, S., Hufford, M. R., & Stone, A. A. (2003). Signaling does not adequately improve diary compliance. *Annals of Behavioral Medicine, 26*, 139–148.

Bryk, A. S., Raudenbush, S. W., & Congdon, R. T. (2000). *HLM* (Version 5.0). Chicago: Scientific Software International.

Collins, R. L. (1993). Drinking restraint and risk for alcohol abuse. *Experimental and Clinical Psychopharmacology, 1,* 44–54.

Collins, R. L., Kashdan, T. B., & Gollnisch, G. (2003). The feasibility of using cellular phones to collect ecological momentary assessment data: Application to alcohol consumption. *Experimental and Clinical Psychopharmacology, 11,* 73–78.

Collins, R. L., & Lapp, W. M. (1991). Restraint and attributions: Evidence of the abstinence violation effect in alcohol consumption. *Cognitive Therapy and Research, 15,* 69–84.

Collins, R. L., & Lapp, W. M. (1992). The Temptation and Restraint Inventory for measuring drinking restraint. *British Journal of Addiction, 87,* 107–115.

Collins, R. L., Lapp, W. M., & Izzo, C. V. (1994). Affective and behavioral reactions to the violation of limits on alcohol consumption. *Journal of Studies on Alcohol, 55,* 475–486.

Collins, R. L., Morsheimer, E. T., Shiffman, S., Paty, J. A., Gnys, M., & Papandonatos, G. (1998). Ecological momentary assessment in a behavioral drinking moderation training program. *Experimental and Clinical Psychopharmacology, 6,* 306–315.

Connor, J. P., Young, R. M., Williams, R. J., & Ricciardelli, L. A. (2000). Drinking restraint versus alcohol expectancies: Which is the better indicator of alcohol problems? *Journal of Studies on Alcohol, 61,* 352–359.

Connors, G. J., Collins, R. L., Dermen, K. H., & Koutsky, J. R. (1998). Substance use restraint: An extension of the construct to a clinical population. *Cognitive Therapy and Research, 22,* 87–99.

Corkrey, R., & Parkinson, L. (2002). A comparison of four computer-based telephone interviewing methods: Getting answers to sensitive questions. *Behavior Research Methods, Instruments and Computers, 34,* 354–363.

Cunningham, J. A., Sobell, M. B., Sobell, L. C., Gavin, D. R., & Annis, H. R. (1995). Heavy drinking and negative affective situations in a general population and a treatment sample: Alternative explanations. *Psychology of Addictive Behaviors, 9,* 123–127.

Curry, S., Southwick, L., & Steele, C. (1987). Restrained drinking: Risk factor for problems with alcohol? *Addictive Behaviors, 12,* 73–77.

Fillmore, M. T., & Vogel Sprott, M. (1998). Behavioral impairment under alcohol: Cognitive and pharmacokinetic factors. *Alcoholism: Clinical and Experimental Research, 22,* 1476–1482.

George, W. H., Phillips, S. M., & Skinner, J. B. (1988). Analogue measurements of alcohol consumption: Effects for task type and correspondence with self-report measurement. *Journal of Studies on Alcohol, 49,* 450–455.

Greeley, J., & Oei, T. (1999). Alcohol and tension reduction. In K. E. Leonard & H. T. Blane (Eds.), *Psychological theories of drinking and alcoholism* (Vol. 2, pp. 14–53). New York: Guilford Press.

Kreft, I. G. G., de Leeuw, J., & Aiken, L. S. (1995). The effects of different forms of centering in hierarchical linear models. *Multivariate Behavioral Research, 30,* 1–21.

Litt, M. D., Cooney, N. L., & Morse, P. (1998). Ecological momentary assessment (EMA) with treated alcoholics: Methodological problems and potential solutions. *Health Psychology, 17,* 48–52.

Marlatt, G. A. (1985). Cognitive factors in the relapse process. In G. A. Marlatt & J. R. Gordon (Eds.), *Relapse prevention* (pp. 128–200). New York: Guilford Press.

Marlatt, G. A., & Gordon, J. R. (1980). Determinates of relapse: Implications for the maintenance of behavior change. In P. O. Davidson & S. Davidson, M. (Eds.), *Behavioral medicine: Changing health lifestyles* (pp. 410–452). New York: Brunner/Mazel.

Muraven, M., & Baumeister, R. F. (2000). Self-regulation and depletion of limited resources: Does self-control resemble a muscle? *Psychological Bulletin, 126,* 247–259.

Muraven, M., Collins, R. L., Morsheimer, E. T., Shiffman, S., & Paty, J. A. (2005a). The morning after: Limit violations and the self-regulation of alcohol consumption. *Psychology of Addictive Behaviors, 19,* 253–262.

Muraven, M., Collins, R. L., Morsheimer, E. T., Shiffman, S., & Paty, J. A. (2005b). One too many: Predicting future alcohol consumption following excessive drinking. *Experimental and Clinical Psychopharmacology, 13,* 127–136.

Muraven, M., Collins, R. L., & Nienhaus, K. (2002). Self-control and alcohol restraint: An initial application of the self-control strength model. *Psychology of Addictive Behaviors, 16,* 113–120.

Muraven, M., Collins, R. L., Shiffman, S., & Paty, J. A. (2005). Daily fluctuations in self-control demands and alcohol intake. *Psychology of Addictive Behaviors, 19,* 140–147.

Muraven, M., Tice, D. M., & Baumeister, R. F. (1998). Self-control as a limited resource: Regulatory depletion patterns. *Journal of Personality and Social Psychology, 74,* 774–789.

Ruderman, A. J., & McKirnan, D. (1984). The development of a restrained drinking scale: A test of the abstinence violation effect among alcohol users. *Addictive Behaviors, 9,* 365–371.

Samo, J. A., Tucker, J. A., & Vuchinich, R. D. (1989). Agreement between self-monitoring, recall, and collateral observation measures of alcohol consumption in older adults. *Behavioral Assessment, 11,* 391–409.

Schwartz, J. E., & Stone, A. A. (1998). Strategies for analyzing ecological momentary assessment data. *Health Psychology, 17,* 6–16.

Searles, J. S., Helzer, J. E., Rose, G. L., & Badger, G. J. (2002). Concurrent and retrospective reports of alcohol consumption across 30, 90 and 366 days: Interactive voice response compared with the timeline follow back. *Journal of Studies on Alcohol, 63,* 352–362.

Searles, J. S., Helzer, J. E., & Walter, D. E. (2000). Comparison of drinking patterns measured by daily reports and timeline follow back. *Psychology of Addictive Behaviors, 14,* 277–286.

Shiffman, S. (2000). Real-time self-report of momentary states in the natural environment: Computerized ecological momentary assessment. In A. Stone, J. Turkkan, C. Bachrach, J. Jobe, H. Kurtzman, & V. Cain (Eds). *The science of self-report: Implications for research and practice* (pp. 49–61). Mahwah, NJ: Lawrence Erlbaum Associates, Inc.

Shiffman, S., & Stone, A. A. (1998). Introduction to the special section: Ecological momentary assessment in health psychology. *Health Psychology, 17,* 3–5.

Singer, J. D., & Willett, J. B. (2003). *Applied longitudinal data analysis: Modeling change and event occurrence.* New York: Oxford University Press.

Sobell, M. B., Bogardis, J., Schuller, R., Leo, G. I., & Sobell, L. C. (1989). Is self-monitoring of alcohol consumption reactive? *Behavioral Assessment, 11,* 447–458.

Stone, A. A., & Shiffman, S. (1994). Ecological momentary assessment (EMA) in behavioral medicine. *Annals of Behavioral Medicine, 16,* 199–202.

Stone, A. A., Shiffman, S., Schwartz, J. E., Broderick, J. E., & Hufford, M. R. (2002). Patient non-compliance with paper diaries. *British Medical Journal, 324,* 1193–1194.

Swendsen, J. D., Tennen, H., Carney, M. A., Affleck, G., Willard, A., & Hromi, A. (2000). Mood and alcohol consumption: An experience sampling test of the self-medication hypothesis. *Journal of Abnormal Psychology, 109,* 198–204.

Vuchinich, R. E., Tucker, J. A., & Harllee, L. M. (1988). Behavioral assessment. In D. M. Donovan & G. A. Marlatt (Eds.), *Assessment of addictive behaviors* (pp. 51–83). New York: Guilford Press.

11

Assessing the Impact of Fibromyalgia Syndrome in Real Time

Dennis C. Turk, Tasha Burwinkle, and Melonie Showlund

This chapter presents preliminary data from a study using real-time data capture (RTDC) in a sample of 201 treatment-seeking fibromyalgia syndrome (FMS) patients. FMS consists of a pervasive set of unexplained physical symptoms with generalized pain and hypersensitivity to palpation at specific body locations ("tender points") as the cardinal features. In addition to pain, FMS patients report a range of functional limitations and psychological dysfunction, including fatigue, sleep disturbance, headaches, irritable bowel disorders, depression, and anxiety (Wolfe et al., 1990). FMS sufferers report that although their pain fluctuates in intensity, it is nearly continuous. They also frequently note that although they are often able to engage in physical activities, they experience pain and excessive fatigue at a later point, either later that day or on a subsequent day, and thus tend to avoid as many activities as possible to prevent exacerbation of pain and exhaustion. The majority of studies of FMS ask patients to provide retrospective reports regarding their pain, fatigue, and mood, among others. Such retrospective reports make it difficult to evaluate the stability of symptoms over time and especially the lagged effect of pain, mood, and fatigue on subsequent pain, mood, and fatigue.

There has been a growing concern about the reliance on patients' retrospective reports and the use of paper-and-pencil instruments and diaries to assess thoughts, feelings, and behavior, in general (Stone, Shiffman, Schwartz, et al., 2003). Concerns regarding the validity of the patient reports using these traditional methods and the availability of sophisticated technology have resulted in studies using computerized data acquisition methods. RTDC methods have been used to assess patients with a wide range of problems, including substance abuse (Collins, Morsheimer, Shiffman, et al., 1998; Litt, Cooney, & Morse, 1998), eating disorders (Hufford, Shields, Shiffman, et al., 2002; LeGrange, Gorin, Dymek, & Stone, 2002; Stein & Corte, 2003), smoking cessation (Catley, O'Connell, & Shiffman, 2000; O'Connell, Gerkovich, Cook, et al., 1998), and chronic pain syndromes (Stone, Broderick, Porter, & Kaell, 1997; Stone, Broderick, Schwartz, et al., 2003; Stone, Broderick, Shiffman, & Schwartz, 2004). Recently, RTDC has been used specifically to assess symptoms in patients with FMS (Affleck, Tennen, Urrows, et al., 1998; Gendreau, Hufford, & Stone, 2003; Peters, Sorbi, Kruise, et al., 2000).

Several RTDC studies have addressed issues of particular relevance to understanding the role of physical symptoms (e.g., pain, mood, and fatigue). For example, Stone, Broderick, Porter, Krupp, and colleagues (1994) explored fatigue, mood, and activities in patients with chronic fatigue syndrome (CFS) and found that fatigue was significantly higher in the morning compared to afternoon and evening hours. Additionally, positive mood increased and negative mood decreased throughout the day. In a study with rheumatoid arthritis (RA) patients, Stone, Broderick, Porter, and Kaeli (1997) found that the presence of some sources of stress was associated with increased pain but not fatigue. There were, however, large individual differences in variations of pain and fatigue. Diurnal cycles of pain and fatigue were identified, but only for a subset of participants. The authors suggest that RTDC methodology may help identify subgroups of patients who are highly "psychoreactive" to environmental stimuli and who have diurnal patterns to their symptoms. These studies offer insights into the associations and patterns of symptoms, mood, activity, fatigue, and sleep as assessed over a period of time using RTDC techniques. They also suggest that different syndromes may have different characteristic diurnal patterns, and there may be subgroups with different associations among these variables.

The results of the RTDC studies, however, have not always been consistent. For example, Peters and colleagues (2000) assessed pain, disability, and psychological adaptation for 4 weeks, with recordings obtained four times per day. In contrast to Affleck and colleagues (1998), Peters and colleagues (2000) found that pain increased over the day and was significantly more severe at night than in the morning. Despite this within-day variability, Peters and colleagues (2000) noted that pain reports across the 4 weeks were stable. This contradicts findings by Stone, Broderick, Shiffman, and Schwartz (2004), who reported that average ratings of pain over a 2-week period changed from Week 1 to Week 2, with 40 percent rating their pain as greater on the second compared to first week.

Although the RTDC studies often used aggregated within-day time periods (e.g., time of day; morning, afternoon, evening) (Affleck et al., 1998; Peters et al., 2000; Stone et al., 1994), daily (O'Connell et al., 1998; Cruise, Broderick, Porter, et al., 1996; Stone et al., 1994), or weekly RTDC scores (Gendreau et al., 2003; Peters et al., 2000; Stone et al., 2004) in the reporting of results, none of these studies reported on the consistency of the patterns of pain, mood, and fatigue over different days (e.g., weekdays vs. weekends; weekday on subsequent weekend days, or weekend day on subsequent weekday) and weeks. However, Peters and colleagues (2000) did examine trends in responding for pain intensity over 4 weeks, and Stone and colleagues (2004) assessed the "consistency" of change scores over 2 consecutive weeks. One advantage of RTDC is that it permits examination of lagged effects both within days and between days (or series of days). Moreover, longitudinal assessment over many days and weeks permits replication of any patterns observed. This is of particular interest in FMS as patients report that activities on one day greatly influence pain and fatigue on subsequent days. Thus, the use of RTDC offers potential to improve the validity of patient reports and provides a useful vehicle for addressing the stability and lagged effects of pain, mood, and fatigue that are particularly important in FMS.

Rationale for a RTDC Approach to Data Collection

With few exceptions, the assessment of FMS patient symptoms has relied on paper-and-pencil questionnaires or patient diaries or journals (daily or weekly). These methods, however, are prone to a number of methodological issues, particularly the influence of recall bias (Gendreau et al., 2003; Stone & Shiffman, 2002). At least one study has reported that 79 percent of paper diaries contain falsified information (Stone & Shiffman, 2002), which calls into question the validity of the results derived from this form of assessment. The advantages of RTDC have been discussed in several papers (Gendreau et al., 2003; Stone & Shiffman, 2002) and in other chapters in this volume; thus, we will not reiterate them here.

In this chapter we report on preliminary results of a subset of data collected as part of an ongoing study designed to address important issues in FMS making use of the RTDC methodology. In particular, what is the pattern of pain, mood, and fatigue scores within days; what are the "lagged" effects of pain, mood, and fatigue over 2 consecutive days; what are the "lagged" effects of pain, mood, and fatigue from weekdays to weekends; and what are the patterns of pain, mood, and fatigue of FMS patients over a 2-week period? We hypothesized that:

- Based on patients' reports, patterns of pain and fatigue would be stable throughout the day and between days, weekends, and weeks both within and between participants, and we hypothesized that mood would be more variable.
- Pain severity and mood would be significantly correlated, both within days and between days, and within and between participants.
- For within-days analysis, greater pain severity at Time 1 (morning) within 1 day would predict more dysphoric mood at Time 2 (afternoon), and more dysphoric mood at Time 2 (afternoon) would predict greater pain severity at Time 3 (evening).
- For between-days analysis, greater pain severity on Day 1 would predict more dysphoric mood and more fatigue on Day 2.
- For weekday–weekend analysis, greater pain severity on weekdays would predict more dysphoric mood and fatigue on weekends. Finally, for Week 1–Week 2 analysis, greater pain severity on Week 1 would predict greater dysphoric mood and fatigue on Week 2.

- There would be a low and nonsignificant correlation between data collected for pain, mood, and fatigue on RTDC and retrospective reports of these variables.

Sample

A potential sample of 201 consecutive women seeking treatment for FMS was invited to participate in this study, which was initiated in November 1998. All participants met the American College of Rheumatology criteria of FMS (i.e., widespread pain of 3 months' duration and pain on palpation of 11 or 18 designated tender points), were between the ages of 18 and 60, were fluent in English, and did not suffer from a major psychiatric disorder.

Eighteen (9%) of the eligible participants refused to participate and 28 (14%) of the eligible sample lived in areas not covered by the paging service (see below) required to receive prompts and thus had to be eliminated from further participation. Aggregating these data, 23 percent of those eligible for participation were lost, resulting in a total sample of 155. The reasons given by those who declined included (1) thought it was too intrusive, (2) thought it was inconvenient to have to return to the research facility twice to upload data, (3) were uncomfortable with the technology, and (4) were unwilling to accept responsibility for the computer.

Because the purpose of this study was to look specifically at consecutive days, only participants who provided data for both consecutive sets of days (weekdays and weekend days) were included. Based on this criterion, six eligible participants (3%) were deleted from the analyses. In sum, the final sample included in the analyses described below is 149 (74% of the original eligible sample). Table 11-1 displays the demographic information for the final sample.

Some of the analyses involved a replication between Week 1 and Week 2. For this set of analyses, it was essential that complete data for 4 days (2 consecutive days on each of 2 consecutive weeks) be available. One hundred nine participants (73% of 149) met this criterion. Thus, for the week-to-week comparisons (reported below) only 109 (54%) of the original 201 eligible participants could be included.

Method

Potential participants were recruited from physicians in the community (FMS) and by media and community announcements (FMS and controls). In addition, a number of FMS sufferers learned of the study by word of mouth. The data were gathered between November 1998 and July 2003. A physician examined all patients to determine whether they met the criteria for FMS (Wolfe et al., 1990). They also completed a medical history and a set of self-report questionnaires

Table 11-1. Sample demographics

	n	percent		n	percent
ETHNICITY			MARITAL STATUS		
White	137	91.9	Married	75	50.3
African American	5	3.4	Separated/Divorced	40	26.8
Native American	1	0.7	Single, Never Married	28	18.8
Latino	1	0.7	Widowed	3	2.0
Other	4	2.7	Missing	3	2.0
Missing	1	0.7			
EDUCATION			ANNUAL HOUSEHOLD INCOME		
Master's degree or higher	12	8.1	$70,000 or more	33	22.1
College degree	51	34.2	$60,000–$69,999	13	8.7
Some college	49	32.9	$50,000–$59,999	22	14.8
Trade/Tech/Voc	19	12.8	$40,000–$49,999	9	6.0
High school graduate	14	9.4	$30,000–$39,999	19	12.8
10th–12th grade completed	4	2.7	$20,000–$29,999	16	10.7
			$10,000–$19,999	15	10.1
			Less than $10,000	16	10.7
MPI SUBGROUP			Missing	6	3.9
Dysfunctional	37	24.8			
Interpersonally distressed	55	36.9	Mean age = 44.58 years (SD = 10.77; Range = 21–65)		
Adaptive coper	38	25.5	Mean Sx months = 127.25 (SD = 110.42;		
Anomalous	12	8.1	Range = 1–532)		
Hybrid	6	4.0			
Missing	1	0.7			

Trade = Trade School; Tech = Technical School; Voc = Vocational School; Mean Sx Months = mean number of months since symptom onset.

(i.e., Multidimensional Pain Inventory [MPI], Kerns, Turk, & Rudy, 1985; Fibromyalgia Impact Questionnaire [FIQ] Burckhardt, Clark, & Bennett, 1991; Center for Epidemiological Studies Depression Scale [CESD], Radloff, 1977).

Palmtop Computer

Participants were provided with a Palm Pilot Professional "Connected Organizer," a commercially available device with a cover and stylus. Software for the palmtop computer was developed by Form Master, Inc., Columbia, Maryland. Patients were asked to complete the following questions: (1) current pain severity, (2) current level of emotional distress, (3) current level of fatigue, (4) current activity (e.g., sitting, standing), (5) category of activity (work-related, leisure), (6) who present at time of responding (spouse, coworker), (7) current state of relaxation, and (8) current level of body tension and stiffness.

Only responses to questions 1 through 3 ("pain," "mood," and "fatigue") are reported here. Each question had a 7-point Likert response scale (e.g., 0 = no pain, 6 = worst pain). The maximum number of questions per screen was two. These questions were derived from previously published pain questionnaires, were specifically prepared to address the questions of interest in the present study, and were based on questions used in previous studies of FMS. The psychometric properties of the set of questions were not specifically tested; however, this approach is commonly reported in other studies using RTDC (e.g., Cruise et al., 1996; Stone et al., 2004). The protocol and methods were pretested on five FMS patients and five healthy controls to test for ease of use and software utility. This process revealed no problems with the methodology.

Training

All participants met with a research associate during scheduled pretreatment evaluations and received approximately 30 minutes of training regarding the procedure involved in operating the computer, changing batteries, strategies to improve the ease and accuracy of the computer, and responding to the paging prompts and questions. During the training, each participant completed the entire set of questions included in each prompted interval during the 2-week trial to confirm that she could use the technology and software and understood the procedure and specific questions.

Participants were provided with a seven-page instructional guide summarizing the procedure covered during the training session and a contact number to call if any problems arose (copies are available upon request). Some have suggested that participants need up to 90 minutes of training (Stone et al., 2004), but we found that they understood the procedures and had sufficient time to practice and ask questions with only 30 minutes of training.

Protocol

Recordings were scheduled three times a day (once in the morning [between 8 a.m. and noon; AM], afternoon [between noon and 4 p.m.; AFT], and evening [between 4 and 8 p.m.; PM], with consecutive ratings scheduled to occur no closer than 2 hours apart) for 14 days. Participants indicated their time of waking and preparing for bed so that no prompts would be provided while they were sleeping. This customization was included in an effort to increase adherence and to prevent premature termination from the study if the prompting was disruptive to usual sleep–wake cycles, a particular problem for FMS patients who indicate problems with sleep. The total number of prompts was 42.

A pager card was installed in each palmtop computer and prompts to respond were administered by a private paging company, Weblink Wireless in Seattle,

Washington. The contracted company was provided with a "prompting" schedule for each participant based on a randomized schedule that took into account participant sleep patterns.

Participants responded to each presented question by using a stylus provided for use with the palmtop computer and pressing down onto the number that corresponded with their selected response. Data from all responses were subsequently stored in the palmtop computer and uploaded (using the hot sync software provided with the Palm Pilot) to an Excel file at the participant's next visit. The software recorded the time and date of each entry. Because averaging of a 7-day period may mask fluctuations in pain, the analyses reported in this chapter were designed so that we could examine within-day (e.g., morning, afternoon, and evening) and between-consecutive-day fluctuations in pain intensity, mood, and fatigue. Analyses of additional days and consecutive weekdays will be examined in the future. The relationships between pain severity, mood, and fatigue from day to day, from weekdays to weekend days, and from one week to the next (e.g., does pain on one day affect mood on the next day, and so on) were also of interest.

The protocol outlined was selected for several reasons. Since the study was particularly interested in the patterns among the variables, a recording period of 14 days was selected. This would permit examination of lagged effects (e.g., day-to-day, weekday-to-weekend, week-to-week) with multiple replications. Moreover, it would permit examination of differences in weekdays, weekends, and the influence of weekdays on weekends and the converse. Only 8 of these 14 days (e.g., 2 consecutive weekdays, and 2 consecutive weekend days for the 2 weeks of the study) are reported in this chapter. Figures 11-1 and 11-2 display the potential

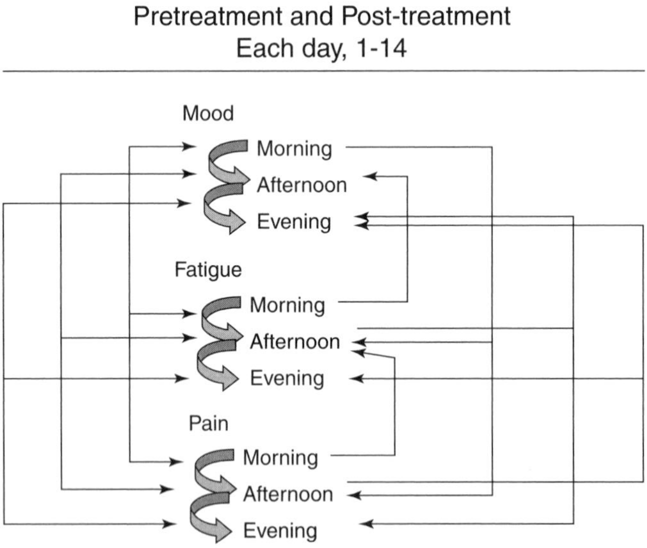

Figure 11-1. Potential comparisons—within days.

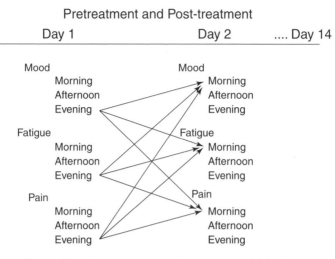

Figure 11-2. Potential comparisons over multiple days.

questions that could be addressed by the design of the study, as noted; however, only selective analyses that address questions of particular interest are reported here.

The interval of three times per day, rather than more frequently, was selected to balance the intrusiveness of the recording with the momentary interest of the associations. The possible reactive effects of repeated assessment was also a consideration. For example, by drawing attention to pain and activity with excessive frequency, the procedure itself might influence responses (e.g., alter activity levels and raise pain severity by repeatedly drawing participants' attention to their pain). There are also some data to suggest that FMS patients believe that their symptoms change at least three times per day (Affleck et al., 1998). Once participants were prompted by the pager signal, they were allowed 5 minutes to respond. If they did not respond in this time period they were prompted a second time. If they failed to respond to the second prompt, they were prompted a third time. If they did not respond to any of the three prompts in the specified time period, the data were treated as missing. A random interval within blocks of time protocol was employed to circumvent patients' expectations about the time approaching for a rating. Patients were permitted to indicate in advance if some times for a particular event were inconvenient (e.g., nap time), and we attempted to accommodate the patients' usual schedules.

Data from the palmtop computer were aggregated over 1-week periods. Participants returned to the Fibromyalgia Research Center at the end of the first and second week of the trial, when data were uploaded from the palmtop computer to the master computer, which contained an Excel database.

Data Reduction

Data were aggregated in several ways to address the questions of interest in this study. Data were initially aggregated within days to examine the patterns of pain, mood, and fatigue over the 14-day period. Data were also aggregated by time of day to identify patterns among morning (AM), afternoon (AFT), and evening (PM) responding. Two weekday intervals and 2 weekend day intervals were selected using the second interval to replicate the patterns observed in the first pair of days.

Two consecutive weekdays and 2 consecutive weekend days were included for purposes of replication. However, an issue encountered was that participants initiated recording on different days of the week. This procedure was implemented to balance this fact with consideration of practice effects—that is, if recordings could not begin until participants had at least 1 full practice day, too large a quantity of data would be lost. Since 2 midweek days (Tuesday and Wednesday) were selected, any participant who began recording on Wednesday, Thursday, or Friday would not have a period of 2 consecutive midweek days. Thus, the 1-day practice criteria were relaxed to permit analyses regarding questions concerning weekday and weekend replications.

The nature of RTDC permits a substantial number of analyses, as there are multiple assessments over time (see Figures 11-1 and 11-2). Prior studies discussed in this chapter and described throughout this volume have used correlations, paired *t*-tests, repeated measures ANOVA, and regression analysis applied to RTDC data, indicating a number of varied approaches to data analysis (Gendreau et al., 2003). These studies were used as models for the data analysis, while we kept in mind that there are limitations to each of the approaches (see Stone & Shiffman, 1994; Gendreau et al., 2003; & Jaccard & Wan, 1993, for more extensive discussion about statistical procedures).

Although an extensive number of analyses could be presented, only an overview of findings for time of day, between 2 consecutive days, between weekdays and weekends, and between Week 1 and Week 2 of the assessment are presented. The data analyses selected modeled techniques described in other studies. These include correlational analyses, paired *t*-tests, repeated measures ANOVA, and regressions for various analyses (each of these is discussed more specifically in the "Results" section). This approach will permit demonstration of various approaches to data analysis using RTDC data. There are of course many other approaches reported in the literature (e.g., multilevel modeling; Singer, 1998).

Results

Availability of Data

One problem encountered in this study was with the contracted paging service. Some participants were prompted inconsistently. For example, on one day, they were prompted to respond at all three time periods (morning, afternoon, and evening), while on another day they were prompted only twice (morning, evening). In addition to the problem of participants receiving the prompts on the predetermined schedule, some participants may have either not heard the prompt or chose not to respond. We could not distinguish between these possibilities in accounting for the missing data. Therefore, caution is necessary so as not to attribute the loss to participant nonadherence.

As a result of these problems, significant amounts of data were unavailable for analysis. For example, of the total number of assessments that were possible (149 participants $\times$ 24 prompts $\times$ 8 days $\times$ 3 times per day = 3,576), participants responded to only 1,776 (49.7%) prompts. Stone and Shiffman (1994) suggest that a criterion of 80 percent should be used for determining that participant responses were valid. Using this criterion, to be an appropriate responder in the present study a participant would have had to respond to at least 19 prompts (24 prompts/day $\times$ 8 days). If that criterion had been used, only 10 of the 149 (7%) of the participants would have been included in the analyses.

The Stone and Shiffman criteria were not used in the analyses reported because had they been, the number of participants included would have been so small and potentially so atypical as to preclude drawing conclusions about FMS patients with any degree of confidence. Consequently, all of the analyses presented are based on the 149 participants, regardless of whether they met the 80 percent criterion. As a result of this decision and the participant attrition previously noted, interpretation of all results should be made with extreme caution. The analyses illustrate some of the potential of RTDC data and a range of strategies that can be used to analyze the data that accrued.

Analyses for Time of Day

Table 11-2 shows ratings for pain, mood, and fatigue during each of the three time periods (AM, AFT, PM) for the 8 days (two each for Wednesday, Thursday, Saturday, and Sunday). Repeated measures ANOVAs revealed no significant differences for time of day for any of the days assessed, except for mood on Thursday (AFT > PM, $p < 0.05$). Given the large number of analyses, this result may be spurious. Thus, it appears that participants' ratings of pain, mood, and fatigue are relatively stable throughout the day.

Correlations between pain, mood, and fatigue for each time period indicate that for every day assessed, and across all time intervals, pain and fatigue were more highly correlated (r range = .39–65) than pain and mood (r range = .22–.48) or mood and fatigue (r range = .20–.47). Additionally, correlations between each time period (e.g., AM–AFT, AFT–PM, AM–PM) for pain, mood, and fatigue were calculated. There were no observable differences among correlations between time periods for AM–AFT (r range = .36–67), AFT–PM (r range = .27 –66), or AM–PM (r range = .30–64).

Multiple regression analyses were also conducted to determine whether morning pain, mood, or fatigue could predict pain, mood, or fatigue in the afternoon.

Table 11-2. Mean pain, mood, and fatigue scores by time of day

	AM	AFT	PM
Pain			
Wednesday	3.26	2.90	3.01
Thursday	2.98	3.08	2.86
Saturday	2.88	2.90	2.75
Sunday	2.94	2.90	3.08
Mood			
Wednesday	1.77	1.96	2.03
Thursday	1.92	2.19	1.75
Saturday	1.61	1.75	1.80
Sunday	1.93	1.81	1.90
Fatigue			
Wednesday	3.68	3.63	3.77
Thursday	3.32	3.42	3.46
Saturday	3.10	3.38	3.70
Sunday	3.22	3.14	3.50

Likewise, morning and afternoon pain, mood, and fatigue were explored to determine if they predicted these variables in the evening—"lagged" effects. In these analyses, pain, mood, and fatigue were entered separately in each predictive model. Table 11-3 lists the significant predictors in each regression, in addition to the cumulative R^2 (to show the amount of variance accounted for by the total model with all predictors) and the R^2 change (to display the amount of variance accounted for by the specific predictor).

In summary, for this subset of analyses, AM pain was a significant predictor of AFT pain, AM mood was a significant predictor of AFT mood, and AM fatigue and pain were significant predictors of AFT fatigue. Both AM and AFT pain predicted PM pain, and AM and AFT mood also predicted PM mood. Somewhat surprisingly, AM and AFT fatigue were not significant predictors of PM fatigue; instead, AM pain, AM mood, and AFT mood all predicted PM fatigue.

Analyses for Days

In addition to within-day time analysis (presented above), scores for pain, mood, and fatigue across days for Week 1 of assessment were examined. Scores for each day represent aggregated scores from all three time periods assessed (AM, AFT, PM). However, daily scores were conducted only for patients who responded to at least two of the possible three prompts throughout the day. If a patient responded to only one prompt (e.g., only the AM prompt), the daily score was not included in the analysis. Figure 11-3 shows the distribution of scores across days.

Repeated measures ANOVAs indicated no significant difference in daily scores for pain ($F = 2.01$, $p = 0.12$; Greenhouse-Geisser corrected F value used

Table 11-3. Regression results– significant predictors

Predictor variables and step	Significant predictors	Cumulative R^2 (total model)	R^2 Change (% accounted for)	Beta	SE
OUTCOME VARIABLES: WITHIN DAY					
AFT Pain	AM Pain	0.38	0.38^3	0.59^3	0.10
AFT Mood	AM Mood	0.14	0.08^1	0.35^1	0.16
AFT Fatigue	AM Fatigue	0.27	0.13^2	0.41^1	0.14
	AM Pain	0.13	0.13^2	0.35^1	0.13
PM Pain	AM Pain	0.21	0.21^2	0.50^2	0.16
	AFT Pain	0.34	0.13^1	0.48^1	0.19
PM Mood	AM Mood	0.26	0.26^2	0.56^2	0.16
	AFT Mood	0.55	0.29^3	0.58^3	0.13
PM Fatigue	AM Pain	0.20	0.17^1	0.62^1	0.24
	AM Mood	0.33	0.13^1	0.52^1	0.22
	PM Mood	0.56	0.23^2	0.57^2	0.15
OUTCOME VARIABLES: BETWEEN DAYS					
THU Pain	WED Pain	0.32	0.32^3	0.62^3	0.08
THU Mood	WED Mood	0.28	0.28^3	0.51^3	0.07
THU Fatigue	WED Fatigue	0.16	0.16^3	0.40^3	0.08
OUTCOME VARIABLES: BETWEEN WEEKDAYS AND WEEKENDS					
WEND Pain	WDAY Pain	0.22	0.22^3	0.42^3	0.07
	WDAY Fatigue	0.26	0.04^1	0.24^1	0.10
WEND Mood	WDAY Mood	0.21	0.21^3	0.48^3	0.09
WEND Fatigue	WDAY Fatigue	0.20	0.20^3	0.50^3	0.09
OUTCOME VARIABLES: BETWEEN WEEK 1 AND WEEK 2					
WK2 Pain	WK1 Pain	0.41	0.41^3	0.65^3	0.08
WK2 Mood	WK1 Mood	0.32	0.32^3	0.76^3	0.11
WK2 Fatigue	WK1 Fatigue	0.35	0.35^3	0.67^3	0.09

[1] $p < 0.05$, [2] $p < 0.01$, [3] $p < 0.001$; B = Beta, SE = Standard Error, AM= morning, AFT = afternoon, PM = evening, WED = Wednesday, THU = Thursday, WDAY = weekday, WEND = weekend, WK1 = week 1, WK2 = week 2.

due to significant Mauchley's test of sphericity) or mood ($F = 1.25$, $p = 0.29$). There was, however, a significant difference in daily scores for fatigue ($F = 6.91$, $p < 0.001$). Post-hoc analysis revealed that fatigue scores on Day 1 (Wednesday) were significantly higher than scores for the other 3 days. Pearson correlations among the three measures for each day were also calculated. As with correlations by time of day (presented above), correlations between pain and fatigue were

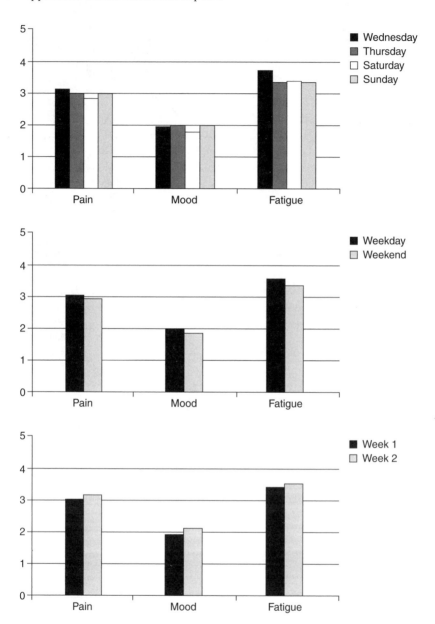

Figure 11-3. Pain, mood, and fatigue across days, weekdays/weekends, weeks.

greater (r range = .55–59) than correlations between pain and mood (r range = .27–.45) and mood and fatigue (r range = .35–.44).

Multiple regression analysis, with daily scores of pain, mood, and fatigue from 1-day predicting scores for the following day (Table 11-3), was also calculated.

Results indicate that Wednesday pain, mood, and fatigue were significant predictors of Thursday pain, mood, and fatigue, respectively.

Analyses for Weekday Versus Weekend

Scores were also evaluated for differences between weekdays and weekends. Wednesday and Thursday scores were aggregated for "weekday" scores; Saturday and Sunday scores were aggregated for "weekend" scores. Weekday ratings preceded weekend ratings in all instances and all scores were from the first week of assessment. Figure 11-3 displays differences for weekdays and weekends.

Paired t-test analysis indicated no significant differences between weekday and weekend scores for pain or mood, although there was a significant difference for fatigue ($t = 3.00$, $p < 0.01$). Although this difference was significant, it is small and is likely not clinically meaningful, as there was only a .20 difference in scores (fatigue = 3.56 for "weekday," 3.36 for "weekend") on a 7-point scale.

Pearson correlations between weekday and weekend scores were for pain, $r = .47$; mood, $r = .46$; and fatigue, $r = .45$. All correlations were significant at $p < 0.001$. Multiple regression analysis to predict weekend scores from weekday scores (Table 11-3) was conducted. Results indicate that weekday pain and weekday fatigue were significant predictors of weekend pain, weekday mood was a significant predictor of weekend mood, and weekday fatigue was a significant predictor of weekend fatigue.

Week 1 to Week 2 Analyses

Differences in scores from Week 1 of assessment to Week 2 were also explored. All scores from weekdays and weekends for Week 1 were aggregated, as were scores for Week 2. Figure 11-3 shows these differences.

Paired t-test analyses indicated significant differences from Week 1 to Week 2 for pain ($t = -2.04$, $p < 0.05$) and mood ($t = -2.46$, $p < 0.05$), with scores for Week 2 being higher than scores for Week 1. However, these differences, although significant, are likely not clinically meaningful, as the difference in mean scores for pain was 0.15 and for mood was 0.26. There were no significant differences between Week 1 and Week 2 for fatigue. Pearson correlations between Week 1 and Week 2 (pain = .64, mood = .57, and fatigue = .59) were all significant at $p < 0.001$. Multiple regression analysis (Table 11-3) to predict Week 2 scores from Week 1 scores indicated that Week 1 pain was a significant predictor of Week 2 pain, Week 1 mood was a significant predictor of Week 2 mood, and Week 1 fatigue was a significant predictor of Week 2 fatigue.

Real-Time Data Capture Versus Retrospective Recall

In an effort to determine whether aggregated daily rating to create weekly scores differed from other weekly recall measures, correlations were calculated between the aggregated weekly RTDC data and responses to other measures of

Table 11-4. RTDC assessment correlated with measures with weekly recall

	MPI Pain	FIQ Pain	FIQ Depress	FIQ Anx	CESD	FIQ Fatigue
WEEK 1						
RTDC						
pain	0.58	0.47				
mood			0.51	0.42	0.42	
fatigue						0.39
WEEK 2						
RTDC						
pain	0.44	0.30				
mood			0.46	0.33	0.39	
fatigue						0.36

pain, mood, and fatigue with a 1-week recall period (MPI Pain Severity Scale, Kerns et al., 1985; FIQ Pain, Anxiety, Depression, and Fatigue Scales, Burckhardt et al., 1991; and the CESD, Radloff, 1977). Table 11-4 presents the correlations between these measures for both Week 1 and Week 2 of assessment with RTDC data.

Paired t-tests between RTDC weekly scores and MPI pain, FIQ depression, and FIQ fatigue (after obtaining standardized z-scores due to different scoring methods for these measures) indicate that RTDC weekly pain (mean = 3.0, SD = 0.88) was significantly different than the retrospective report (MPI Pain Severity scale mean = 3.84, SD = 1.00) for pain severity, paired t-test: $t = -11.72$, $p < 0.001$. Since the FIQ and CESD data use a different scale than used for the question presented on the computers, we converted the scores on mood and fatigue to standard scores. The results for mood and fatigue were not significantly different.

Multiple regression analysis was used to explore whether scores from Week 1 would predict scores from Week 2. Results from the regression indicate that Week 1 pain was a significant predictor of Week 2 pain (R^2 change = .41, $p < 0.001$), Week 1 mood was a significant predictor of Week 2 mood (R^2 change = .32, $p < 0.001$), and Week 1 fatigue was a significant predictor of Week 2 fatigue (R^2 change = 0.35, $p < 0.001$).

Discussion

The results of this study confirmed only one of the original six hypotheses concerning the relationships among pain, mood, and fatigue across time in FMS patients. The first hypothesis was based on FMS patient reports that their pain and fatigue were relatively stable. The results confirmed that not only pain and fatigue but also mood was relatively stable within days, between days, and between weeks. Scores for these variables were not significantly different (e.g., they were stable) across time, regardless of whether the time period assessed was within 1 day, between 2 consecutive days, between weekdays and weekends, or between 2 consecutive weeks.

The results of the within-day analyses differed from findings in other studies. Peters and colleagues (2000), for example, found that pain in chronic pain patients increased over the day and was significantly more severe at night than in the morning. In a study with RA patients, Stone and colleagues (1994) also found diurnal cycles of pain and fatigue, but only for a subset of participants. Stone and colleagues (1994) also found in a sample of patients with CFS that fatigue was significantly higher in the morning compared to afternoon and evening hours. Furthermore, positive mood increased and negative mood decreased from morning to evening hours.

The between-day and between-week findings are similar to those reported by Cruise and colleagues (1996), who demonstrated no significant differences in pain or mood across a series of days for RA patients, and Peters and colleagues (2000), who found stable pain reports across a 4-week period in chronic pain patients. These findings, however, contradict other studies of chronic pain populations. Stone and colleagues (2004), for example, reported that pain intensity the second week was higher than ratings obtained during the first week for a significant proportion of chronic pain patients.

It may be that the sample of FMS patients in the present study reported more stability in physical and psychological symptoms than patients with other chronic pain conditions that may have more symptom variability. For example, there is likely more variability in pain severity for patients with chronic headache or RA, for whom symptoms fluctuate throughout the day. On the other hand, Cruise and colleagues (1996) postulated that certain subsets of patients may be so accustomed to their pain that attending to it exerts little, if any, influence in their experiences of pain or mood. This may very well be the case for patients with FMS, who are known to experience widespread, generalized pain on a consistent basis.

At minimum, our results suggest that the FMS patients included in the current study are reasonably accurate when they state that their pain is relatively stable. These patients report that they frequently are fatigued and they may avoid activities that they believe will produce incapacitating fatigue. This may result in fairly stable levels of fatigue. The associations between fatigue and activities in future analyses of the data that have been collected will be examined in the future. The stability in mood was less expected. We expected that mood would be more situationally dependent. It appears that FMS patients' mood remains fairly consistent and they are moderately distressed most of the time—within days, over consecutive days, and across weeks.

The results failed to confirm the hypothesis that pain severity and mood would be significantly correlated. The results are, however, consistent with a study reported by Rudy, Kearns, and Turk (1988) showing that the association between pain and depression was mediated by chronic pain patients' perceptions regarding the impact of pain on their activities and their sense of control over their pain. Potential mediators of this association were not examined but will be in future analyses.

Larger, significant correlation coefficients were found between pain and fatigue than between pain and mood, both for scores within 1 day and for scores between 2 consecutive days. These results are consistent with Nicassio, Moxham, Schuman, and Gevirtz (2002), who used patient diaries and determined that although pain was correlated with fatigue, it did not independently contribute to fatigue.

The results of the multiple regression analysis failed to confirm the third hypothesis regarding the predictive nature of pain severity on mood and fatigue. At least in this sample, it does not appear that pain severity predicts either mood or fatigue, across all time conditions (within 1 day, between 2 consecutive days, between weekdays and weekends, and between Week 1 and Week 2). These findings can be contrasted with those of Nicassio and colleagues (2002), who found that the previous day's pain and sleep quality in patients with RA predicted fatigue the next day. These inconsistent results require further investigation and may be accounted for by the methods used to assess pain, fatigue, and mood, the nature of the symptoms in the samples included, and the wording of the questions.

One benefit of this study was the exploration of differences across time of day. Only one other study of which we are aware (Stone et al., 1994) investigated diurnal patterns in outcome variables (in this case, mood), although there were only 8 CFS patients and 15 controls. A novel approach to the data analytic strategy was undertaken in this report. No other study reviewed used regression analysis to predict pain, mood, or fatigue scores at a future time period (whether later in the day, subsequent days, subsequent weekends, or subsequent weeks) using earlier scores. Affleck and colleagues (1998) used regression to predict goal processes on future days using earlier sleep, pain, and fatigue as predictors. Although we found little meaningful information from this approach (likely due to the stability of scores in this population), it suggests yet another way to conceptualize RTDC data.

Missing Responses

We emphasized throughout this chapter that we had a great deal of missing data, so interpretation of all of the results must be done with caution. Stone and Shiffman (2002) suggested that a criterion of 80 percent should be used to determine the validity of the data. The data from any participant who fails to meet this criterion should, therefore, be excluded from the analyses. In this study the number of possible ratings was 72 (8 days × 3 prompts/day × 3 questions). Using the 80 percent criterion, only participants who responded to 58 percent or more of the potential questions in this study should be included. If the 80 percent criterion was used, only 10 of the original 149 eligible participants would have been included. It is important to note that the large percentage of missing data is unusual when compared to other studies that have used RTDC. The explanation for this discrepancy is unclear.

The reasons for missing data may be associated with the paging service, malfunctioning hardware, the inability to detect the prompt, or a conscious decision on the part of the patient not to respond. To reiterate a previous comment, since we cannot distinguish among these possibilities, we cannot infer that patient nonadherence accounted for any or even a significant amount of the missing data.

The number of missing responses for each day and time period in which data were collected was examined. In general, there was no distinct pattern of missing responses detectable (e.g., there was no statistically larger percentage of missing responses during weekdays vs. weekends).

Insights Gained from a Real-Time Approach

Perhaps the most surprising finding in this study was the statistically significant correlations between the RTDC data and the retrospective reports of pain, fatigue, and mood. The correlational results are consistent with an earlier study using daily ratings and retrospective reports of a heterogeneous sample of chronic pain patients (Salovey, Sieber, Smith, & Turk, 1992). Nevertheless, the magnitude of correlations suggests that RTDC assessment and retrospective methods are not interchangeable. In fact, Stone and colleagues (2004) suggest that momentary measures of change may not be measuring the same construct as recall measures. Stone and colleagues (2004) also state, however, that validation studies of each method need to be conducted, although they acknowledge that this will be a "complex difficult task, involving discriminant and convergent validation with other measures (behavioral, physiological, observer) that are related in various ways to the construct." Thus, additional work is needed to evaluate the differences between RTDC assessment and retrospective assessment.

There was also a significant difference between the retrospective ratings and mean RTDC ratings of pain severity, with the retrospective pain ratings on average 27 percent higher than the RTDC data, supporting the concerns raised about the validity of such recall measures. However, this conclusion must be tempered once again by the observation that there was an extensive amount of missing data that may have underestimated the actual pain experienced. For example, as Stone and Shiffman (2002) noted, when patients' levels of pain are high, they may ignore prompts; as a result, their average ratings will appear to be lower than their actual pain experienced. In contrast to the pain data, no significant differences between the RTDC and retrospective ratings of mood or fatigue were found in the current study.

Based on the RTDC approach, it appears that the sample of FMS patients included in the current study does, in fact, have stable symptoms across time. If scores for FMS patients are stable across time, then the time and effort expended to use RTDC methods may be less beneficial than for other populations. The observation that on average the retrospective reports rated pain as 27 percent greater does support the concerns raised about the validity of such recall measures. However, this conclusion must be tempered by the fact that the data presented are aggregated over the entire sample. It is possible that the stability observed was not consistent across all participants. Future analyses should examine individual participant stability, as there may be different patterns detected. The data on the stability must also be mitigated by the observation that there was an extensive amount of missing data that may have underestimated the actual pain experienced. In contrast to the pain data, no significant differences between the RTDC and retrospective ratings of mood or fatigue were found.

There are some controversial findings regarding RTDC versus weekly ratings. One study with a small sample ($n = 14$) of FMS patients (Gendreau et al., 2003) found variability in pain scores from day to day, and the authors advocate for the use of RTDC data, arguing that creating a weekly aggregated score will likely be inaccurate, resulting in errant conclusions based on this score. Significant variability in pain severity within day, between days, or between weeks, was not found in the current study using a much larger sample. Consistent with the results of the current study, Jamison, Raymond, Levine, and colleagues (2001) found that in a sample of chronic pain patients, there was a high correlation ($r = .88$) between averaged weekly RTDC data and weekly pain reports.

Peters and colleagues (2000) observed that in a sample of 12 participants whose weekly MPI and RTDC scores were assessed in the same week, nearly every participant reported higher pain severity on the MPI than on the RTDC pain assessment. Stone and colleagues (2004) also found considerably different levels of pain reports between RTDC and weekly recall assessment. The data from the present study, again with a much larger sample, are consistent with both of these studies. Peters and colleagues (2000) speculated that retrospection bias (where participants overestimate negative events in the process of recollection) might account for the results.

Successes and Challenges

SOFTWARE PROBLEMS

A number of problems were encountered with the software used in the project. In several instances, the software "skipped" screens so that participants were not presented with all of the questions. At times, the programming routine also skipped questions and participants could not return to those inadvertently missed. Problems with batteries also resulted in lost data.

HARDWARE PROBLEMS

Problems encountered with hardware can be grouped into two general types: (1) technology and (2) the computers. The most significant problem with the technology was associated with the decision to use a professional paging service. Since the study recruited people in a wide geographic area, a significant number of potential participants were lost because they lived outside the range of the paging service. A number of participants were also lost because of unreliability of the paging service. An additional technological problem was related to malfunctioning of the master computer transmitting the pager requests.

It is unfortunate that we could not determine whether all prompts were, in fact, administered and whether they were administered at each scheduled time. We are, therefore, unable to estimate the number of prompts that were not sent or were not received. It is important to note, however, that this study was conducted when using palmtop computers for data collection was relatively novel; it is likely that current methodologies (e.g., computer prompting) are more reliable and would result in more accurate information about the administration of prompts.

One of the most significant causes of the loss of data was that the sound card used was too quiet and participants often had difficulty hearing the page. This problem was especially acute when the pager was placed in a woman's purse, even if it was a short distance away.

A number of problems evolved over the course of the project as the aging palmtop computers were passed from participant to participant. Problems encountered included (1) touch screen malfunctions, (2) inability to turn on the computer, (3) failure of the computer to receive or accept prompting signals, (4) the computer turned on randomly, depleting the batteries, and (5) problems with batteries (short life, corrosion). After a period of 4 years and 149 participants (use for 2 consecutive weeks), none of the 16 original computers was still fully functional. This resulted in an inability to include the complete set of participants proposed.

Participant/Operator Problems

In addition to the problems already outlined, a large number of participant/ operator problems throughout this project were also identified. Some of the most common problems were (1) difficulty changing batteries, resulting in lost data (only given 90 seconds to change battery), (2) failure to keep computer accessible, (3) the process was perceived as inconvenient, and (4) placement of Palm computer near electrical equipment, resulting in loss of pager capacity.

Issues of Data Analysis

As discussed by Stone and Shiffman (2002), there is a lack of consensus about how best to analyze RTDC data. Strategies such as regression analysis (Affleck et al., 1998; Peters et al., 2000; Stone et al., 1994), repeated measures analysis of variance (Cruise et al., 1996; Peters et al., 2000), paired t-tests (Gendreau et al., 2003; Stone et al., 2004), and correlations (Cruise et al., 1996; Jamison et al., 2001; Stone et al., 2004) have all been used to explain findings in studies using RTDC procedures. The issue becomes even more complicated at varying levels of analysis (e.g., time of day vs. day to day vs. week to week, which can all be aggregated in different ways).

Figures 11-1 and 11-2, presented earlier, depict the various ways that RTDC data assessment can be conceptualized, resulting in a large number of potential analyses. The more analyses one conducts, the more one has to consider the influence of type 1 errors, which is a consideration for investigators. The use of multilevel modeling has gained increasing attention as a model for data analyses that can estimate both random and fixed effects simultaneously and does not omit all of the data for a participant if there are missing data. By retaining participants in the analysis and using all possible observations for all participants, the analysis yields findings based on the maximum amount of information available (e.g., Singer, 1998).

Prospects for Application of RTDC Methods

Despite the problems with RTDC methods discussed in this chapter, the use of the methodology enabled by the availability of RTDC has important implications for understanding the associations among variables that are important in the assessment and treatment of patients with chronic health conditions. This technique has a number of advantages over recall and paper-and-pencil measures. For example, RTDC allows for the assessment of information as it occurs in real time, providing more accuracy in responses. It also allows for careful evaluation of patient data so as to explore trends over time, lagged relationships, and so forth. Moreover, the availability of this sophisticated source of data will permit better assessment of treatment outcomes than can be obtained by retrospective reports, which may be biased for a number of reasons. The methodology afforded by the technology of RTDC can also contribute to the understanding of the interactions among important variables to determine the associations among pain, mood, activity, fatigue, and contextual factors. The sample of FMS patients in the current study, however, appeared to have stable symptoms across time. Given the previous cautions, if scores for FMS patients are determined to be stable across time, then the time and effort involved in using RTDC methods may be less beneficial than for other populations.

Limitations of the Study Reported

Some barriers to the use of RTDC should be noted: (1) technological or computerized tools are expensive to buy, replace, and maintain and are not completely reliable; (2) if participants forget to change batteries (such as on Palm Pilots), data may easily be lost; and (3) the amount of data obtained by RTDC is enormous; this can create difficulties in database management and analysis.

An important limitation of the study was the declining sample size from the time of invitation to participate to the assessment period. Figure 11-4 shows the declining trajectory of accrual. For purposes of comparison, however, the numbers from other RTDC studies are included to demonstrate that this trajectory is common. The rates of complete data in the current study were extremely low. If we used the 80 percent criterion suggested by Stone and Shiffman (2002),

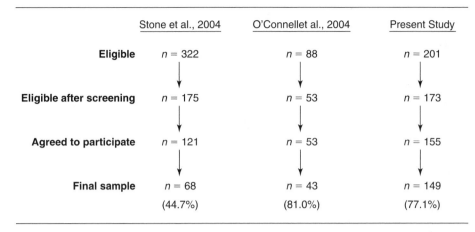

	Stone et al., 2004	O'Connellet al., 2004	Present Study
Eligible	*n* = 322	*n* = 88	*n* = 201
Eligible after screening	*n* = 175	*n* = 53	*n* = 173
Agreed to participate	*n* = 121	*n* = 53	*n* = 155
Final sample	*n* = 68	*n* = 43	*n* = 149
	(44.7%)	(81.0%)	(77.1%)

Figure 11-4. Reduction in sample size across studies. After patients agreed to participate, further reduction in sample size was due to having too much missing data for analysis, assignment to control group (for Stone et al. study, 23 of those eligible were assigned to a not-RTDC control group), having schedules that did not permit participation, withdrawal, losing equipment, and being unable to remain abstinent (O'Connell et al., 2004).

we would have had to eliminate 93 percent of the eligible participants. Because of these limitations, the results reported must be interpreted cautiously, as they may be biased and unrepresentative of all patients with FMS. For example, the fact that the paging service coverage was not sufficiently broad, causing the loss of participants, may have resulted in eliminating some from outlying areas. The results may be flawed, furthermore, by the inclusion of a large number of participants who provided "invalid" data (Stone & Shiffman, 2002).

One possible explanation for the refusal rate may be that, in this study, the RTDC protocol was described as a voluntary addition to the treatment study. There were no consequences for refusal to participate in the RTDC protocol. In the present study, the addition of the RTDC protocol was "extra" and unrelated to the provision of treatment. Furthermore, there may have been limited motivation for patients to participate, as they were not given any incentive (e.g., financial) for participating or adhering to the repeated prompts. One strategy to remedy this would be to offer a financial incentive for participating, with a bonus available for achieving over 80 percent response.

It is important to try to understand what contributed to refusal to participate, as this may serve as the basis for developing strategies to increase the rate of those willing to respond. It also might be possible to identify what characterizes those who refuse, as it would be possible to customize information to address specific contributors to refusal. Software and hardware advances should reduce many of the problems encountered.

The limitations of RTDC technology, procedures, and data analytic challenge need to be acknowledged. Strategies to address these limitations need to be developed to maximize the potential of RTDC. The advantages of RTDC must be tempered with the problems confronted in the present study and the limitations on the representativeness of the sample persons who volunteer to participate and the significant loss of data encountered. The excessive loss of data encountered in this study may even have challenged the interpretations based on multilevel modeling.

The difficulties in acquiring data using RTDC in this study present an opportunity to provide recommendations for researchers who wish to employ this methodology in future studies. First, researchers should critically evaluate the various available palmtop computers, selecting for use those that are easiest to maintain and are most cost-effective for their study. Problems such as equipment breakage might be minimized if participants were better trained about the handling of the equipment or if they were provided with damage-resistant holding cases for the palmtop computer. Lost data due to battery drainage might be alleviated if participants were provided with a longer-life battery, if they were provided with a second replacement battery, or if they were prompted by the computer to change the battery when it becomes low. Data analysis problems might be mediated by the use of preexisting databases, into which participant data can automatically be uploaded (perhaps via wireless technology). Furthermore, investigators might benefit from consultation with individuals skilled in the management of RTDC data. Such consultation can aid researchers in forming hypotheses, creating syntax to aggregate data appropriately, and analyzing findings. Finally, participant accrual might be strengthened by offering incentives or by providing ongoing training to alleviate any technological difficulties that might prevent regular recording of responses.

ACKNOWLEDGMENT

Preparation of this manuscript was supported in part from NIH grant AR 44724, awarded to the first author.

References

Affleck, G., Tennen, H., Urrows, S., Higgins, P., Abeles, M., Hall, C., Karoly, P., & Newton, C. (1998). Fibromyalgia and women's pursuit of personal goals: A daily process analysis. *Health Psychology, 17,* 40–47.

Burckhardt, C. S., Clark, S. R., & Bennett, R. M. (1991). The Fibromyalgia Impact Questionnaire: Development and validation. *Journal of Rheumatology, 18,* 728–733.

Catley, D., O'Connell, K. A., & Shiffman, S. (2000). Absentminded lapses during smoking cessation. *Psychology of Addictive Behaviors, 14,* 73–76.

Collins, R. L., Morsheimer, E. T., Shiffman, S., Paty, J. A., Gnys, M., & Papandonatos, G. D. (1998). Ecological momentary assessment in a behavioral drinking moderation training program. *Experimental and Clinical Psychopharmacology, 6,* 306–315.

Cruise, C. E., Broderick, J., Porter, L., Kaell, A., & Stone, A. A. (1996). Reactive effects of diary self-assessment in chronic pain patients. *Pain, 67,* 253–258.

Gendreau, M., Hufford, M. R., & Stone, A.A. (2003). Measuring clinical pain in chronic widespread pain: Selected methodological issues. *Best Practice and Research Clinical Rheumatology, 17,* 575–592.

Hufford, M. R., Shields, A. L., Shiffman, S. I., Paty, J., & Balabanis, M. (2002). Reactivity to ecological momentary assessment: An example using undergraduate problem drinkers. *Psychology of Addictive Behaviors, 16,* 205–211.

Jaccard, J., & Wan, C. K. (1993). Statistical analysis of temporal data with many observations: Issues for behavioral medicine data. *Annals of Behavioral Medicine, 15,* 41–50.

Jamison, R. N., Raymond, S. A., Levine, J. G., Slawsby, E. A., Nedeljkovic, S. S., & Katz, N. P. (2001). Electronic diaries for monitoring chronic pain: 1-year validation study. *Pain, 91,* 277–285.

Kerns, R. D., Turk, D. C., & Rudy, T. E. (1985). The West Haven-Yale Multidimensional Pain Inventory (WHYMPI). *Pain, 23,* 345–356.

LeGrange, D., Gorin, A., Dymek, M., & Stone, A.A. (2002). Does ecological momentary assessment improve cognitive behavioural therapy for binge eating disorder? A pilot study. *European Eating Disorders Review, 10,* 316–328.

Litt, M. D., Cooney, N. L., & Morse, P. (1998). Ecological momentary assessment (EMA) with treated alcoholics: Methodological problems and potential solutions. *Health Psychology, 17,* 48–52.

Nicassio, P. M., Moxham, E. G., Schuman, C. E., & Gevirtz, R. N. (2002). The contribution of pain, reported sleep quality, and depressive symptoms to fatigue in fibromyalgia. *Pain, 100,* 271–279.

O'Connell, K. A., Gerkovich, M. M., Cook, M. R., Shiffman, S., Hickcox, M., & Kakolewski, K. E. (1998). Coping in real time: Using Ecological Momentary Assessment techniques to assess coping with the urge to smoke. *Research in Nursing and Health, 21,* 487–497.

Peters, M. L., Sorbi, M. J., Kruise, D. A., Kerssens, J. J., Verhaak, P. F. M., & Bensing, J. M. (2000). Electronic diary assessment of pain, disability and psychological adaptation in patients differing in duration of pain. *Pain, 84,* 181–192.

Radloff, L. (1977). The CES-D Scale: A self-report depression scale for research in the general population. *Applied Psychological Measurement, 3,* 385–401.

Rudy, T. E., Kerns, R. D., & Turk, D. C. (1998). Chronic pain and depression: Toward a cognitive-behavioral mediation model. *Pain, 35,* 129–140.

Salovey, P., Sieber, W. J., Smith, A. F., & Turk, D. C. (1992). Reporting chronic pain episodes on health surveys. *National Center for Health Statistics: Vital and Health Statistics,* Series 6, No. 6, 1992.

Singer, J. D. (1998). Using SAS PROC MIXED to fit multilevel models, hierarchical models, and individual growth models. *Journal of Educational and Behavioral Statistics, 23,* 323–355.

Stein, K. F., & Corte, C. M. (2003). Ecologic Momentary Assessment of eating-disordered behaviors. *International Journal of Eating Disorders, 34,* 349–360.

Stone, A. A., Broderick, J. E., Porter, L., & Kaell, A. (1997). The experience of rheumatoid arthritis pain and fatigue: Examining momentary reports and correlates over one week. *Arthritis Care and Research, 10,* 185–193.

Stone, A. A., Broderick, J. E., Porter, L. S., Krupp, L., Gnys, M., Paty, J.A., & Shiffman, S. (1994). Fatigue and mood in chronic fatigue syndrome patients: Results of a momentary assessment protocol examining fatigue and mood levels and diurnal patterns. *Annals of Behavioral Medicine, 16,* 228–234.

Stone, A. A., Broderick, J. E., Schwartz, J. E., Shiffman, S., Litcher-Kelly, L., & Calcanese, P. (2003). Intensive momentary reporting of pain with an electronic diary: Reactivity, compliance, and patient satisfaction. *Pain, 104,* 343–351.

Stone, A. A., Broderick, J. E., Shiffman, S. S., & Schwartz, J. E. (2004). Understanding recall of weekly pain from a momentary assessment perspective: Absolute agreement, between- and within-person consistency, and judged change in weekly pain. *Pain, 107,* 61–69.

Stone, A. A., & Shiffman, S. (1994). Ecological momentary assessment (EMA) in behavioral medicine. *Annals of Behavioral Medicine, 16,* 199–202.

Stone, A. A., & Shiffman, S. (2002). Capturing momentary, self-report data: A proposal for reporting guidelines. *Annals of Behavioral Medicine, 24,* 236–243.

Stone, A. A., Shiffman, S., Schwartz, J. E., Broderick, J. E., & Hufford, M. R. (2003). Patient compliance with paper and electronic diaries. *Controlled Clinical Trials, 24,* 182–199.

Wolfe, F., et al. (1990). The American College of Rheumatology 1990 criteria for the classification of fibromyalgia: Report of the multicenter criteria committee. *Arthritis and Rheumatism, 33,* 160–172.

12

Evaluating Fatigue of Ovarian Cancer Patients Using Ecological Momentary Assessment

Karen Basen-Engquist and Carl de Moor

Fatigue has been defined as "a general feeling of debilitating tiredness or loss of energy" (Vogelzang, Breitbart, Cella, et al., 1997). People with cancer experience fatigue much differently than do healthy individuals. For healthy people, fatigue is experienced as a normal, even pleasant consequence of hard work or exercise that is ameliorated by rest and sleep. Fatigue as experienced by people with cancer is a chronic, distressing lack of energy that severely limits activity and is not relieved by sleep or rest (Glaus, Crow, & Hammond, 1996).

Previous research has shown that a high proportion of people being treated for cancer report problems with fatigue (Chang, Hwang, Feuerman, & Kasimis, 2000; Portenoy, Thaler, Kornblith, et al., 1994; Vogelzang et al., 1997; Winningham, Nail, Burke, et al., 1994), and those receiving chemotherapy for treatment report worse fatigue than people without a history of cancer (Hann, Garovoy, Finkelstein, et al., 1999; Jacobsen, Hann, Azzarello, et al., 1999). Fatigue was the most frequently endorsed symptom in a study of individuals with cancer of the prostate, colon, breast, or ovary. Nearly three fourths of the respondents reported a lack of energy; of these, 80 percent rated it as moderate to severe, and approximately one third were bothered by fatigue "quite a bit" or "very much" (Portenoy et al., 1994).

Cancer survivors who have completed their treatment continue to experience fatigue to a greater extent than healthy comparison groups (Andrykowski, Curran, & Lightner, 1998; Bower, Ganz, Desmond, et al., 2000; Broeckel, Jacobsen, Horton, et al., 1998; Cella, Lai, Chang, et al., 2002; Hann, Jacobsen, Martin, et al., 1997). Cancer-related fatigue is more common among women (Akechi, Kugraya, Okamura, et al., 1999; Pater, Zee, Palmer, et al., 1997; Vogelzang et al., 1997), in younger patients (Lakusta, Atkinson, Robinson, et al., 2001; Pater et al., 1997; Schwartz, 2000; Vogelzang et al., 1997), and those who live alone (Akechi et al., 1999). Cancer survivors who are employed and have higher educational levels also report more fatigue (Akechi et al., 1999). Fatigue is more commonly reported among those who have advanced or metastatic disease (Pater et al., 1997), poor performance status (Jacobsen et al., 1999; Pater et al., 1997), and additional symptoms such as dyspnea, pain, anxiety, and depression (Hann et al., 1997, 1999; Irvine, Vincent, Graydon, & Bubela, 1998; Jacobsen et al., 1999; Loge, Abrahamsen, Ekeberg, & Kaasa, 2000; Okuyama, Akechi, Kugaya, et al., 2000; Stone, Hardy, Broadley, et al., 1999; Stone, Richards, Hern, & Hardy, 2001).

There are few effective interventions for cancer-related fatigue. Health care providers sometimes recommend energy conservation strategies, which involve limiting patients' energy expenditure and prioritizing activities in an attempt to reduce fatigue. There is not a large evidence base for this strategy, but a recent clinical trial of an energy conservation intervention demonstrated positive effects on fatigue during cancer treatment (Barsevick, Dudley, Beck, et al., 2004). In contrast, a growing body of research suggests that physical activity may ameliorate fatigue. Randomized and quasi-experimental studies of exercise interventions have demonstrated reductions in fatigue (Courneya, Mackey, Bell, et al., 2003; Dimeo, Rumberger, & Keul, 1998; Dimeo, Stieglitz, Novelli-Fischer, et al., 1999; Mock, Burke, Sheehan, et al., 1994; Mock, Dow, Meares, et al., 1997). These studies have primarily focused on structured exercise programs and have not studied the relationship between fatigue and lifestyle activity—that is, moderate or more intense activity that takes place during a patient's usual activities (e.g., household chores, work-related activity, yard work).

Cancer-related fatigue does not maintain a steady level over time, but varies with treatment-related variables. For example, patients receiving radiation therapy appear to have steadily increasing fatigue over the treatment course (Irvine et al., 1998; Monga, Kerrigan, Thornby, & Monga, 1999; Smets, Visser, Willems-Groot, et al., 1998). The pattern of fatigue in patients receiving chemotherapy is more complex and may depend on the cancer site, type of chemotherapy, and the way it is administered (Richardson, Ream, & Wilson-Barnett, 1998). Studying the variability of fatigue over a chemotherapy cycle can uncover patterns that might provide clues to the causes of fatigue. Several studies have measured fatigue at multiple points during a chemotherapy cycle using pencil-and-paper diaries, with assessment time frames ranging from several days (Berger, 1998) to daily (Richardson et al., 1998; Schwartz, 2000). These studies indicate that, at least when the chemotherapy is administered in a traditional short-term infusion, fatigue is worst during the days after chemotherapy administration and then improves (Berger, 1998; Richardson et al., 1998; Schwartz, 2000; Schwartz et al., 2000). One study using daily diaries to measure fatigue also found a slight rise in fatigue around the time of the hematologic nadir (Richardson et al., 1998). However, most studies have not included a sufficient number of patients in the study who were receiving the same kind of chemotherapy to study between-patient differences in the patterns of fatigue.

Rationale for Momentary Data Collection

Most research on cancer-related fatigue has used retrospective questionnaires to measure fatigue (Bower et al., 2000; Broeckel et al., 1998; Hann et al., 1997,

1999; Servaes, van der Werf, Prins, et al., 2000; Servaes, Verhagen, & Al, 2002; Servaes, Verhagen, & Bleijenberg, 2002). This research has been useful in determining the prevalence of fatigue among cancer patients and the predictors of who will develop fatigue. However, retrospective data are subject to a number of errors and recall biases that may distort the data and affect conclusions made about the data (Shiffman, 2000). For example, in remembering events or behaviors, highly salient or unusual events are more likely to be recalled, and retrospective reports of symptoms are influenced by the respondent's experience of the symptom at the time of reporting or recent extreme levels of the symptom (Redelmeier & Kahneman, 1996; Redelmeier, Katz, & Kahneman, 2003). Furthermore, retrospective questionnaires make it difficult to study patterns of change over short periods of time.

Ecological Momentary Assessment (EMA) enables investigators to study questions that are difficult to examine with traditional retrospective questionnaires, such as variability of symptoms, mood states, or behaviors over time; cyclical patterns such as diurnal or weekly patterns; and covariation of symptoms and environmental conditions or psychological states, such as an increase in pain following high-stress situations, or the effect of negative mood on subsequent coping responses (Stone, Broderick, Porter, & Kaell, 1997).

A few studies have used daily (or less frequent) diaries to describe patterns of fatigue among patients receiving treatment, but the variability in disease sites and treatment types in these studies has limited their ability to identify patient characteristics and behaviors that predict or explain different patterns of fatigue. The data from these studies are considerably more detailed than studies that use retrospective questionnaires covering longer time periods, but the diary data still may be subject to recall biases because participants are asked to respond to questions about fatigue over the course of a day retrospectively at bedtime.

Stone and colleagues (1997) have found that fatigue in patients with rheumatoid arthritis has a diurnal pattern. Thus, respondents completing diaries at the end of the day are required to reflect on and aggregate their changing fatigue experiences from throughout the day. As mentioned above, this aggregation process is subject to recall error and biases. In contrast, EMA of fatigue requires the participant to quantify only the fatigue he or she is experiencing at the moment of the assessment; recall of information is not required, and the participant does not have to aggregate multiple levels of fatigue over time. In addition, paper-and-pencil diary measures do not enable the investigator to know with certainty when the assessments are completed. The instruction may be given to complete the diary daily, but a participant who misses a night may complete assessments for 2 days on the second night, or worse yet, complete the entire diary the day before returning it to investigators (Stone, Shiffman, Schwartz, et al., 2003).

We conducted a pilot study using EMA methods to study cancer-related fatigue of ovarian cancer patients during chemotherapy. Our primary aim was to test the feasibility of collecting EMA data from cancer patients using hand-held computers as data prompting and entry devices. To assess feasibility, we examined recruitment rates, participant retention, data completeness, and feedback obtained in semi-structured interviews with a subsample of participants. Secondarily, we aimed to assess the patterns of fatigue occurring over a chemotherapy cycle and evaluate whether physical activity predicts fatigue. We hypothesized that there would be a negative relationship between physical activity and fatigue, consistent with studies showing that exercise ameliorates cancer-related fatigue (Courneya et al., 2003; Dimeo et al., 1998, 1999; Mock et al., 1994, 1997).

Method

Sample

Our study population was women who were being treated with carboplatin and/or paclitaxel for advanced (FIGO stage III or IV) ovarian cancer. Combination therapy with carboplatin and paclitaxel is the chemotherapy regimen typically given to newly diagnosed ovarian cancer patients. Single-agent therapy with carboplatin (or sometimes paclitaxel) is given to women who have recurrent ovarian cancer if they responded to it previously and have a disease-free interval of at least 6 months. Patients receive the chemotherapy by intravenous infusion over several hours every 3 to 4 weeks.

Thirty-three patients participated in the study and provided sufficient data for analysis. Table 12-1 provides data on the demographic and medical characteristics of the sample. Nineteen of the 33 patients were newly diagnosed with ovarian cancer and 14 had persistent or recurrent disease. Their average age was 58.5, and their ages ranged from 27 to 81. The sample was predominantly White, non-Hispanic/Latino; approximately one third had at least a college degree. Most were receiving carboplatin and paclitaxel, but a few were receiving single-agent therapy.

Momentary Data Collection

Palm m100 and m105 computers (palmOne, Inc., Milipitas, CA) were used for the study. These computers are small (4.7 × 3.1 × 0.7 inches) and light (4.4 oz) and run on two AAA batteries. The m100 has two megabytes of RAM, and the m105 has eight megabytes of RAM.

An application, titled the Personalized Assessment of Cancer Experience (PACE), was developed to prompt the participants and record data. Our first decision in the design of the PACE application was whether to use event-contingent, random, or scheduled assessments. We considered using event-contingent assessments, such as having participants complete assessments when their fatigue was at its worst. We decided not to use this type of assessment because we expected compliance to be low (we would be asking participants to respond when they were feeling least able to do so) and because fatigue is not generally experienced as a discrete event with a starting and ending time. We wanted to capture fatigue as it changed throughout the day, so we chose to assess fatigue and other variables at random times during the day.

Table 12-1. Demographic and medical characteristics of the sample

Variable	Category	n	Percent
Age	<50	6	18
	50–59	12	36
	60–69	9	27
	≥70	6	18
Ethnicity	White	29	88
	Black/African–American	2	6
	Asian	2	6
Marital status	Married	22	67
	Single	2	6
	Divorced	5	15
	Widowed	4	12
Employment	Full-time	7	21
	Part-time	2	6
	Not employed	24	73
Education (highest level)	<High School	1	3
	High School	6	20
	Technical/ Vocational school	4	13
	Some College	8	27
	College graduate	5	17
	Postgraduate	6	20
	Missing	3	
Children <19 living at home	Yes	6	19
	No	26	81
	Missing	1	
Body Mass Index	Underweight (<18.5)	0	0
	Normal (18.5–24.9)	17	52
	Overweight (25–29.9)	8	24
	Obese (>30)	8	24
Disease status	Newly diagnosed	19	58
	Persistent disease	4	12
	Recurrent disease	10	30
Stage	III	26	79
	IV	5	15
	Unstaged	2	6
Chemotherapy regimen	Carboplatin and paclitaxel	21	64
	Carboplatin	9	27
	Paclitaxel	3	9

(Continued)

Table 12-1. Demographic and medical characteristics of the sample (Continued)

Variable	Category	n	Percent
Cycle length	21 days	21	64
	28 days	12	36
Cycle of chemo	Second	3	9
during participation	Third	13	39
	Fourth	7	21
	Fifth	5	15
	Sixth	2	6
	Eighth	1	3
	Ninth	1	3
	Eleventh	1	3
Previous	0	16	48
chemotherapy regimens	1	4	12
	2	6	18
	3	4	12
	4	2	6
	5	1	3

In choosing the number of assessments, we had to balance the need to detect changes during the day with participant burden, keeping in mind that these patients were experiencing disease- and treatment-related symptoms. We chose a schedule for the random assessments similar to that used by Affleck and colleagues (Affleck, Tennen, Urrows, et al., 1998) in their study of fibromyalgia patients. They had high completion rates with this schedule in a sample of chronically ill individuals who experienced considerable symptoms. In the PACE application the random assessments were spaced throughout the day; the first random assessment took place between waking time and noon, two additional random assessments were between noon and 6 p.m., and the fourth random assessment took place between 6 p.m. and the participant's bedtime. Because a secondary goal of the study was to explore the effect of sleep on the presence of fatigue, the participants completed scheduled assessments at waketime and bedtime, using measures similar to those used in studies that use sleep diaries.

The computer sounded an alarm when it was time for the participant to complete the assessment. If the patient did not respond to the alarm, she received repeated alarms every 3 to 5 minutes. If she did not enter her information within 30 minutes of the first alarm, the program did not allow her to enter information and recorded this as a missed assessment.

The purpose of the waketime assessment was to provide information about the participants' sleep quantity and quality. Questions from the Pittsburgh Sleep Diary (Monk, Reynolds, Kupfer, et al., 1994) were used to assess the time they went to bed and turned the lights out, the time of waking, the number of times and the amount of time they were awake during the night, whether sleep medications were used, and subjective ratings of sleep quality, current mood, and alertness. The assessment was scheduled at the participant's usual waking time, identified by the participant at the beginning of her participation in the study. The waketime assessment was the only assessment that participants could do more than 30 minutes after the assessment time. This was allowed because they were reporting retrospective, rather than momentary, data at this assessment. If participants had not completed the waketime assessment by the time their first random assessment alarm sounded, they were prompted to complete the waketime assessment first.

The scheduled bedtime assessment provided information on current fatigue, fatigue throughout the day, and fatigue interference with activities, as well as behaviors during the day that could interfere with sleep (caffeine consumption, naps, smoking, and alcohol use). To assess fatigue and fatigue interference, participants completed the nine-item Brief Fatigue Inventory (Mendoza, Wang, Cleeland, et al., 1999) on the computer. Questions from the Pittsburgh Sleep Diary were used to evaluate behaviors that could interfere with sleep.

The random assessments measured current fatigue, pain, nausea, trouble concentrating, and mood. Questions were also asked about physical activity since the last assessment. Current fatigue, pain, nausea, and trouble concentrating were rated on a 0-to-10 scale similar to the one used in the Brief Fatigue Inventory, the Brief Pain Inventory, the M.D. Anderson Symptom Inventory, and other symptom measures (Cleeland, 1991; Cleeland, Mendoza, Wang, et al., 2000; Mendoza et al., 1999). Mood was measured with the 16-item mood adjective checklist used by Affleck and colleagues (Affleck, Apter, Tennen, et al., 2000). The checklist was based on the mood circumplex model and included two adjectives at each end of four dimensions: positive/negative, high arousal/low arousal, positive and high arousal/negative and low arousal, positive and low arousal/negative and high arousal.

Physical activity was assessed using two types of questions. The first asked participants to report how much time they spend sleeping/resting, in sitting activity, or doing light, moderate, or hard activity. Examples of activities at each intensity level could be accessed by the participant by tapping on the word describing intensity (e.g., tapping on the phrase "moderate activity"). Examples for each level were based on the metabolic equivalent (MET) values of the activity (Ainsworth, Haskell, Whitt, et al., 2000). Hard activities (jogging, aerobics, conditioning exercises, swimming laps) were 6.0 to 8.4 METs; moderate activities (brisk walking, mowing, washing a car, bicycling for leisure) were 4 to 5.9 METs; light activities (dressing, washing dishes, driving, showering, strolling) were 2 to 3.9 METs; sitting activities (desk work, eating, playing cards, talking) were 1.1 to 1.9 METS; and sleeping/resting activities (reading or watching television while lying down, riding in a car, sleeping) were approximately 1 MET. The program also calculated the amount of time that had elapsed since the last assessment, displayed it at the top of the screen, and summed the amount of time reported by the participants as they entered their information. It did not, however, require the total amount of time entered by the participant to equal the time that had elapsed since the last assessment. The second type of question asked participants to report how much time since the last assessment they spent "doing activity vigorous enough to make you breathe heavily and make your heart beat fast."

Procedures

Participants for the study were recruited at two sites, the M.D. Anderson Gynecologic Oncology Center and a private gynecologic oncology practice. Participants were recruited at a clinic appointment, generally at a chemotherapy clearance appointment at which they had blood tests to determine whether their blood counts were high enough to receive their next infusion. If they consented to participation, they were contacted approximately 4 to 7 days before their next chemotherapy infusion to begin the study. The data collection was started several days before the chemotherapy infusions so that patients could learn to use the computers when they were experiencing relatively few side effects.

The research coordinator met with the patients either in their homes or at the clinic. Patients filled out several retrospective questionnaires to measure quality of life, depression, sleep, and medication use. The research coordinator entered a participant profile into the PACE computer program that specified the patient's personal identification number, usual waking time and bedtime, whether she smoked (questions on tobacco use were presented only to patients who reported being smokers), the scheduled date of her chemotherapy infusion, and the beginning and ending dates of the assessment period. The program then generated the alarms for the patient's assessments. Then the research coordinator demonstrated each of the assessments to the patient, allowing her to respond to each type of question to ensure that she understood how to register her response. The coordinator explained the assessment schedule and alarms to the patient and helped her select an alarm sound that would be tolerable and easy for her to hear. A manual explaining the PACE program, including basic care of the computer, how to respond to each type of question, and the research coordinator's contact information, was also given to each participant. The patient began using the PACE program that day. As a final step in the training, the research coordinator called the participant each of the next 3 days to answer questions and troubleshoot any problems she might be having.

The patients continued to use the computers throughout their chemotherapy cycle, a period lasting approximately 4 weeks. Because chemotherapy administration was sometimes delayed due to low blood cell counts, some patients used the computer for a longer period. In this chapter we present data from the 21-day period starting the day the patient received chemotherapy. The research coordinator met with each patient once a week, usually at her home, to upload the data to a laptop computer and to administer questionnaires. Patients received compensation each week for participation, based on the percentage of assessments they completed. Compensation was in the form of gift cards from several national retail chains. Patients received gift cards worth $50 for 85 percent completion or better, $30 for 70 to 84 percent completion, $20 for 55 to 69 percent completion, and $10 for 40 to 54 percent completion. If they provided any data during the study and returned the computer at the conclusion of their participation, they received an additional $50.

Patients also completed retrospective questionnaires to measure quality of life, depression, sleep, and medication use. At baseline (4 to 7 days before the chemotherapy infusion) they completed the Functional Assessment of Cancer Therapy—Ovarian (FACT-O) (Basen-Engquist, Bodurka-Bevers, Fitzgerald, et al., 2001), the Center for Epidemiologic Studies—Depression Questionnaire (CESD) (Radloff, 1977), and the Pittsburgh Sleep Quality Index (PSQI) (Buysse, Reynolds, Monk, et al., 1989). Each week during the study the patients completed the FACT-O, CESD, and a record of the medications taken in the past week; however, only results involving the baseline questionnaires are presented in this chapter.

Analysis

The analyses in this chapter use the mean rating of current fatigue during the day (averaged over up to five time points) as the main outcome measure. The overall pattern of fatigue during the chemotherapy cycle was examined by plotting the mean fatigue score for each day, for days 0 (day of chemotherapy infusion) to 20. While participants started using the computer before the day of the chemotherapy infusion, we did not include these data in the analysis because the number of days on which data were provided varied a great deal among participants, and because these data do not truly provide a "baseline" measure, as all participants had received at least one cycle of chemotherapy before starting the study.

To explore whether there were subgroups of patients with different patterns of fatigue over the chemotherapy cycle, we developed a regression model for each patient that regressed fatigue on number of days since chemotherapy. We then conducted a cluster analysis of the intercepts (indicating average level of fatigue for the patient) and slopes (representing change over time) from the regression models for each patient. Demographic and medical differences between clusters of participants were tested using chi-square statistics and one-way analysis of covariance. Differences between the groups in baseline quality of life, sleep, and depression were tested using one-way univariate analysis of covariance, controlling for body mass index (BMI) and the number of days that elapsed between baseline questionnaire completion and the start of the chemotherapy cycle. Differences in physical activity were tested using mixed model linear regression. For pairwise comparisons of psychosocial and physical activity variables a Bonferroni correction was applied to avoid inflating type I error.

Results

Feasibility

Patients were recruited from two clinical sites: the M.D. Anderson Gynecologic Oncology Center and Gynecologic Oncology of Houston, a private clinic. At the M.D. Anderson site we were able to carefully track the number of patients approached about the study, the number who refused, and their reasons for refusing. At M.D. Anderson, a total of 59 patients were approached about the study and 30 enrolled (51%). Of the 29 patients who refused participation, only 10 cited concerns about the study demands, disruptiveness, or using the computer. At the private gynecologic oncology clinic, patients were first told a little about the study by the clinic nurse, who obtained their verbal consent for our research coordinator to meet with them and explain the study in more detail. Of the 12 patients who met with our research coordinator, all agreed to participate. We do not know exactly how many women did not agree to meet with the research coordinator, but the chemotherapy nurse said that most of them agreed.

A total of 42 patients enrolled in the study (30 from M.D. Anderson and 12 from the private clinic). Four of the women were taken off the study because their chemotherapy regimen changed, making them ineligible for the study. Five women dropped out of the study before completing. Three of these women dropped out before they started the data collection, and only two dropped out after beginning the study. These two women reported that they wanted to discontinue participation because the computer was too disruptive (one of the women had extraordinarily severe nausea and vomiting after her chemotherapy infusion, making it difficult for her to complete assessments). Compliance with the assessments was high; patients completed an average of 86 percent of their assessments during participation. Twenty of the 33 women completed over 90 percent of the assessments.

To obtain their feedback, the first five patients who were enrolled in the study completed open-ended interviews with the research coordinator about the PACE program. They were interviewed each week about their experiences with the assessment program. Their feedback related to the PACE program is summarized in Table 12-2.

Patterns of Fatigue

Figure 12-1 displays the daily means for ratings of fatigue, nausea, pain, and trouble concentrating. Fatigue was reported at a higher level than the other symptoms throughout the chemotherapy cycle and showed a more distinct pattern of change. There was an increase in fatigue starting on day 2 after chemotherapy administration, with a peak on day 3. Fatigue then decreased until about day 7 and was level until day 14, when it decreased further. The other symptoms increased slightly in the days after chemotherapy and peaked around day 3, but the change was not as large.

The cluster analysis yielded three clusters of patients with distinct patterns of fatigue during the chemotherapy cycle. The low fatigue group ($n = 13$) had low levels of fatigue throughout most of the cycle; their fatigue increased slightly after chemotherapy and then decreased after the first week. The declining fatigue group ($n = 8$) reported sharply rising fatigue in the 3 to 4 days after chemotherapy and then it declined to the level of patients in the low fatigue group. The high fatigue group ($n = 12$) had consistently high levels of fatigue

Table 12-2. Feedback on PACE program from interviews with first five participants

Positive comments	Problems with PACE program	Suggested changes
• "Interesting, new, and different"	• Had to "study a bit" to understand the on-screen instructions at times	• Use a smaller/lighter computer
• Questions easy to read and understand	• Glare on the screen made it hard to read at times	• Add a backlight feature for low light conditions
• On-screen instructions easy to read and understand	• Questions repetitious • Randomly timed daytime assessments felt like interruptions or "a distraction"	• Have an optional vibrating (vs. auditory) prompt
• Alarms easily audible, even when in a purse	• Difficult to keep track of computer	• Add capability to go back and check/change answers
• "Like a game," "fun"	• Preset waketime and bedtime prompts don't allow for variability in daily schedule	• Tailor questions more to each participant's functional status
• Liked knowing when to expect waketime and bedtime alarms	• Often too tired mentally and physically to answer questions	• Add questions on appetite and diet
• Computer began to feel "like my partner"	• Did not understand distinction between similar mood adjectives	• Add the adjective "angry" to mood questions
	• Inconvenient to take to friend's house, worried about leaving it behind	• Eliminate similar mood adjectives
	• Got "not time for assessment message" after prompt had sounded/computer wouldn't let participant do assessment	• Include more information in the manual on how to resolve problems
	• Questions were a "constant reminder" of the cancer	• Have one fewer assessment per day

through the chemotherapy cycle. Figure 12-2 shows the average daily fatigue scores for the participants in each cluster.

We examined the number of days during the cycle that each group experienced moderate (4 to 6 on 10-point scale) and severe (7 to 10 on 10-point scale) fatigue, as defined by the developers of the Brief Fatigue Inventory (Mendoza et al., 1999). The high fatigue group experienced an average of 15.8 days (SD = 6.8) with moderate fatigue and 4.7 days (SD = 6.8) with severe fatigue. The low fatigue group reported no days with severe fatigue and 0.4 days, on average (SD = 0.7), of moderate fatigue. As expected, the declining fatigue groups reported intermediate

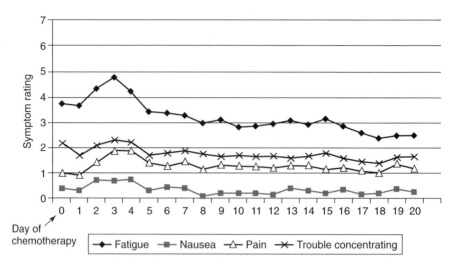

Figure 12-1. The average daily fatigue and other symptoms are presented by day in the chemotherapy cycle. Day 0 denotes the day patients received a chemotherapy infusion.

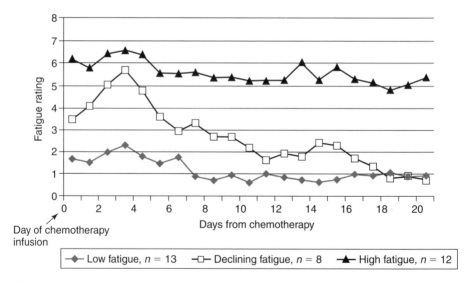

Figure 12-2. The average daily fatigue scores for each day in the chemotherapy cycle are displayed for three clusters of patients with unique patterns of fatigue.

values; they had 1.5 days (SD = 2.8) of severe fatigue and 5.0 days (SD = 2.8) of moderate fatigue.

Differences among the Clusters

There were few differences among the clusters in demographic and medical characteristics. The high fatigue cluster had a higher BMI (M = 29.3, SD = 4.9) than the low fatigue (M = 24.6, SD = 4.9) and declining fatigue (M = 24.7, SD = 3.2; p = 0.020) clusters. The high fatigue cluster was more likely to be taking antidepressants or anxiolytics (p = 0.009) than the other two groups. While not significant at the p = 0.05 level, a few other findings were suggestive of differences between the groups. Patients in the clusters with higher fatigue were more likely to be unmarried (p for linear trend = 0.07) and older (p for linear trend = 0.10). The declining fatigue cluster had a higher proportion of women with newly diagnosed disease (p = 0.119). Seven of the eight women in this cluster had newly diagnosed disease and one had progressive disease, suggesting that perhaps this pattern is unusual for women with recurrent ovarian cancer.

Controlling for BMI and the number of days between baseline and chemotherapy infusion, the high fatigue cluster had the poorest quality of life at baseline in physical well-being and ovarian cancer-specific concerns (Table 12-3). On these quality of life scores, the declining fatigue cluster scores were similar to those of the high fatigue cluster. The clusters also differed significantly in overall sleep (p = 0.001) and several of the sleep subscales; subjective sleep quality, sleep latency, and sleep disturbance were related to cluster membership, but sleep duration, sleep efficiency, use of sleep medication, and daytime dysfunction were not. For most of the subscales with significant differences, the high and declining fatigue groups had worse sleep than the low fatigue group. Baseline depression was also strongly associated with cluster, with the high fatigue group reporting a higher level of depressive symptoms than the low fatigue group.

To evaluate the effect of physical activity on fatigue, we first examined physical activity during the week after chemotherapy administration, when the level of chemotherapy side effects was highest. We reasoned that if fatigue was related to a physical deconditioning caused by inactivity, patients who stayed more active during the week after chemotherapy would be less likely to be fatigued during the rest of the chemotherapy cycle. The proportion of each day that women engaged in moderate or hard physical activity was calculated, and we examined the differences among the three fatigue clusters in the proportion of the day spent in moderate or hard activity. As Figure 12-3 shows, women in the high fatigue cluster spent a greater proportion of their day in moderate or more intense activity than the low fatigue and declining fatigue cluster (p = 0.016 after controlling for obesity; adjusted means presented in Figure 12-3). The percentage of the day patients reported spending in activity that increased heart rate and respiration also differed among the clusters (p = 0.027). Interestingly, while both the low and declining fatigue clusters reported less moderate or more intense physical activity than the high fatigue cluster, only the low fatigue cluster differed from the high fatigue

Table 12-3. Differences in quality of life, sleep, and depression among fatigue clusters

Variable	Low fatigue Adj. Mean (SE)	Declining fatigue Adj. Mean (SE)	High fatigue Adj. Mean (SE)	p value, overall difference
Physical well-being	25.3 (1.21)[a]	23.9 (1.46)[ab]	19.18 (1.31)[b]	0.011
Social well-being	25.9 (1.21)[a]	25.3 (1.46)[a]	21.4 (1.31)[a]	0.063
Emotional well-being	21.1 (1.23)[a]	17.6 (1.48)[a]	18.6 (1.33)[a]	0.183
Functional well-being	23.1 (1.36)[a]	20.7 (1.65)[a]	17.6 (1.54)[a]	0.063
Ovarian-specific subscale	37.9 (1.14)[a]	31.4 (1.38)[b]	29.5 (1.29)[b]	0.000
Subjective sleep quality	0.4 (0.20)[a]	0.9 (0.24)[ab]	1.3 (0.22)[b]	0.042
Sleep latency	0.8 (0.29)[a]	2.0 (0.35)[b]	1.0 (0.33)[b]	0.022
Sleep duration	0.4 (0.24)[a]	0.8 (0.29)[a]	1.2 (0.27)[a]	0.132
Sleep efficiency	0.5 (0.26)[a]	0.8 (0.32)[a]	1.4 (0.30)[a]	0.141
Sleep disturbance	1.3 (0.12)[a]	1.8 (0.14)[b]	1.9 (0.13)[b]	0.002
Sleep medication	0.7 (0.35)[a]	1.4 (0.42)[a]	1.5 (0.37)[a]	0.270
Daytime dysfunction	0.6 (0.18)[a]	0.9 (0.22)[a]	1.1 (0.20)[a]	0.283
PSQI Global Score	4.6 (0.85)[a]	8.6 (1.03)[b]	9.3 (0.97)[b]	0.003
Depression	4.9 (1.84)[a]	9.5 (2.21)[ab]	14.8 (1.99)[b]	0.008

Means adjusted for BMI and number of days between baseline and chemotherapy infusion. Adjusted means with different superscript letters are significantly different, $p < 0.05$.

cluster in the proportion of the day spent in activity that increased heart rate and respiration, a more subjective measure of activity intensity.

Moderate or more intense activity in Weeks 2 and 3 was not significantly related to cluster membership ($p = 0.213$; adjusted means presented in Figure 12-4). However, the proportion of the day spent in activity that increased perceived heart rate and respiration had a marginal relationship with cluster ($p = 0.054$), with the women in the low fatigue cluster reporting less of their day spent in such activity.

Discussion

Results of this study indicate that EMA is feasible for studying symptoms in cancer patients undergoing treatment. Furthermore, using EMA to measure fatigue, we were able to identify patterns of fatigue during chemotherapy and subgroups of patients with differing patterns. The results suggest that patients with a higher

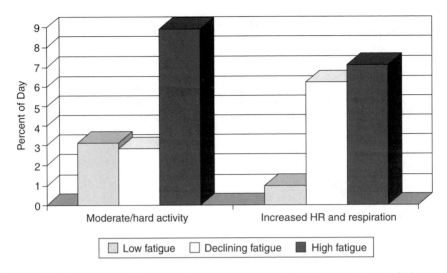

Figure 12-3. Percentage of day spent in moderate or hard activity across low, declining, and high fatigue clusters. In the week after the chemotherapy infusion, the three fatigue pattern clusters differed significantly in percentage of day spent in moderate and hard activity ($p = 0.007$; controlling for BMI, $p = 0.016$) and in percentage of day spent in activity that increased heart rate and respiration ($p = 0.016$; controlling for BMI, $p = 0.027$). Those in the high fatigue cluster reported more activity than those in the low and declining fatigue clusters.

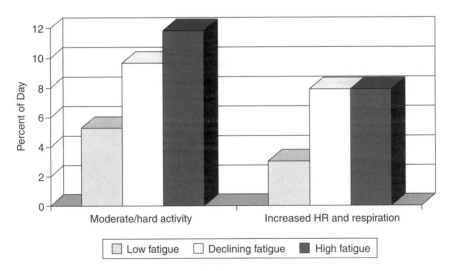

Figure 12-4. Relationship between cluster membership and moderate or more intense activity in weeks 2 and 3. Clusters did not differ significantly in the percentage of day spend in moderate and hard activity ($p = 0.230$; controlling for BMI, $p = 0.213$) during weeks 2 and 3 of the chemotherapy cycle. Percentage of day spend in activity that increased heart rate and respiration did not differ significantly by cluster ($p = 0.112$), but this difference was significant after controlling for BMI ($p = 0.054$).

BMI and those receiving psychoactive medication experience the most fatigue. Those with high fatigue also have more disrupted sleep, more depression, and poorer quality of life. A fatigue pattern characterized by a sharp increase in fatigue after chemotherapy administration, but low fatigue in Weeks 2 and 3 of the cycle, appears to be associated with quality of life and sleep difficulties similar to women with consistently high fatigue. A surprising finding was that the high fatigue group reported the highest level of physical activity during the week after chemotherapy. This was counter to expectations, because studies have shown that exercise and physical activity in cancer patients are associated with reduced symptoms, lower fatigue, and improved quality of life (Courneya et al., 2003; Dimeo et al., 1998, 1999; Mock et al., 1994, 1997; Pinto, Trunzo, Rabin, et al., 2003). These results raise the possibility that an energy conservation approach to managing fatigue would be beneficial (Barsevick, Dudley, Beck et al., 2004), at least at certain times during the treatment process. It is possible that remaining active during the week after chemotherapy administration, when the side effects of chemotherapy are most intense, would be detrimental rather than beneficial to fatigue.

Insight Gained from a Real-Time Approach

The EMA methods were successful in capturing data related to fatigue patterns over time in ovarian cancer patients receiving chemotherapy. A limited number of studies have done frequent assessment of fatigue during cancer treatment using patient diaries or repeated retrospective questionnaires. However, this was the first study to evaluate a "momentary" approach, in which patients reported their fatigue several times a day. This allowed us to identify patterns of fatigue during the chemotherapy cycle and in the future will enable us to study within-day patterns. Using handheld computers to prompt assessments and enter data allowed us to conduct the assessment on a random basis rather than at a time of the patient's choosing, which might bias the results. Furthermore, we were able to ascertain the extent to which participants complied with the assessments by limiting the times patients could access the assessment and by time-stamping data entry. Paper diaries do not have this advantage.

The real-time assessment of fatigue and physical activity led to some conclusions that were counter to our original expectations. Most notably, we found that patients who were more active during the week after chemotherapy were more likely to be fatigued throughout the cycle. This result runs counter to other studies that have found a significant negative association between fatigue and physical activity. There could be several explanations for this result. First, most studies of physical activity and fatigue have been conducted with patients who had a better prognosis than the ovarian cancer patients in this study. It is possible that having more advanced disease and a poorer prognosis could moderate the effects of physical activity or exercise on fatigue.

A second explanation for the unexpected direction of the relationship between physical activity and fatigue could be related to the type of activity assessed. The EMA allowed us to measure lifestyle physical activity, which includes activity related to work, transportation, household chores, and so forth, in addition to intentional exercise. Lifestyle physical activity is more difficult than intentional exercise to measure retrospectively because short bouts of activity, and activities that are engaged in for another purpose, are difficult for respondents to remember when queried about their activity.

Most of the extant literature on fatigue and physical activity assesses the relationship between planned intentional exercise and fatigue. There may be something unique about engaging in exercise, specifically, that provides greater relief from fatigue than physical activity more broadly defined. For example, going for a walk may distract a cancer survivor from worry about her next treatment and thus improve her mood. In walking to improve fitness, a person may be more likely to sustain activity continuously, but more likely to stop and rest while gardening or doing housework. The few trials that have tested the effect of exercise on fatigue have been small, have confounded attention/social support with the exercise intervention, and have tested a limited range of activities and cancer survivor populations. The question of whether specific exercise or general moderate physical activity affects fatigue needs to be studied more thoroughly.

It was curious that our analysis of physical activity in the week after chemotherapy found that the declining fatigue cluster differed from the high fatigue cluster in the amount of time spent in moderate or hard activity but not in the amount of time spent in activity that increased respiration and heart rate. We examined the correlation between these two variables for the declining fatigue group and found a high correlation ($r = .69$). However, the correlation was also high between time spent in activities increasing heart rate and respiration and time spent in light-intensity activity ($r = .49$). The high correlation with light activity was not observed in Weeks 2 and 3 of the cycle. This indicates that in the week after chemotherapy, patients in the declining fatigue group perceived more exertion during activities that are typically considered to be of light intensity, perhaps due to the same physiologic mechanisms that are causing their fatigue to increase. However, because the declining fatigue group did not differ significantly from the low fatigue group in any of the pairwise comparisons, another explanation for the apparent similarity to the high fatigue group on the heart rate and respiration variable is that it was due to random variation. The size of the cluster was small and we may not have had sufficient power to determine the level of physical activity of the declining fatigue group relative to the other two clusters on this variable.

Successes and Challenges

The use of EMA was fairly well received by patients and their compliance rates with data collection were high. Interviews with a subsample of patients revealed positive and negative aspects of the EMA study. Several patients reported that using the computer was interesting and fun. However, they also identified a number of problems with the hardware, software, and study design, including glare on the screen, no flexibility in the scheduled assessments, defects in the software that occasionally prevented them from completing assessments, excessive repetition in the assessments, and the inconvenience of keeping the computer with them.

Although the interview results need to be interpreted with caution because of the small sample size and the potential selection bias of interviewing the first five patients, the information provided and reasons given by nonparticipants for refusing the study provide some indication of changes that should be implemented in future studies. With regard to hardware, for example, the device we used did not have a vibrating alarm, which several patients said they would prefer. They considered the vibrating alarm to be less disruptive, and it would be helpful to patients who had difficulty hearing the alarms. The computer screen was difficult for some patients to see, so a device with a backlit screen and better resolution would be helpful for future studies. Font sizes should be sufficiently large for people to see easily, particularly if the sample includes older people who may have visual problems. Regarding software and EMA design, more research is needed on the optimal number of assessments for studying cancer-related fatigue during chemotherapy. Finally, we need additional development of measures that are as brief as possible while maintaining adequate reliability and validity.

An additional hardware issue was related to project implementation. The device we used had the advantage of being lightweight and inexpensive, but it also had several disadvantages. The computer runs on two AAA batteries, which we initially thought would be an advantage because patients would not have to charge the devices and the battery power was sufficient to last the 1 week between visits from the research coordinator. When the computers were new we could change batteries without the loss of data; however, as the computers aged they lost this ability to retain the data during brief power losses, such as occur with battery changes. When we changed the batteries we found that not only the data but also the entire application would be erased from the computer. Even more troubling, if a patient dropped a computer and the batteries were momentarily jarred, resulting in a loss of power, the data and the computer application would be erased. Given these limitations with battery power, it seems better to use a device with rechargeable batteries.

Prospects for Application of EMA Methods

The results of this pilot test indicate that real-time assessment of cancer-related symptoms is feasible and provides information that cannot be obtained using more retrospective questionnaires. Such an approach is applicable to studying cancer-related symptoms to better understand them and to identify causes and remedies. This approach shows promise in its ability to reveal patterns in outcomes that are not apparent in retrospective reports. Using EMA to study a complex symptom such as fatigue can advance the science of fatigue management by revealing information on the antecedents of peak fatigue episodes and uncovering patterns that may point to causes of fatigue. Such information could support the development of effective fatigue interventions that would greatly improve quality of life for people with cancer. It can also be applied to monitoring symptoms for which we have treatment (e.g., pain, vomiting) to optimize timing of treatment and to evaluate its effectiveness. In addition to monitoring the symptoms and use of treatment, EMA methods can be extended to provide feedback to both patients and health care providers in order to improve symptom management and overall patient care.

References

Affleck, G., Apter, A., Tennen, H., Reisine, S., Barrows, E., & Willard, A. (2000). Mood states associated with transitory changes in asthma symptoms and peak expiratory flow. *Psychosomatic Medicine, 62*, 61–68.

Affleck, G., Tennen, H., Urrows, S., Higgins, P., Abeles, M., & Hall, C. (1998). Fibromyalgia and women's pursuit of personal goals: A daily process analysis. *Health Psychology, 17*(1), 40–47.

Ainsworth, B. E., Haskell, W. L., Whitt, M. C., Irwin, M. L., Swartz, A. M., & Strath, S. J. (2000). Compendium of physical activities: An update of activity codes and MET intensities. *Medicine and Science in Sports and Exercise* (Supplement), S498–S516.

Akechi, T., Kugraya, A., Okamura, H., Yamawaki, S., & Uchitomi, Y. (1999). Fatigue and its associated factors in ambulatory cancer patients: A preliminary study. *Journal of Pain and Symptom Management, 17*(1), 42–48.

Andrykowski, M. A., Curran, S. L., & Lightner, R. (1998). Off-treatment fatigue in breast cancer survivors: A controlled comparison. *Journal of Behavioral Medicine, 21*(1), 1–18.

Barsevick, A. M., Dudley, W., Beck, S., Sweeney, C., Whitmer, K., & Nail, L. M. (2004). A randomized clinical trial of energy conservation for patients with cancer-related fatigue. *Cancer, 100*, 1302–1310.

Basen-Engquist, K., Bodurka-Bevers, D., Fitzgerald, M., Webster, K., Cella, D., & Hu, S. (2001). Reliability and validity of the Functional Assessment of Cancer Therapy-Ovarian (FACT-O). *Journal of Clinical Oncology, 19*(6), 1809–1817.

Berger, A. M. (1998). Patterns of fatigue and activity and rest during adjuvant breast cancer chemotherapy. *Oncology Nursing Forum, 25*(1), 51–62.

Bower, J. E., Ganz, P. A., Desmond, K. A., Rowland, J. H., Meyerowitz, B. E., & Belin, T. R. (2000). Fatigue in breast cancer survivors: Occurrence, correlates, and impact on quality of life. *Journal of Clinical Oncology, 18*(4), 743–753.

Broeckel, J. A., Jacobsen, P. B., Horton, J., Balducci, L., & Lyman, G. H. (1998). Characteristics and correlates of fatigue after adjuvant chemotherapy for breast cancer. *Journal of Clinical Oncology, 16*(5), 1689–1696.

Buysse, D. J., Reynolds, C. F., 3rd, Monk, T. H., Berman, S. R., & Kupfer, D. J. (1989). The Pittsburgh Sleep Quality Index: A new instrument for psychiatric practice and research. *Psychiatry Research, 28*(2), 193–213.

Cella, D., Lai, J. S., Chang, C. H., Peterman, A., & Slavin, M. (2002). Fatigue in cancer patients compared with fatigue in the general United States population. *Cancer, 94*(2), 528–538.

Chang, V. T., Hwang, S. S., Feuerman, M., & Kasimis, B. S. (2000). Symptom and quality of life survey of medical oncology patients at a Veterans Affairs medical center. *Cancer, 88*(5), 1175–1183.

Cleeland, C. S. (1991). Pain assessment in cancer. In D. Osoba (Ed.), *Effect of cancer on quality of life* (pp. 293–305). Boca Raton: CRC Press, Inc.

Cleeland, C. S., Mendoza, T. R., Wang, X. S., Chou, C., Harle, M. T., & Morrissey, M. (2000). Assessing symptom distress in cancer patients: The M.D. Anderson Symptom Inventory. *Cancer, 89*(7), 1634–1646.

Courneya, K. S., Mackey, J. R., Bell, G. J., Jones, L. W., Field, C. J., & Fairey, A. S. (2003). Randomized controlled trial of exercise training in postmenopausal breast cancer survivors: Cardiopulmonary and quality of life outcomes. *Journal of Clinical Oncology, 21*(9), 1660–1668.

Dimeo, F., Rumberger, B. G., & Keul, J. (1998). Aerobic exercise as therapy for cancer fatigue. *Medicine and Science in Sports and Exercise, 30*(4), 475–478.

Dimeo, F. C., Stieglitz, R., Novelli-Fischer, U., Fetscher, S., & Keul, J. (1999). Effects of physical activity on the fatigue and psychologic status of cancer patients during chemotherapy. *Cancer, 85*(10), 2273–2277.

Glaus, A., Crow, R., & Hammond, S. (1996). A quantitative study to explore the concept of fatigue/tiredness in cancer patients and in healthy individuals. *Supportive Care in Cancer, 4*, 82–96.

Hann, D. M., Garovoy, N., Finkelstein, B., Jacobsen, P. B., Azzarello, L. M., & Fields, K. K. (1999). Fatigue and quality of life in breast cancer patients undergoing autologous stem cell transplantation: A longitudinal comparative study. *Journal of Pain and Symptom Management, 17*(5), 311–319.

Hann, D. M., Jacobsen, P. B., Martin, S. C., Kronish, L. E., Azzarello, L. M., & Fields, K. K. (1997). Fatigue in women treated with bone marrow transplantation for breast cancer: A comparison with women with no history of cancer. *Supportive Care in Cancer, 5*, 44–52.

Irvine, D., Vincent, L., Graydon, J., & Bubela, N. (1998). Fatigue in women with breast cancer receiving radiation therapy. *Cancer Nursing, 21*(2), 127–135.

Jacobsen, P. B., Hann, D. M., Azzarello, L. M., Horton, J., Balducci, L., & Lyman, G. H. (1999). Fatigue in women receiving adjuvant chemotherapy for breast cancer: Characteristics, course, and correlates. *Journal of Pain and Symptom Management, 18*(4), 233–242.

Lakusta, C. M., Atkinson, M. J., Robinson, J. W., Nation, J., Taenzer, P. A., & Campo, M. G. (2001). Quality of life in ovarian cancer patients receiving chemotherapy. *Gynecological Oncology, 81*, 490–495.

Loge, J. H., Abrahamsen, A. F., Ekeberg, O., & Kaasa, S. (2000). Fatigue and psychiatric morbidity among Hodgkin's disease survivors. *Journal of Pain and Symptom Management, 19*(2), 91–99.

Mendoza, T. R., Wang, X. S., Cleeland, C. S., Morrissey, M., Johnson, B. A., & Wendt, J. K. (1999). The rapid assessment of fatigue severity in cancer patients. *Cancer, 85*(5), 1186–1196.

Mock, V., Burke, M. B., Sheehan, P., Creaton, E. M., Winningham, M. L., & McKenney-Tedder, S. (1994). A nursing rehabilitation program for women with breast cancer receiving adjuvant chemotherapy. *Oncology Nursing Forum, 21*(5), 899–908.

Mock, V., Dow, K. H., Meares, C. J., Grimm, P. M., Dienemann, J. A., & Haisfield-Wolfe, M. E. (1997). Effects of exercise on fatigue, physical functioning, and emotional distress during radiation therapy for breast cancer. *Oncology Nursing Forum, 24*(6), 991–1000.

Monga, U., Kerrigan, A. J., Thornby, J., & Monga, T. N. (1999). Prospective study of fatigue in localized prostate cancer patients undergoing radiotherapy. *Radiation Oncology Investigations, 7*, 178–185.

Monk, T. H., Reynolds III, C. F., Kupfer, D. J., Buysse, D. J., Coble, P. A., & Hayes, A. J. (1994). The Pittsburgh Sleep Diary. *Journal of Sleep Research, 3*, 111–120.

Okuyama, T., Akechi, T., Kugaya, A., Okamura, H., Imoto, & S., Nakano, T. (2000). Factors correlated with fatigue in disease-free breast cancer patients: Application of the Cancer Fatigue Scale. *Supportive Care in Cancer, 8*, 215–222.

Pater, J. L., Zee, B., Palmer, M., Johnston, D., & Osoba, D. (1997). Fatigue in patients with cancer: Results with National Cancer Institute of Canada Clinical Trials Group studies employing the EORTC QLQ-C30. *Supportive Care in Cancer, 5,* 410–413.

Pinto, B. M., Trunzo, J., Rabin, C., Bucknam, L., Cram, R., & Marcus, B. (2003). Moving Forward: A randomized trial of a home-based physical activity program for breast cancer patients. *Annals of Behavioral Medicine, 25*(Suppl.), 53.

Portenoy, R. K., Thaler, H. T., Kornblith, A. B., Lepore, J. M., Friedlander-Klar, H., & Coyle, N. (1994). Symptom prevalence, characteristics and distress in a cancer population. *Quality of Life Research, 3*(3), 183–189.

Radloff, L. S. (1977). The CES-D scale: A self-report depression scale for research in the general population. *Applied Psychological Measurement, 1*(3), 385–401.

Redelmeier, D. A., & Kahneman, D. (1996). Patients' memories of painful medical treatments: Real-time and retrospective evaluations of two minimally invasive procedures. *Pain, 66,* 3–8.

Redelmeier, D. A., Katz, J., & Kahneman, D. (2003). Memories of colonoscopy: A randomized trial. *Pain, 104,* 187–194.

Richardson, A., Ream, E., & Wilson-Barnett, J. (1998). Fatigue in patients receiving chemotherapy: Patterns of change. *Cancer Nursing, 21*(1), 17–30.

Schwartz, A. (2000). Daily fatigue patterns and effect of exercise in women with breast cancer. *Cancer Practice, 8*(1), 16–24.

Schwartz, A. L., Nail, L. M., Chen, S., Meek, P., Barsevick, A. M., & King, M. E., (2000). Fatigue patterns observed in patients receiving chemotherapy and radiotherapy. *Cancer Investigation, 18*(1), 11–19.

Servaes, P., Van Der Werf, S., Prins, J., Verhagen, S., & Bleijenberg, G. (2000). Fatigue in disease-free cancer patients compared with fatigue in patients with Chronic Fatigue Syndrome. *Supportive Care in Cancer, 9,* 11–17.

Servaes, P., Verhagen, C., & Al, E. (2002). Fatigue in cancer patients during and after treatment: Prevalence, correlates, and interventions. *European Journal of Cancer, 38*(1), 27–43.

Servaes, P., Verhagen, S., & Bleijenberg, G. (2002). Determinants of chronic fatigue in disease-free breast cancer patients: A cross-sectional study. *Annals of Oncology, 13,* 589–598.

Shiffman, S. (2000). Real-time self-report of momentary states in the natural environment: Computerized Ecological Momentary Assessment. In A. Stone, J. S. Turkkan, C. A. Bachrach, J. B. Jobe, H. S. Kurtzman, and V. S. Cain (Eds.), *The science of self-report: implications for research and practice* (pp. 277–296). Mahwah, NJ: Lawrence Erlbaum Associates.

Smets, E. M. A., Visser, M. R. M., Willems-Groot, A. F. M. N., Garssen, B., Oldenburger, F., & Van Tienhoven, G. (1998). Fatigue and radiotherapy: (A) experience in patients undergoing treatment. *British Journal of Cancer, 78*(7), 899–906.

Stone, A. A., Broderick, J. E., Porter, L. S., & Kaell, A. T. (1997). The experience of rheumatoid arthritis pain and fatigue: Examining momentary reports and correlates over one week. *Arthritis Care and Research, 10*(3), 185–193.

Stone, A. A., Shiffman, S., Schwartz, J. E., Broderick, J. E., & Hufford, M. R. (2003). Patient compliance with paper and electronic diaries. *Controlled Clinical Trials, 24*(2), 182–199.

Stone, P., Hardy, J., Broadley, K., Tookman, A.J., Kurowska, A., & Hern, R. A. (1999). Fatigue in advanced cancer: A prospective controlled cross-sectional study. *British Journal of Cancer, 79*(9/10), 1479–1486.

Stone, P., Richards, M., Hern, R. A., & Hardy, J. (2001). Fatigue in patients with cancers of the breast or prostate undergoing radical radiotherapy. *Journal of Pain and Symptom Management, 22*(6), 1007–1015.

Vogelzang, N. J., Breitbart, W., Cella, D., Curt, G. A., Groopman, J. E., & Horning, S. J. (1997). Patient, caregiver and oncologist perceptions of cancer-related fatigue: Results of a tripart assessment survey. *Seminars in Hematology, 34*(3), 4–12.

Winningham, M. L., Nail, L. M., Burke, M. B., Brophy, L., Cimprich, B., & Jones, L. S. (1994). Fatigue and the cancer experience: The state of the knowledge. *Oncology Nursing Forum,* 21, 23–36.

13

Personality, Mood States, and Daily Health

Randy J. Larsen

In this chapter I present an example of the use of Ecological Momentary Assessment (EMA) methods to study health and emotion. In this context, the questions I pursue are not as important as the examples they provide of the different ways that EMA can be used to open up new areas for investigation. Previously I have illustrated the use of experience sampling to study such diverse processes as emotional variability (Larsen, 1987), the within-subject linkage between life events and moods (Larsen & Cowan, 1988), the existence of weekly cycles in moods (Larsen & Kasimatis, 1990), and the within-subject factor structure of emotions over time (Larsen & Cutler, 1996). None of these topics can be adequately addressed without the use of intensive time sampling through some form of real-time EMA data capture.

My intention here is to inspire enthusiasm for the unique questions that can be addressed by these techniques. When time is included in data capture, by intensively sampling experience over many occasions, then time becomes an inherent structural component of the data. As such, it can be analyzed in unique ways that reveal specific processes (Larsen, 1989, 1990). In particular, processes that involve patterns of change, such as cycles or rhythms, or that involve duration or rate of change, or that involve covariation of change, either at the same time (co-occurrence) or across time (lagged-covariation, such as in incubation periods), are all ideal questions for study with these methods. In fact, only intensive time-sampling methods can be used to adequately address such questions about process.

In the example described in this chapter (drawn from Larsen & Kasimatis, 1991), I started out with a main concern about the personality–health relationship. Many psychologists have investigated the link between personality dispositions and health (e.g., Carson, 1989; Rodin & Salovey, 1989). The dominant question in this area is whether or not personality factors foster an increased proneness for specific illnesses—that is, whether personality predicts who gets sick. Results have been mixed (Depue & Monroe, 1986; Friedman & Booth-Kewley, 1987).

One might turn the personality–health question around and ask whether personality predicts who gets better—that is, when it comes to common daily illnesses (e.g., stomachaches, headaches, respiratory infections), everyone gets ill from time to time. The personality effects may occur not so much in who gets ill, but in who gets better faster. Said differently, personality may predict the within-subject duration of common illnesses more than the frequency or occurrence of those illnesses. To examine duration we must study people over time, and so intensive real-time repeated samples of health status are necessary to quantify duration.

There are many models of how personality may work to produce greater frequency of illnesses, such as health behavior models, or stress and coping models (Larsen & Buss, 2002). However, all would predict that certain personality traits should relate to the greater frequency of specific illnesses. Most research along these lines relies on assessing health through retrospective self-reports (e.g., Aldwin, Levenson, Spiro, & Bosse, 1989). We know that people's retrospective reports of illness frequency contain specific biases and are prone to error (Larsen, 1992). Real-time measures of symptom occurrence are thus essential to assess the personality–symptom relationship uncontaminated by memory bias. As in the present study, researchers who employ on-line measures of health status avoid the contaminating effects of memory biases in the recall of health information (Gorin & Stone, 2001).

When we focus on health and illness as a process that occurs over time, alternative formulations of the link with personality become available. Personality may relate not so much to the occurrence of illness as to the course that an illness takes once it does occur. Attempting to understand the course of illness demands that we study persons over time and include the temporal dimension in data on illness.

Other researchers have examined the duration of illnesses, or at least have discussed the theoretical implications of this conception. For example, Akiskal, Hirschfeld, and Yerevanian (1983) suggested that personality may play a negligible role in the **onset** of depression, but it may play a large role in determining who is likely to **recover** from depression once it occurs. Another example is work on recovery rates from coronary artery bypass surgery and dispositional optimism (e.g., Scheier, Matthews, Owens, et al., 1989). Here the researchers found that several indicators of faster recovery from surgery (e.g., postsurgical days in the hospital) were related to dispositional optimism.

In the present study, I examine the duration of common illnesses, using real-time assessments, over a 2-month period in the lives of the participants. While I quantify occurrence, I also make the case that occurrence and duration of illnesses should be distinct processes—that is, what causes a person to, say, catch a cold (a virus) is quite different from what "causes" the person to recover (rest, plenty of fluids). As such, different personality factors may be involved in the onset and recovery rate or duration of common illnesses.

In addition to occurrence and duration, a third parameter of daily illness concerns the emotional concomitants of becoming ill. Many researchers consider emotions and moods to function something like a signal system (Larsen & Prizmic, 2004), revealing to the person his or her state of affairs. These signals may be important in self-regulation behaviors necessary to cope with illness. For example, if an individual does not feel "down" during a cold, then he or she may not engage in the self-regulatory behaviors necessary to recover efficiently from the cold. If one is stoically unresponsive to illness symptoms, then one is disconnected from a source of information useful in guiding self-regulatory behaviors.

The third parameter thus examined in this study concerns the linkage between changes in a person's health status and his or her daily moods. This parameter will be operationalized as a within-subject correlation between daily mood ratings and daily symptom ratings computed across occasions for each subject. We then examine whether some people show a diminished or enhanced emotional consequence of becoming ill.

Rationale for a Momentary Approach to Data Collection

One important aspect of life that changes from day to day is ongoing health status. The onset of a stomachache, a sore throat, or a strained back can represent an important change in health status that may, in turn, influence other aspects of a person's ongoing life, such as work, relationships, or recreational activities. And this influence may cascade across days and across other life domains, perhaps exacerbating the effects of stress from other areas of a person's life. Moreover, this influence may differ for different health problems, for different people, and for different life domains. Health is a changing process embedded in and fluctuating over time, and to fully understand health and its implications we need to study it over time in the ongoing lives of people. This necessitates that we take an intensive time-sampling approach to the study of health.

Many researchers who have employed on-line or experience sampling methods in the study of health nevertheless maintain a focus on the occurrence of illness (e.g., Clark & Watson, 1988; Watson, 1988), which is a static conception of health. Even though this formulation of relating personality to illness occurrence is widely used, Holroyd and Coyne (1987) suggest that this model "oversimplifies the role of personality variables in illness" (p. 367). Researchers need to expand their conception of health by examining different mechanisms and processes that may link personality to illness, rather than continuing to simply correlate traits with illness. In this chapter I present three distinct models of the link between personality and health that rely on the unique properties of data resulting from EMA.

Method

Sample

Participants were 46 undergraduates enrolled in a semester-long course on personality research. The only requirement for participation was completion of an introductory psychology course. Subjects received a letter grade based on attendance and participation in weekly class meetings and completion of assignments and a written report. As is typical in this area of research, three subjects dropped out of the study after only a few weeks, leaving an effective sample size of 43. Partial data sets from these three subjects were not included in any of the analyses.

Momentary Data Collection

Subjects completed a mood and symptom report three times a day for 2 consecutive months (8 weeks). They completed a report at noon each day to rate their moods and symptoms that morning, at dinnertime to report on their moods and symptoms in the afternoon, and again at bedtime to report their evening moods and symptoms. Paper diaries were used, primarily for convenience and because of the fixed reporting times.

The issue of reporting periods and type of report format used (paper vs. electronic) is a complicated judgment call in designing such EMA protocols. Paper format is convenient for subjects, immune to technical failures, and suitable when the questions ask subjects to integrate their experiences or reports over some extended time period (in our case, participants integrated over about a 6-hour period for each report). This format is also convenient when the reporting period is fixed instead of random, as participants can simply put the reports in their pockets, purses, or book binders and not have to worry about hearing the beep signal or breaking an electronic device.

The choice of reporting periods has to be driven by some consideration of the phenomenon under investigation and how quickly it changes. We felt that moods and physical symptoms do fluctuate within days, but that the major fluctuations could be captured in 6-hour increments. Faster-changing phenomena (e.g., strong emotions) might need to be sampled more frequently. Or, if the idea were to capture states (e.g., are you in a social interaction right now) versus more trait-like variables (e.g., how much social interaction did you engage in today), then one would alter the sampling period accordingly.

The daily mood and symptom report consisted of 9 emotion adjectives and 25 symptoms. For the emotion adjectives, subjects responded to the following: "Use a number from this scale to indicate how much of each mood you experienced during the time period." Responses were made on a 7-point scale ranging from 0 (not at all) to 6 (extremely much). The nine emotion adjectives used are presented in the reproduction of the research form in Table 13-1. This set of adjectives represents the pleasantness–unpleasantness or hedonic tone dimension of affective space (Larsen & Diener, 1992). On each occasion a mood score was calculated by subtracting the average response to the pleasant adjectives from the average response to the unpleasant adjectives. High scores thus indicate unpleasant affect.

To help increase compliance, reports were returned to the experimenter on a daily basis, except for weekends, where reports for Friday, Saturday, and Sunday were turned in on Monday. Participants were required to drop off the completed forms each weekday at specially designated drop boxes on campus. Compliance was excellent, with only 6.65 percent of the possible reports missing (i.e., we obtained a total of 7,225 reports out of a possible 7,740).

Table 13-1. The daily mood and symptom report

Pseudonym _____ ID # ____ Report # (circle one) 1 2 3 Date _____ Time _____ a.m. p.m.

Use a number from this scale to indicate how much of each mood you experienced during the time period.

NOT AT ALL 0	VERY SLIGHTLY 1	SOME-WHAT 2	MODERATE AMOUNT 3	MUCH 4	VERY MUCH 5	EXTREMELY MUCH 6

_____ happy   _____ joyful   _____ depressed/blue   _____ unhappy
_____ frustrated   _____ worried/anxious _____ enjoyment/fun   _____ pleased
_____ angry/hostile

Consider whether or not you had any of the following symptoms during the time period on which you are reporting. If you experienced a symptom during the reporting period, place an X in the box in front of that symptom.

☐ Upset stomach   ☐ Vomiting   ☐ Took medications   ☐ Fever/chills
☐ Back pain   ☐ Muscle cramps   ☐ Headache   ☐ Blurred vision
☐ Dizziness   ☐ Runny nose   ☐ Run down, exhausted   ☐ Trouble concentrating
☐ Poor appetite   ☐ Skin rash   ☐ Ringing in ears   ☐ Cough/sore throat
☐ Sinus pain   ☐ Nervous/sweaty   ☐ Constipation   ☐ Diarrhea
☐ Short of breath   ☐ Muscle or joint aches ☐ Racing or pounding heart
☐ Sore feet   ☐ Eye strain   ☐ Other _____

Compliance is a complex issue, and it has different facets. For example, compliance can refer to completing the forms at the requested time, or it can refer to completing the forms conscientiously. Monetary reward may influence the former more than the latter. However, having the participants engaged in the project, with frequent feedback on performance, and with commitment to the project fostered by good rapport with the investigators, can work to increase both forms of compliance. We worked to increase rapport with the participants and to foster their commitment to the project. For example, in weekly meetings we read and discussed published reports that used momentary assessment to illustrate to the participants that the data they were generating were likely to also enter the scientific literature. We also provided frequent feedback on reporting compliance and tried to make it easy to return reports daily by providing multiple drop boxes around campus. Of course, we have no objective way to assess whether a particular morning report was actually completed at noon on the particular day. We only know that the day's reports together were, for the most part, completed on the day requested. Nevertheless, our subjective confidence in the overall compliance, both reporting compliance and conscientiousness, is high, mainly due to the efforts we put into building working relationships with the participants.

Symptom reports were in the form of a checklist, where subjects indicated whether each of 25 symptoms was felt during the report period. The daily form is reproduced in Table 13-1. The 25 symptom reports were factored across the 7,225 observations and resulted in the following four factors: distress (loss of interest, trouble concentrating, urge to cry, low energy), aches (headache, backache,

SUB: 54

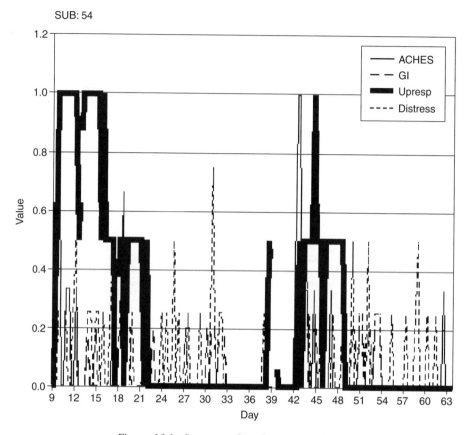

Figure 13-1. Symptom data from one subject.

muscle soreness), gastrointestinal (poor appetite, nausea/upset stomach, consti-
pation/diarrhea, trembling, dizziness), and upper respiratory (sore throat, runny
nose, congestion). These factors are the health dimensions that are used in the
primary analyses.

Figure 13-1 presents the EMA data on the four health factors for a single subject.
Upper respiratory infection symptoms are highlighted with a bold line, showing
that this particular subject suffered two bouts of upper respiratory symptoms
during the 2 months of the study. This graph is also typical in that the upper respiratory symptoms tended to have a longer duration than the other symptoms.

Procedure

Several weeks before the daily report phase of the study, subjects completed a
variety of personality questionnaires. We focused on three variables due to their
utility in health psychology research. Neuroticism was selected for its history of
being associated with psychosomatic complaints. We assessed neuroticism with

the Eysenck Personality Inventory-Revised (Eysenck, Eysenck, & Barrett, 1985). The hypothesis was that neuroticism should correlate with symptom frequency.

The second personality variable of interest was anger/hostility, which we assessed with Roger and Nesshoever's (1987) Emotional Control Questionnaire. The authors speculated that a high potential for aggressive responding may "be associated with delayed recovery from illness through the reactivation of emotional responses" (p. 533)—that is, individuals prone to aggressive responses may be more likely to experience reactivated arousal responses to stressful or frustrating events, implying a slower recovery from stress-induced symptoms. The hypothesis was that anger/hostility should predict longer-duration illnesses.

The third personality variable of interest was the Type A behavior pattern, which was assessed with the Jenkins Activity Survey (JAS; Jenkins, Zyzansk, & Rosenman, 1979). This measure assesses the Type A syndrome mainly as a behavior pattern characterized by impatience, excessive drive, competitiveness, and exaggerated achievement motives (Friedman & Booth-Kewley, 1987). The hypothesis was that this combination of traits might foster an inattention to the emotional concomitants of physical symptoms due to exaggerated drive and a focus on external achievements.

Results

Temporal parameters of daily symptoms were extracted for each subject for each of the four symptom factors. The three parameters were occurrence frequency, duration, and mood–illness linkage.

Occurrence Frequency of Daily Symptoms

Frequency measures of the four symptom factors were computed by counting, for each subject, how often symptoms from each factor were reported over the 180 occasions of observation. Descriptive statistics on all parameters—occurrence frequency, duration, and mood–illness linkage—are reported in Table 13-2. More details, including the rationale for using these parameters, their specific calculation, and the software used, can be found in Larsen and Kasimatis (1991). In terms of occurrence, the most frequently reported symptom was upper respiratory problems, though there was wide variability on the total number of occasions on which respiratory symptoms were reported. The least frequently reported symptom factor was gastrointestinal, with distress and aches falling in between in terms of frequency.

Duration of Daily Symptoms

For duration scores we wanted to quantify the probabilistic degree to which symptoms persisted over contiguous observation periods for each subject. To do this we calculated, for each person, the degree to which current symptoms predicted

Table 13-2. Descriptive statistics for the parameters of daily symptoms

Occurrence	Mean	SD	Range
Distress	15.66	12.93	2–59
Aches	12.04	11.63	1–72
Gastrointestinal	6.06	6.42	1–36
Upper respiratory	24.64	24.48	0–106
Duration			
Distress	1.81	1.85	0–7
Aches	2.77	2.39	0–9
Gastrointestinal	1.58	1.81	0–7
Upper respiratory	5.40	3.67	0–12
Covariation with mood*			
Distress	2.40	1.46	.02–4.06
Aches	1.30	2.50	.03–4.10
Gastrointestinal	1.78	4.41	.05–8.72
Upper respiratory	.14	1.21	.04–3.21

* The covariation with mood score is the mean of the unstandardized beta weights (β_4) from the regression equation described in the analytic plan section.

symptoms on future occasions, across increasing time lags. The autocorrelation of a variable with itself, at increasing time lags, can be displayed as a correlogram. In Figure 13-2 are two idealized correlograms created to illustrate differences in duration. In panel A is a correlogram of a process that has longer duration than that in panel B. In panel A the autocorrelation remains significant out to lag 8, whereas in panel B the autocorrelation is significant out to only lag 3. Autocorrelation is computed by correlating a variable with itself in the future. As an example, respiratory infection at Time T was correlated with respiratory infection at Times T+1, T+2, T+3 . . . If symptom occurrence tends to be followed in time by further symptom occurrence, then significant lagged autocorrelations will be found.[1]

Autocorrelations were computed separately for each subject for each of the four symptom factors to model individual differences in the duration of symptoms over time. For each subject and symptom factor, we determined the maximum lag at which the autocorrelation remained significantly different from zero. The "symptom duration" variable thus represents the largest number of lags at which the autocorrelation remains significant for each symptom factor for each subject. A larger number means a longer duration of symptom.

In terms of duration, the upper respiratory factor had the longest average duration, with the average autocorrelation staying significant out to over 5 lags forward in time. Since 3 lags covers a full day in the data set, this implies that, on average, if we know a person has respiratory symptoms on one occasion, we are able to significantly predict the occurrence of symptoms almost 48 hours later. This finding does not mean that respiratory infections last only 2 days; rather, the meaning of this lag variable is that respiratory symptoms persist in a probabilistic way that allows significant predictability almost 2 days into the future, on average.

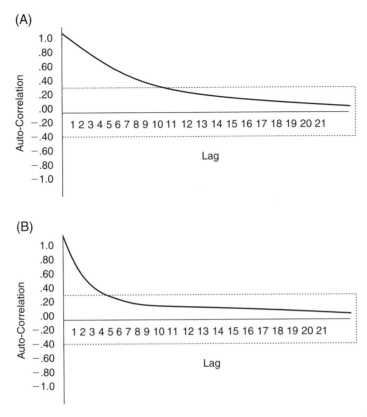

Figure 13-2. Hypothetical correlograms illustrating a long-duration symptom with significant autocorrelation out to lag 8 (A) and a shorter-duration symptom with significant autocorrelation out to lag 3 (B).

By contrast, the shortest-duration symptom was found for the gastrointestinal factor. The finding of a significant autocorrelation of only 1.58 lags into the future (on average) suggests that such symptoms do not last long (about 6 to 9 hours in this sample).

It is noteworthy that the distress symptom factor had a very short duration, with significant autocorrelation slightly less than 2 lags into the future. The symptoms reported on in this factor probably have to do with intense but temporary negative affect associated with acute stress, which is common enough among college students to produce a distinct symptom factor.

Emotional Concomitants of Daily Symptoms

To assess the linkage between daily mood and daily symptoms, we regressed daily mood on each symptom score over the occasions of observation for each subject. In this time–series correlation between mood and symptoms we controlled for the previous three mood scores. This has the effect of removing any autocorrelation in mood that might contribute to the mood–symptom correlation, as in the following equation:

$$Mood_t = a + \beta_1 Mood_{t-3} + \beta_2 Mood_{t-2} + \beta_3 Mood_{t-1} + \beta_4 Symptom_t$$

The parameter used as an indicator, for each subject, of the linkage between mood and symptoms is the β_4 parameter in the above equation. If a subject has a large β_4 parameter, it means that his or her negative emotions co-vary strongly with the presence of symptoms, even after controlling for autocorrelation in the mood measure. Such a subject displays affective changes that co-occur with changes in health status.

In terms of the linkage between illness and moods, respiratory infections were the least linked to day-to-day moods. Apparently, when someone catches a cold, it has little impact on daily moods. The distress factor was the symptom with the strongest linkage to daily mood. This stands to reason, given that the items that went into this symptom are relevant to strong negative emotions, including "urge to cry" and "trouble concentrating." However, as with all the parameters, there was a large range across persons in the linkage between distress and daily affect. Finally, moderate levels of linkage were found between aches and gastrointestinal symptoms, on the one hand, and daily mood on the other. This suggests that these symptoms are frequently accompanied by greater-than-chance levels of negative affect.

So far, only mean levels of the different temporal parameters have been discussed. However, of equal or even more interest is the range across subjects in each of the symptom parameters. We turn now to an examination of individual differences in each of the parameters, starting with the relationship between individual differences in occurrence and duration of symptom reports.

Covariation of Occurrence and Duration

Given the findings on duration and occurrence, we might ask whether these represent two distinct parameters in symptom reporting. Do people who get sick frequently also suffer from the symptoms longer? Or alternatively, could there be a spurious relationship suggesting that the two parameters—occurrence and duration—are necessarily correlated? For example, in order to have a long duration a symptom must occur frequently, but does the frequency of occurrence imply longer duration or "runs" of symptoms?

The correlations between occurrence and duration are presented in Table 13-3. There was a large correlation between occurrence and duration for the upper respiratory factor. This means that frequency and duration are highly intertwined for this symptom factor; if a person gets a cold or respiratory infection, it must run its course. Said differently, respiratory symptoms, when they occur, tend to last over time. The other symptom factors showed more modest correlations between duration and occurrence, suggesting that these two aspects of illness could have differential correlates with personality.

Table 13-3. Correlations between occurrence and duration
parameters for each of the four symptoms

Occurrence	Duration
Distress	.16
Aches	.40**
Gastrointestinal	.31*
Upper respiratory	.71**

* $p < 0.05$.
** $p < 0.01$.

Personality Correlates of the Parameters of Daily Symptoms

The correlations between the three personality variables and the three parameters
of daily symptom reports—occurrence, duration, and linkage with mood—are
reported in Table 13-4. In terms of occurrence of symptoms, the strongest correlations are with neuroticism, especially for the frequency of distress and gastrointestinal symptoms. Type A also correlated significantly with the occurrence of
distress. It is interesting to note that the occurrence of respiratory symptoms did
not correlate with any of the personality variables examined in this study. This
may mean that respiratory infections represent the symptom that was most
caused by factors outside of a person's influence (e.g., microbes) rather than
being caused by specific behaviors.

In terms of duration, a pattern emerged such that, with the exception of respiratory symptoms, the duration of all other symptoms correlated significantly

Table 13-4. Correlations between personality variables and occurrence, duration, and
linkage with mood for each of the four symptom factors

	Distress	Aches	Gastrointestinal	Upper respiratory
Occurrence of Symptoms				
Type A	.31*	.05	.16	.06
Anger control	.05	.12	−.24	.07
Neuroticism	.47**	.15	.44**	.08
Duration of Symptoms				
Type A	.37**	.13	−.12	.06
Anger control	−.40**	−.41**	−.26*	.05
Neuroticism	.15	.21	−.07	.23
Covariation with Mood				
Type A	−.34**	−.26*	−.38**	−.52**
Anger control	−.02	.13	.18	.10
Neuroticism	.01	.06	−.09	.21

* $p < 0.05$.
** $p < 0.01$.

(and negatively) with anger control. Individuals who are less likely to act aggressively when frustrated report illness symptoms that tend to be of shorter duration compared to the more aggressive subjects. The one other significant correlation with the duration parameter is with Type A for the distress symptom factor. This implies that when Type A persons suffer from distress, their symptoms are of longer duration than for persons lower on the Type A dimension. Neuroticism showed no correlation with duration, even though it was significantly related to two out of the four symptom occurrence factors. Interestingly, the respiratory duration parameter did not correlate with any personality variable, even though the duration scores on this symptom factor had the largest range of between-subjects scores of all the parameters. Recovery rate from respiratory symptoms was unrelated to any of the personality dimensions.

In terms of the linkage between mood and symptoms, a very consistent pattern emerged with Type A personality. The negative correlations in this row of Table 13-4 indicate that subjects high on the Type A dimension reported lower linkages between negative moods and symptoms than subjects low on this personality measure. The within-subject regression coefficients—the temporal parameter indexing linkage—ranged from essentially zero to strongly positive in this sample. The larger this linkage, the more likely it is that negative moods co-occur with symptoms for that person. The results in Table 13-4 thus indicate that Type A individuals tend to have negative moods when they are ill much more than persons low on Type A—that is, episodes of illness are more likely to be accompanied by bouts of negative affect (feeling blue, unhappy, frustrated, worried, anxious, and angry) for high Type A individuals but less so for persons low on this personality variable.

Discussion

When it comes to the relationship between health and personality, most researchers focus on personality in relation to illness onset, using personality to predict who gets sick. However, if we take a more dynamic, real-time view of health, we can ask a variety of new questions about health as a process that fluctuates over time. Such questions are simply unassailable with traditional cross-sectional, retrospective or even pre–post research designs.

Insights Gained from a Real-Time Approach

In the present study an intensive time-sampling method was used to develop temporal models of the course of several common illness symptoms. Three temporal parameters were extracted from the stream of 180 symptom reports for each person. These parameters represent individual differences in the occurrence frequency, the duration, and the affective concomitants of illness symptoms.

The three illness parameters had fairly distinct personality correlates. For occurrence frequency, the personality variable of neuroticism showed the most consistent relationships. This finding replicates what has been widely found using retrospective reports of health (Larsen, 1992), but does so using a prospective methodology. Such a real-time methodology allows us to have more confidence that the link between neuroticism and illness frequency is not simply a memory bias for persons high in neuroticism to simply recall more episodes of illness (Schwarz & Sudman, 1994). Instead, persons high on neuroticism report more on-line episodes of illnesses, especially distress and gastrointestinal symptoms, on a prospective basis as well.

The duration of symptoms correlated most consistently with anger control, in the direction that persons low on anger control—those who respond aggressively when frustrated—were more likely to have longer-duration illnesses (with the exception of respiratory symptoms, which most likely run their course in a fashion unrelated to the individual differences studied here). And in terms of the emotional concomitants of daily illnesses, the only significant personality correlate was with the Type A behavior pattern, with persons high on this dimension exhibiting more co-occurrence between being ill and bouts of negative mood. It may be that, for high Type A persons, becoming ill is an impediment to their drive to accomplish as much as possible in the least amount of time. They may respond to illness with frustration and anger, and thus create this pattern of covariation between being ill and reports of negative affect.

Successes and Challenges

On-line or intensive time sampling of data allows the researcher to examine different formulations of the personality–health relationship. The example in this chapter was successful to the extent that it replicated prospectively what is often found retrospectively. It also characterized two aspects of the course of illnesses that, while important to our daily lives, have been relatively neglected by researchers to date. The temporal models used in this study allowed for an examination of the duration of these common illnesses and for an estimate of the impact of illnesses on another aspect of the subjects' daily lives—their emotions.

Such a research strategy is not without its challenges, however. One challenge is to appreciate the size of the data sets and the myriad analytic possibilities that are inherent in data gathered on-line or intensively over time. An important logistic issue is to keep from being overwhelmed by the magnitude of data. The size of the final data set grows geometrically, not algebraically, such that the final size of the data set is the product of the number of subjects times (not plus) the number of occasions. Many researchers will be tempted to simply average over the temporal dimension to get more reliable estimates on a particular variable. While this averaging strategy is appropriate for some research questions (e.g., Zelenski & Larsen, 2000), it discards all temporal variation in the data and precludes any further investigation of temporal processes.

One needs only to look at Figure 13-1, the display of raw symptom data for only one subject, to appreciate the magnitude and complexity of the data gained through EMA. It looks chaotic, but our research questions can ask whether there are patterns in such data and whether those patterns differ for different people or tell us something about different conditions or illnesses. For example, we discovered that respiratory infection symptoms are of a longer duration than the other symptoms, that longer-duration illnesses (except for respiratory infections) are associated with being anger-prone, and that part of being a Type A personality is to be less affected by one's physical symptoms. These insights, specific to the findings of this study, are possible only through extracting the information inherent in EMA data.

The type of within-subject analyses that are possible can result in a large number of models potentially open to investigation. One lesson I have learned is the importance of having substantive research questions dictate the analytic strategy, rather than the other way around. In contemplating whether to gather such data in the first place, and in deciding how to analyze them in the second, one simply has to keep the research questions in clear focus as a guiding principle throughout the design and analysis of the project. If the researcher were to proceed on a purely inductive path, he or she would be quickly overwhelmed by analytic possibilities. In the present example, the research question was on the course of illnesses and, specifically, on the duration and affective concomitants of illnesses as they are experienced. This focus led to a consideration of the within-subject parameters that might best serve as indicators to characterize these two processes. Lagged autocorrelations were used to model the duration of symptoms and bivariate autoregressive beta weights to model the affective concomitants of symptoms.

Other researchers have described other challenges for users of online intensive time-sampling methods, including the problems of compliance (Stone, Shiffman, Schwartz, et al., 2002), deciding on a proper sampling frequency (Reis & Gable, 2000), the issue of measurement reactivity (Shiffman, Hufford, & Paty, 2001), and the unique technical and statistical issues in the analysis of such data (Boker & Nesselroade, 2002; Michela, 1990; Schwartz & Stone, 1998; West & Hepworth, 1991). One of the larger challenges of this type of research is becoming familiar with time-series statistics (e.g., Chatfield, 1996; Gottman, 1981; Warner, 1998), as well as other statistical techniques not traditionally covered in graduate training in the behavioral sciences, such as hierarchical linear models (Raudenbush & Bryk, 2002).

Prospects for Applications of Intensive Time-Sampling Methods

Traditional research questions, those answerable with cross-sectional methods, can also be addressed with intensive time-sampling methods. However, the real power of real-time EMA data collection is gained when these methods are used to leverage the temporal dimension into the research questions under investigation. This truly opens up processes to investigation. Intensive time sampling, where investigators can pinpoint the size and shape of changes in various phenomena, is increasingly being used by researchers (Khoo, West, Wu, & Kwok, 2006). Standards are being proposed for the application, analysis, and reporting of data so gathered (Stone & Shiffman, 2002). As attested to by other chapters in this volume, the technology for efficient and creative data gathering is growing by leaps and bounds.

Given these developments, it is likely that the prospects for future applications of EMA data-gathering techniques will be limited only by the creativity and ingenuity of researchers. Any researcher who is seriously interested in studying a phenomenon over time, "catching it in the act" as a temporal process, would benefit from adopting this method of investigation.

ACKNOWLEDGMENT

Preparation of this manuscript was supported by grant RO1-MH63732 from the National Institute of Mental Health.

Note

1. The autocorrelation function is a probabilistic indicator of duration. It does not tap uninterrupted symptom episodes as much as it assesses the stochastic nature of symptoms over time. The autocorrelation in general provides a probabilistic index for predicting event sequences, from time (T-k) to times (T), where k represents the time lag. In this application it reflects the degree to which the probability of a symptom occurring at Time T is a function of whether symptoms occurred previously in the series (e.g., T-1, T-2, T-3). The autocorrelation also indicates the degree of predictability of symptoms over multiple contiguous reporting occasions. It thus is a probabilistic indicator of contiguity, not mere predictability. This operationalization of duration represents this construct as the probabilistic sequencing of symptoms across contiguous reporting occasions.

References

Akiskal, H. S., Hirschfeld, R., & Yerevanian, B. I. (1983). The relationship of personality to affective disorders: A critical review. *Archives of General Psychiatry, 40,* 801–810.

Aldwin, C. M., Levenson, M. R., Spiro, A., & Bosse, R. (1989). Does emotionality predict stress? Findings from the normative aging study. *Journal of Personality and Social Psychology, 56,* 618–624.

Boker, S. M., & Nesselroade, J. R. (2002). A method for modeling the intrinsic dynamics of intraindividual variability: Recovering the parameters of simulated oscillators in multi-wave data. *Multivariate Behavioral Research, 37,* 127–160.

Carson, R. C. (1989). Personality. *Annual Review of Psychology, 40,* 227–248.

Chatfield, C. (1996). *The analysis of time series: An introduction* (5th ed.). London: Chapman and Hall.

Clark, L. A., & Watson, D. (1988). Mood and the mundane: Relations between daily life events and self-reported mood. *Journal of Personality and Social Psychology, 54,* 296–308.

Depue, R. A., & Monroe, S. M. (1986). Conceptualization and measurement of human disorder in life stress research: The problem of chronic disturbance. *Psychological Bulletin, 99,* 36–51.

Eysenck, S. B. G., Eysenck, H. J., & Barrett, P. (1985). A revised version of the psychoticism scale. *Personality and Individual Differences, 6,* 21–29.

Friedman, H. S., & Booth-Kewley, S. (1987). The "disease-prone personality:" A meta-analytic view of the construct. *American Psychologist, 42,* 539–555.

Gorin, A. A., & Stone, A. A. (2001). Recall biases and cognitive errors in retrospective self-reports: A call for momentary assessments. In A. Baum, T. Revenson, & J. Singer (Eds.), *Handbook of health psychology* (pp. 405–413). Mahwah, NJ: Lawrence Erlbaum.

Gottman, J. M. (1981). *Time-series analysis: A comprehensive introduction for social scientists.* New York: Cambridge University Press.

Holroyd, K. A., & Coyne, J. (1987). Personality and health in the 1980's: Psychosomatic medicine revisited? *Journal of Personality, 55,* 359–375.

Jenkins, C. D., Zyzansk, S. J., & Rosenman, R. H. (1979). *Jenkins Activity Survey.* New York: Psychological Corp.

Khoo, S., West, S. G., Wu, W., & Kwok, O. (2006). Longitudinal methods. In M. Eid & E. Diener (Eds.), *Handbook of multimethod measurement in psychology* (pp. 301–317). Washington, DC: American Psychological Association.

Larsen, R. J. (1987). The stability of mood variability: A spectral analytic approach to daily mood assessments. *Journal of Personality and Social Psychology, 52,* 1195–1204.

Larsen, R. J. (1989). A process approach to personality: Utilizing time as a facet of data. In D. Buss & N. Cantor (Eds.), *Personality psychology: Recent trends and emerging directions* (pp. 177–193). New York: Springer-Verlag.

Larsen, R. J. (1990). Spectral analysis of psychological data. In A. Von Eye (Ed.), *Statistical methods in longitudinal research, Volume II: Time series and categorical longitudinal data* (pp. 319–349). Boston: Academic Press.

Larsen, R. J. (1992). Neuroticism and selective encoding and recall of symptoms: Evidence from a combined concurrent-retrospective study. *Journal of Personality and Social Psychology, 62,* 480–488.

Larsen, R. J., & Buss, D. M. (2002). *Personality psychology: Domains of knowledge about human nature.* New York: McGraw-Hill.

Larsen, R. J., & Cowan, G. S. (1988). Internal focus of attention and depression: A study of daily experience. *Motivation and Emotion, 12,* 237–249.

Larsen, R. J., & Cutler, S. (1996). The complexity of individual emotional lives: A within-subject analysis of affect structure. *Journal of Social and Clinical Psychology,* 15, 206–230.

Larsen, R. J., & Diener, E. (1992). Problems and promises with the circumplex model of emotion. *Review of Personality and Social Psychology, 13,* 25.

Larsen, R. J., & Kasimatis, M. (1990). Individual differences in entrainment of mood to the weekly calendar. *Journal of Personality and Social Psychology, 58,* 164–171.

Larsen, R. J., & Kasimatis, M. (1991). Day-to-day physical symptoms: Individual differences in the occurrence, duration, and emotional concomitants of minor daily illnesses. *Journal of Personality, 59,* 387–423.

Larsen, R. J., & Prizmic, Z. (2004). Affect regulation. In R. Baumeister & K. Vohs (Eds.), *Handbook of self-regulation research* (pp. 40–60). New York: Guilford.

Michela, J. (1990). Within-person correlational design. In C. Hendrick & M. Clark (Eds.), *Review of Personality and Social Psychology Series,* 279–311.

Raudenbush, S. W., & Bryk, A. S. (2002). *Hierarchical linear models: Applications and data analysis methods* (2nd ed.). Thousand Oaks, CA: Sage.

Reis, H., & Gable, S. (2000). Event-sampling and other methods for studying everyday experience. In H. Reis & C. Judd (Eds.), *Handbook of research methods in social and personality psychology* (pp. 190–223). Cambridge, England: Cambridge University Press.

Roger, D., & Nesshoever, W. (1987). The construction and preliminary validation of a scale for measuring emotional control. *Personality and Individual Differences, 8,* 527–534.

Rodin, J., & Salovey, P. (1989). Health psychology. *Annual Review of Psychology, 40,* 533–579.

Scheier, M. F., Matthews, K. A., Owens, J. F., Magovern, G. J., Lefebvre, R. C., Abbott, R. A., & Carver, C. S. (1989). Dispositional optimism and recovery from coronary artery bypass surgery: The beneficial effects on physical and psychological well-being. *Journal of Personality and Social Psychology, 57,* 1024–1040.

Schwartz, J., & Stone, A. (1998). Data analysis for EMA studies. *Health Psychology, 17,* 6–16.

Schwarz, N., & Sudman, S. (1994). *Autobiographical memory and the validity of retrospective reports.* New York: Springer-Verlag.

Shiffman, S., Hufford, M., & Paty, J. (2001). Subject experience diaries in clinical research. Part 1: The patient experience movement. *Applied Clinical Trials, 10,* 46–56.

Stone, A. A., Shiffman, S. S., Schwartz, J. E., Hufford, M., & Broderick, J. B. (2002). Patient non-compliance with paper diaries. *British Medical Journal, 324,* 1193–1194.

Warner, R. M. (1998). *Spectral analysis of time-series data.* New York: Guilford.

Watson, D. (1988). Intraindividual and interindividual analyses of positive and negative affect: Their relation to health complaints, perceived stress, and daily activities. *Journal of Personality and Social Psychology, 54,* 1020–1030.

West, S., & Hepworth, J. (1991). Statistical issues in the study of temporal data: Daily experiences. *Journal of Personality, 59,* 609–662.

Zelenski, J. M., & Larsen, R. J. (2000). The distribution of emotions in everyday life: A state and trait perspective from experience sampling data. *Journal of Research in Personality, 34,* 178–197.

14

Ecological Momentary Assessment as a Resource for Social Epidemiology

Thomas W. Kamarck, Saul Shiffman,
Matthew F. Muldoon, Kim Sutton-Tyrrell,
Chad J. Gwaltney, Denise L. Janicki,
and Joseph E. Schwartz

Over the past several decades, behavioral scientists have identified several social–environmental characteristics that appear to be linked with enhanced risk for premature morbidity or mortality (Hemingway & Marmot, 1999; Rozanski, Blumenthal, & Kaplan, 1999). As with other environmental risk factors (for example, passive smoking; Hackshaw, Law, & Wald, 1997), the impact of such characteristics on health should be expected to vary as a function of the frequency, duration, or intensity of daily exposure. Documenting the extent of environmental risk exposure (e.g., Fehrenbacher & Hummel, 1996) is a challenge for epidemiologists who study the risk factors related to disease (see Labarthe, 1998), and all the more so when such risk factors involve psychosocial processes. Here we examine the potential benefits of Ecological Momentary Assessment (EMA) as a strategy for measuring exposure to social environments that may increase health risk. As a case in point, we discuss the relationship between occupational stress and cardiovascular disease.

A prominent model in the literature on occupational stress posits a link between exposure to job strain and the development of cardiovascular disease (Karasek, 1979). In this model, "job strain" is said to occur in a workplace characterized by high "psychological demands" and low "decision latitude" or control, and a deleterious impact on health is hypothesized primarily for those exposed to environments that are characterized jointly by high demands and low control. Studies that have tested the job strain model in the context of cardiovascular health outcomes have frequently demonstrated main effects for one or both of these two dimensions (Bosma, Marmot, & Hemingway, 1997; Karasek, Baker, Marxer, et al., 1981), rather than the predicted interaction effect (greatest impact in the high demand/low control group) per se. Although the specific predictions of the model are not always borne out, a majority of studies, including at least 10 prospective or cohort reports, show partial support for this model, in that indices of job strain or its components are associated with an increased risk for cardiovascular morbidity (e.g., heart attack, angina) or mortality (Belkic, Landsbergis, Schnall, et al., 2000; Brisson, 2000).

Although workplace characteristics are frequently shown to be associated with health outcomes, the mechanisms by which such characteristics may promote disease development have not been widely examined. Daytime ambulatory blood pressure (ABP) has been hypothesized as a mediator explaining the deleterious effects of job strain (Schnall, Schwartz, Landsbergis, et al., 1992), the assumption being that high demand/low control environments may increase blood pressure because they may activate nervous system processes (e.g., sympathetic nervous system) that are responsible for blood pressure regulation (Fossum, Hoieggen, Moan, et al., 2000). A number of studies, including two prospective reports, have demonstrated relationships between global ratings of demand and control at the workplace and average workday ABP (Belkic et al., 2000; Schnall, Schwartz, Landsbergis, et al., 1998; Theorell, Perski, Akerstedt, et al., 1988). There have been few efforts made, however, to explore the effects of job strain experiences on moment-to-moment fluctuations in blood pressure during daily life, as a means of examining how such relationships may unfold in real time. Moreover, one of the merits of the study we describe here involves our ability to examine the inter-relationships among job strain characteristics, ABP, and measures of cardiovascular disease within a single sample.

Findings from the job strain literature may lead us to assume that transactions in the work environment are unique with respect to their impact on cardiovascular health outcomes. Demand and control, for example, are typically assessed using workplace ratings derived from individuals or from normative survey reports across occupational groups (Landsbergis, Theorell, Schwartz, et al., 2000). While it is possible that the findings in these studies reflect the effects of characteristics that are specific to the workplace, it is also possible that the research on job strain may be capturing important characteristics of individuals' transactions with the environment, more generally, that are associated with health. From this perspective, it would be productive to examine the effects of demand and control in settings outside of the workplace as well as on the job, and in individuals who are not employed as well as in workers.

Rationale for a Momentary Approach to Data Collection

How might EMA methods contribute to our efforts to understand the association between social environmental characteristics and disease? First, with respect to the measurement of risk exposure, questionnaires and interview reports designed to assess the frequency or duration of daily experiences require the use of estimation heuristics that may be inaccurate or biased (Stone, Turkkan, Bacharch, et al., 1999). A person asked about work strain, for example, is faced with the task of summarizing daily experiences at the workplace. Retrieval and summary processes of this sort are both subject to bias. In contrast, use of immediate or momentary reports, sampled frequently throughout the day, should allow us to reduce measurement errors in estimates of exposure that are attributable to problems with memory accessibility and distortion.

Secondly, EMA methods may be particularly well suited for assessing differences in the experience of demand and control across settings, using comparable rating formats—that is, rather than asking people to use global ratings to estimate the degree to which their work and non-work lives are demanding and uncontrollable (a format that may not invoke comparable decision rules for weighing different types of activities across settings), we may get more accurate reports of setting differences in demand and control by drawing upon average ratings of representative activities as they unfold during daily life, both inside and outside of the workplace.

A third rationale for using EMA methods for answering social epidemiological questions is that they may provide an opportunity to examine mechanistic hypotheses linking social environmental factors with disease risk. Even relatively stable environmental characteristics should be expected to vary in intensity over the course of daily living. Such variability in the experience of the social environment in the short run (over minutes, hours, or days) is measurable using EMA methods and provides us with an opportunity to examine potential links between the social environment and biological processes within persons. If job strain is hypothesized to be associated with heart disease over the course of years by virtue of its impact on ABP, then we might expect to observe changes in job strain to also be associated with concomitant fluctuations in ABP during daily life. In the long run (months or years), such effects are proposed to exert a cumulative impact on the pathophysiology of disease. The EMA methods give us an opportunity to examine how such processes may unfold in the natural environment. This rationale for using EMA methods relies on our ability to link momentary self-reports, within each person, to relevant measures of biological function.

We recently reported on our efforts to examine the relationship between daily experiences of demand and control and cardiovascular disease, using EMA assessments of biology and behavior. As highlighted above, our work has focused on the determinants of short-term fluctuations in ABP (within-person), as well as individual differences in health outcomes (between-person; see Kamarck, Muldoon, Shiffman, et al., 2004). The purpose of this chapter is to summarize these findings and to describe some of the methodological considerations that went into the design of this research. We address four questions here. First, can we observe effects of demand and control on ABP during daily life? These effects are examined at the level of momentary observations (within-person) as well as individual differences (between-person, using averaged momentary scores). Second, are mean daily experiences of demand and control related to individual differences in carotid artery atherosclerosis? Third, does mean ABP mediate the observed relationship between individual differences in demand/control and atherosclerosis? And fourth, are the effects of demand and control specific to, or independent of, the job environment?

Method

The Pittsburgh Healthy Heart Project (PHHP) is an ongoing prospective epidemiological study designed to examine the role of psychosocial factors in the development of early signs of cardiovascular disease. Our most recent reports from this study to date have involved initial cross-sectional findings. Along with a variety of other assessments, each subject was trained to use electronic diary units and automated ABP monitoring methods for two 3-day periods at the beginning of this study (see Kamarck et al., 2004).

Our major outcome measure in the PHHP involved a measure of artery wall thickness frequently used as an index of atherosclerosis, the lesion that causes heart disease. This measure, which is referred to as "intima-medial thickness," or IMT, can be measured in the large carotid arteries along the neck using ultrasound techniques (Devereux, Waber, & Roman, 1992). Because atherosclerosis tends to develop at a fairly uniform rate across different artery beds, measures of carotid artery IMT are also associated with atherosclerosis in the arteries that feed the heart (Pignoli, Tremoli, Poli, et al., 1986; Wong, Edelstein, Wollman, & Bond, 1993). Such measures have been shown to predict future development of heart attack and stroke in community samples (e.g., O'Leary, Polak, Kronmal, et al., 1999). Because carotid artery IMT can be measured in asymptomatic adults who have no history of heart disease, it is a good measure for documenting early signs of cardiovascular disease.

Sample

We recruited 337 healthy participants, ages 50 to 70, using mass mailing and media announcements. Participants of this age range were selected because of the increasing risk for subclinical cardiovascular disease associated with aging. Only healthy, unmedicated individuals were included in order to reduce confounding effects of symptoms or treatment on measures of psychosocial risk. For further information about this sample, see Kamarck and colleagues (2004).

Momentary Data Collection

ABP and electronic diary assessments were collected over two 3-day intervals, 4 months apart. During each of these monitoring periods, assessments were collected every 45 minutes throughout the waking day. We monitored at equal intervals in order to ensure that our data would best represent the average experience of our participants (a "sampling strategy" using intensive sampling at regular intervals; see Shiffman, Chapter 3, this volume). We chose 45 minutes rather than a more frequent interval because of the time-consuming nature of each assessment. We avoided a strict hourly interval for monitoring in order to reduce synchronization with daily activities, such as classes or meetings, that typically start and stop on the hour.

We chose a continuous 3-day monitoring interval because our previous work suggested that 3 or more days of monitoring with these methods may be required in order to reliably discriminate differences in daily experience. Generalizability data from a previous sample showed that the median reliability across 11 different self-report measures collected in this manner was .65 (range of .55 to .80) when based on 1 day of monitoring (approximately 15 observations), .79 (range of .71 to .89) when each measure was based on the average of 2 days of monitoring (approximately 30 observations), and .85 (.79 to .92) when each measure was based on the average across 3 days (approximately 45 observations; Kamarck, Shiffman, Smithline, et al., 1998). Keep in mind that each of these observations involved momentary assessments, which can be quite variable, explaining the large number of observations required to obtain estimates of stable individual differences. We opted for two (rather than one) 3-day periods of data collection, 4 months apart, in order to enhance the stability and representativeness of our estimates.

We used an Accutracker DX monitor (SunTech, Raleigh, NC) for ABP assessment (Goodie & Kamarck, 1996). These devices are designed for repeated nonobtrusive blood pressure assessment in the natural environment. A motorized unit, which controls cuff inflation and stores the data, is worn on a belt around the waist. This unit is attached to an arm cuff on the nondominant arm using an air hose extending up the back and down the arm. The cuff is programmed to inflate automatically on a predetermined schedule. The cuff surrounds a microphone attached to the skin surface over the brachial artery. All of this equipment (cuff, microphone wire, and air hose) is designed to be worn under the clothing. Arm cuffs were equipped with a D-ring and a Velcro strip to facilitate self-instrumentation each morning. Custom-fitting Lycra sleeve cuffs, containing a mesh pocket for microphone placement, were custom designed for this study for enhanced comfort during the prolonged monitoring intervals (see O'Brien, Coats, Owens, et al., 2000, for more information about ABP monitoring).

We used a Palm Pilot Professional (Palm, Inc., Santa Clara, CA) for presentation of diary items following each cuff inflation. The Palm Pilot is a microcomputer equipped with a clock, a miniature screen for item presentation, a stylus for response selection, and auditory prompting capabilities. Programming for this device was conducted by invivodata, inc. (Pittsburgh, PA), which specializes in electronic diary methods for research. A carrying case for the unit was custom designed for this study. Participants were instructed to carry the Palm Pilot with them throughout the day, on their belt, in a pocket, or in their briefcase or purse.

Several considerations led us to adopt an electronic rather than a paper-and-pencil diary for this study. First, the internal clock associated with the electronic device, along with the time stamp provided in the resulting output data stream, allowed us to verify the timing of each assessment. (In contrast, the timing of paper-and-pencil diary records has not been shown to be reliable [Stone, Shiffman, Schwartz, et al., 2002].) The diary was programmed to accept data for only 9 minutes after each ABP inflation was initiated (and 1 minute before), and to reject attempts to initiate interviews that were "out of window."

Second, use of the electronic diary allowed us to coordinate prompting cues provided by each of the two assessment devices. In most cases, participants used the inflation of the cuff (every 45 minutes) as a cue to begin each diary entry. The diary was programmed to administer an auxiliary auditory reminder 6 minutes after each scheduled cuff inflation (e.g., if cuff inflation began at 9:45 a.m., subjects received the auditory prompt at 9:51) in the event that no diary entry had yet begun. If the diary entry was initiated within the 6-minute time window, the auxiliary auditory prompt was cancelled. Because the prompting took place at a fixed-interval schedule and at the same times each day, no formal interface was required between the electronic diary and the ABP monitor in order to permit this synchronization.

In addition to facilitating coordination with the ABP monitor, use of the electronic diary permitted us to adopt several flexible data collection features as part of the protocol that we assumed would enhance compliance, and to carefully monitor their use. The electronic diary included an alarm clock feature that participants were encouraged to use each morning, and a "sleep" feature that was used to designate the end of the day. They were allowed to sleep and awaken according to their usual routines. Upon awakening, they were given 45 minutes to wash themselves and to instrument the monitor, and data collection began at the next designated prompting period. The alarm feature, then, allowed us to tailor data collection to suit the subject's schedule, and as an alternative to a standard start time for each participant, use of this feature allowed us to maximize the number of diary entries recorded each day. For example, using a standard 9 a.m. start time for the whole sample would have missed early morning assessments for subjects who tend to awaken earlier than 9 a.m.

In addition to maximizing our observations, tailoring our data collection to the participant's preferred schedule was expected to reduce systematic biases introduced by differentially sampling in the middle of the waking day. To test this hypothesis, we compared the data collected within a standard 12-hour window (9 a.m. to 9 p.m.) to the data collected outside of this window (before 9 a.m. or after 9 p.m.). "Out-of-window" data constituted 16 percent of valid observations for the average person. ABP was significantly lower during out-of-window periods (representing evenings and early mornings) when compared to the standard sampling interval (for systolic blood pressure [SBP], mean of 128.7 mmHg within window and 127.3 outside of window; t (336) = 4.99, $p < 0.0001$; for diastolic blood pressure [DBP], mean of 78.8 within window and 77.1 outside of window; t (336) = 9.2, $p < 0.0001$).

Additional program features associated with the electronic diary allowed participants to delay their responses to an interview prompt for up to 20 minutes when activities (e.g., driving) might not permit timely responding. Interviews completed following a delay were designed to capture activities and mood at the time the original blood pressure was taken. Participants were also permitted by design to suspend auditory prompting during activities (e.g., during religious services) that might require restrictions on noise or sound. Finally, they were permitted to suspend prompting during daytime naps, and a means of recording this was provided. Participants were encouraged to use these program features if necessary but to avoid them whenever possible. When offered in this manner, these features were assumed to increase flexibility and thereby to enhance compliance. Importantly, the program allowed us to record each instance of delay, suspend, and naps so that we could monitor the use of these features (see "Results").

Given the large number of assessments associated with this project (over 35,000 data points during ABP monitoring), eliminating the need for manual data entry was an attractive feature of the electronic diary format. Programming features with an electronic diary can reduce data entry errors as well, by eliminating missed questions or out-of-range responses. Because electronic data can be readily downloaded, moreover, we could provide timely feedback to participants about the patterns of their responding (e.g., frequency of inconsistent or repetitive responses), a practice that we assumed would have a favorable effect on compliance.

Assessment Content

Task demand and decisional control were assessed using two multi-item scales (Table 14-1). Each time the questions were presented, subjects were asked to consider reactions to their activities during the 10 minutes prior to the cuff inflation. We used visual analogue scales for each item; we made the simplifying assumption that subjects were not likely to parse these scales into more than 10 units, so scores were translated to 0-to-10 integer scales and then averaged across items within each scale. We have shown that scores on these two scales are reliable within and between persons. Such measures have also been shown to be valid, insofar as they differ, in the expected direction, across work and home settings within subjects (Kamarck et al., 1998). Moreover, workplace ratings on these scales are associated, as expected, with global ratings of demand and control at work (Kamarck et al., 1998, 2004).

The demand and control scales were one part of a larger 45-item instrument that also measured activity, posture, substance use, and other factors affecting blood pressure during daily life (see Kamarck et al., 1998). These additional items were used as covariates to control for influences that we considered to be extraneous for the purpose of this study.

Procedures

Prior to the first 3-day assessment period, subjects participated in a 2-hour group-based training session in the laboratory on a Monday morning, focused on the use

Table 14-1. Diary of ambulatory behavioral states: measures of task demand and decisional control

Task demand	Decisional control
Required working hard?	Could change activity if you chose to?
Required working fast?	Choice in scheduling this activity?
Juggled several tasks at once?	

of the electronic diary and ABP devices. The training session involved opportunities to practice the assessment questions and the program features associated with the Palm Pilot, as well as the instrumentation procedures associated with the ABP. Participants took the equipment home and began a practice data collection period ("shakedown day") during the morning following training (Tuesday). They were encouraged to call if they ran into technical problems; a staff member wore a beeper to facilitate contact during each of the assessment periods.

Participants returned to the laboratory on Tuesday afternoon for individual feedback sessions. We downloaded the data and prepared individualized reports to facilitate a discussion of data quality, as well as any remaining questions about the procedures. Participants who showed low variability in their responses, who showed unusual patterns of response (e.g., endorsing extreme scores for "alert" and "tired" at the same time), or who had missed too many interviews were identified at this time and were offered additional training. Payment for the upcoming monitoring period was contingent upon completing at least 15 interviews per day, on average. We also offered positive feedback for successful interview completion. The intention was to emphasize the importance of the monitoring and to enhance compliance.

Data from the shakedown day were not used as part of the study. The assessment period officially began on Wednesday morning upon awakening and ended Friday evening at bedtime. Each evening before bedtime during the assessment period, participants set their electronic diaries to "sleep" using a programmed hibernation mode. They removed the ABP cuff at this time and placed it around a storage tube provided to them (the alternative, turning off the monitor, would have evoked a recalibration routine, which requires staff assistance). Upon awakening Wednesday through Friday morning, the electronic diary was reactivated and the cuff was re-instrumented as per instruction. After the assessment period was complete, participants returned the equipment to the laboratory, at which point they received payment for this portion of the study. Except in unusual cases, all assessments took place during weekdays. This procedure was designed to maximize our ability to characterize participants' experiences during the work week and to minimize staff overtime demands.

Participants were invited back to the laboratory for a second 3-day assessment period approximately 4 months (median of 101 days) after the first. A training review was offered, along with a shakedown day and feedback session, as before. The second 3-day assessment period was scheduled to encompass a Monday through Wednesday. Once again, our emphasis was on weekday assessments.

Approximately 1.5 months after the initial ABP assessment, participants attended an appointment with the ultrasound research laboratory affiliated with this project. We used B-mode ultrasound (Toshiba SSA-270A and SSA-140A scanners; Toshiba American Medical Systems, Tustin, CA) to identify the borders of the intima and medial layers of the left and right carotid arteries. Mean IMT was calculated for each participant, using the mean interface distance within each of eight identified segments, averaged across segments (for more information, see Kamarck et al., 2004).

For the ABP analyses that involved multiple observations on each participant, we used multilevel modeling with SAS Proc Mixed. Advantages of multilevel modeling include its ability to handle time-varying covariates, to model autocorrelation effects, and to tolerate unbalanced designs (Schwartz & Stone, 1998). In contrast, use of a more conventional procedure for these analyses would have required throwing out an entire case whenever one or more data points were missing, resulting in an unwarranted loss of data.

Results

Of the 454 participants who were eligible and enrolled in the study, 44 (10%) dropped out before the initial monitoring period. Of the 410 participants who began the first 3-day monitoring interval, 384 (94%) completed the monitoring. Twenty-five (6.5%) of the 384 participants who completed the first monitoring period declined to participate in the second 3-day assessment period. An additional two (5.2%) were dropped for reasons of ineligibility. Finally, 357 participants completed the second 3-day monitoring period, representing an overall retention rate (357/454) of 79 percent.

The average participant completed diary interviews for 82 percent of all possible intervals during the waking hours throughout the monitoring period (for most, this was a 6-day period). This suggests that we were successful in our efforts to characterize a representative "slice of life" of the participants in this sample. With respect to the blood pressure assessments, an average of 81 percent of all possible observations were valid. Here, missing data were attributed to error codes, outlying values, or removal of the blood pressure cuff during the day. In sum, the average participant produced 105 complete observations (representing 75% of possible observations) involving matched diary and ABP assessments over the 6-day period.

Electronic diary entries were missing due to the use of the *suspend* feature, daytime naps, noncompliance (missed prompts or abandoned interviews), and occasional equipment problems. The average participant used the *suspend* feature an average of 2.6 times during the 6 days of monitoring (range of 0 to 21), for an average of 70 minutes during each suspend for those who used this feature ($n = 241$). The *delay* feature was used, on average, 3.7 times over the monitoring periods, a range of 0 to 58 times, with a maximum delay of 20 minutes per use. Daytime naps occurred, on average, less than once per person (mean of 0.70, range = 0 to 12 times), with an average naptime of 80 minutes for those who used this feature ($n = 121$). Missed prompts were infrequent: participants responded to the auditory prompt on the electronic diary within 3 minutes an average of 98 percent of the time. (Note, however, that prompts were not presented during suspend or nap periods, so this figure underrepresents missed prompts that may have been planned in advance.) Finally, abandoned interviews were very uncommon and occurred less than once per person (mean = 0.28, range of 0 to 9 times): Once participants started a given diary assessment, they tended to complete it.

After eliminating participants who had fewer than 30 complete observations during each of the monitoring periods ($n = 11$), those who were on medication during one or both of the monitoring periods ($n = 7$), and those who were missing one or more measures of carotid ultrasound data ($n = 2$), the sample size was 337. This final sample ($n = 337$) was 51 percent (173/337) female and 16 percent (53/337) nonwhite (48 Black/African-American, 2 Asian/Pacific Islander, 3 Hispanic/Latino), with a mean age of 60 (SD = 4.7). Eighty-four (25%) said they had a high school education or less and 174 (52%) reported they had a bachelor's degree or greater. Within this group, we had an average of 106 complete observations with matched diary and ABP assessments over the 6 days of monitoring.

Results for the major hypotheses are presented elsewhere (Kamarck, Janicki, Shiffman, et al., 2002; Kamarck, Muldoon, Shiffman, et al., 2004) and summarized below.

Can We Observe Effects of Demand and Control on ABP During Daily Life?

We used multilevel models to examine these relationships, controlling for posture, activity, and substance use in each model. First, we examined whether our two psychosocial measures were related, within-person, with fluctuations in blood pressure. Our results demonstrate that blood pressure is relatively elevated during periods of the day that are rated as more demanding and less controllable. Partial regression coefficients associated with demand and control in covariate-adjusted models were .30 and −.13 for SBP, and .36 and −.21 for DBP, respectively. These results suggest that each exposure to a moderately demanding and uncontrollable situation during daily life (movement of 5 points on each scale) is associated with a transient blood pressure increase of approximately 2 mmHg SBP and 3 mmHg DBP, on average, independent of its effects on posture, activity, or health behaviors (see Kamarck et al., 2002, in which these findings are presented in the context of other psychosocial measures).

Second, we examined whether daily experiences of demand and control, between-person, are also associated with mean differences in ABP. In contrast to the within-person analyses described above, here we examined whether people who generally report their lives as more demanding or less controllable show elevated mean ABPs. Once again, we controlled for posture, activity, and substance use as well as demographic differences and conventional blood pressures taken in the clinic. Results suggest that average daily experiences of demand and control are, in fact, associated with ABP, with pressures being higher for those who rate their lives as more demanding (approximately 3 mmHg difference between those in top and bottom quartiles for SBP) and lower for those whose lives are more controllable (approximately 4 mmHg difference between those in top and bottom quartiles for SBP; data presented in Kamarck et al., 2002).

Are Mean Daily Experiences of Demand and Control Related to Carotid Artery Atherosclerosis?

Mean ratings of demand were, in fact, significantly associated with carotid IMT after adjustment for demographic factors and clinic blood pressure, with higher ratings of demand associated with greater IMT, as hypothesized ($r^2 = .02$; Figure 14-1). In contrast with the ratings for demand, mean ratings for decisional control showed only a marginally significant inverse association with mean IMT (data presented in Kamarck et al., 2004).

Does Mean ABP Mediate the Observed Relationship Between Demand/Control and Atherosclerosis?

In separate models that included reader effects, demographic covariates, and clinic SBP and DBP along with task demand, we added measures of mean daytime ambulatory SBP. The effects associated with task demand were reduced, becoming only marginally significant after adjustment for daytime ambulatory SBP. The indirect effect (MacKinnon, Lockwood, Hoffman, et al., 2002) of demand on IMT through ambulatory SBP was significant. This suggests that the relationship between perceived demands and atherosclerosis may be accounted for, at least in part, by an effect of demand on daytime ABP (see Kamarck et al., 2004).

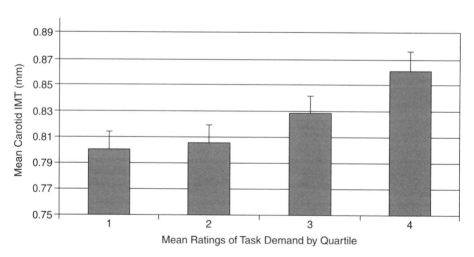

Figure 14-1. Association between mean diary ratings of task demand and mean carotid artery intima-medial thickness (N = 337) (Reprinted with permission from Kamarck, T.W., Muldoon, M.F., Shiffman, S., Sutton-Tyrrell, K., Gwaltney, C., & Janicki, D.L. (2004) Experiences of demand and control in daily life as correlates of subclinical carotid atherosclerosis in a healthy older sample. *Health Psychology* 23: 24-32. Copyright American Psychological Association.)

Are the Effects of Demand and Control Specific to, or Independent of, the Job Environment?

Interestingly, associations between task demand and carotid atherosclerosis did not differ as a function of employment status. Task demand ratings were associated with atherosclerosis even among those who were not employed during the study ($r^2 = .03$). This association was comparable in magnitude to that shown among those who were employed ($r^2 = .02$). Moreover, among employed individuals, relationships between demand and carotid disease did not differ as a function of whether ratings were derived from inside or outside of the workplace.

It was also surprising that the more conventional questionnaire measures of job strain from the Karasek Job Content scale were not significantly associated with IMT in this sample. We showed no significant gender differences in the association between task demand and carotid atherosclerosis (see Kamarck et al., 2004).

Discussion

Our findings are consistent with a model whereby daily activities perceived as demanding may trigger momentary elevations in blood pressure, that these momentary elevations may result in mean overall pressure elevations during daily life for those whose demand ratings are consistently highest, and that such mean overall pressure elevations may lead to an increased risk of atherosclerosis. Forthcoming prospective analyses will help us to examine the implications of these findings for ABP changes and atherosclerotic progression over time. Our ratings of decisional control were related to momentary blood pressure fluctuations and mean blood pressure differences, but, in contrast with the measures of demand, they were not associated with increased carotid artery atherosclerosis.

The job strain model in its strictest form (with greatest effects for high demand/low control conditions) was not confirmed in this study. Moreover, our results call into question the assumption that previously observed associations between measures of job strain and disease are best attributed to characteristics that are unique to the work environment.

Insights Gained from a Real-Time Approach

In a broader sense, our findings support the utility of momentary assessment methods as a strategy for characterizing exposure to psychosocial risk characteristics. What are the insights that we have gained through application of these methods? Most broadly, we discovered that we can collect multiple days of ABP data on a large community-based sample with an acceptable level of compliance. Moreover, we have determined that self-report and physiological data may be successfully linked using EMA methods in such an investigation, allowing us to examine some of the behavioral determinants of rapidly fluctuating physiological processes.

With respect to specific hypotheses, the EMA data from this study allowed us to examine links between task demand and cardiovascular risk using a similar rating format across settings and individuals. The diary-based measure was more strongly associated with carotid disease than was the global questionnaire assessment in this sample. This result might be attributed, in part, to the positive features of diary measures in terms of their ability to capture daily life experiences. To the extent that some of the ill effects of psychological stress on health are cumulative over the course of daily life, it is possible that EMA methods may capture the frequency and duration of such effects more effectively than standard measurement methods that rely on retrospective self-report. Moreover, use of EMA methods in this study allowed us to broaden the scope of the questions that are generally asked about job strain and cardiovascular health, examining demand and control as dimensions of daily experience; in this context, we learned that these dimensions appeared to have relevance across a variety of different life settings, not simply in the workplace.

This is the first study, to our knowledge, that examined ABP as a potential mediator accounting for the relationship between measures of demand and control and increased cardiovascular risk. Prospective analyses examining these and other psychosocial variables should help us to better characterize the potential merits of EMA as a social epidemiology tool.

Successes and Challenges

The ambulatory monitoring portion of this study represents a substantial effort for the participants. These study methods are more burdensome than typical protocols that are used for epidemiological samples, and many of those who dropped out of the study initially cited time constraints as the major obstacle to their participation. On the positive side, the compliance data look quite promising, and the vast majority of these participants (>90%) who completed both sessions of monitoring have continued in the study throughout the initial 3-year follow-up. Participants who were retained in the sample remain a socioeconomically diverse group, with 25 percent of them reporting a high school education or less. Our experience suggests that the use of electronic diary monitoring can be mastered even among those with little education or computer experience. Nevertheless, it is important to note that EMA methods of this sort do systematically exclude those whose daily routines cannot handle interruption, such as fast-food vendors, assembly line workers, or surgeons. We need to further investigate the extent to which such limitations may affect our interpretation of these results. Strategies for streamlining our data collection procedures in the field setting should continue to be investigated.

We encountered a number of challenges with respect to maintaining participant comfort while wearing the monitor over several consecutive daytime periods. In particular, the arm cuff and the microphone pad were sources of discomfort. We were successful in surmounting some of these difficulties, as noted above, with the use of custom-designed Lycra sleeve units. In the future, we will consider the use of cuffs with embedded microphone units, the use of non-microphone-based or oscillometric blood pressure systems, and the use of breathable nylon cuffs and bladders, all of which should increase participant comfort, especially in hot weather. Such innovations may make it feasible to extend our ABP monitoring overnight in our sample, to examine the role of nocturnal blood pressure changes as markers of disease progression (Pickering & Kario, 2001).

The EMA methods in studies such as this can be time-consuming to the staff as well as to the participants. For example, training and feedback sessions require considerable dedication and orientation to detail and a great deal of staff time as well. We need to further investigate the potential for streamlining these methods; for example, we may want to consider the use of video-based training to orient participants to these methods in future studies. On the other hand, any efforts to reduce staff burden will need to consider potential side effects in terms of participant compliance. We attribute our success in this area to the positive relationships we were able to develop with the participants and to the health information (e.g., cholesterol, blood pressure screening) that we were able to provide them.

Any data collection system such as ours that is so heavily dependent on technology will suffer from occasional technical difficulties, such as program bugs, battery failure, and even an exploding blood pressure bladder or two. Although we did not find these problems to be a major source of data loss in this study, working with such a protocol does require vigilance. We found it helpful to have an on-call staff member during each of the monitoring periods so that participants could reach someone after hours if they encountered technical problems. In the majority of cases, such problems were dealt with successfully over the phone. Occasionally, they required the participant to stop in the following day to pick up replacement equipment.

We have found that rapid advances in technology in these areas have made data collection increasingly user-friendly. For example, in a previous study in the mid-1990s, we used a Psion handheld computer as our electronic diary (PSION, Ltd., London, England); this first-generation device was more bulky, less flexible, and more prone to data loss than the more recently designed palmtop units.

Prospects for Application of EMA Methods

Because they can provide valuable information about person–environment transactions in daily life that are not accessible from interviews or questionnaires, we anticipate that intensive sampling strategies such as these will find an important place in the future of social epidemiological research. In addition to assisting us in interpreting the literature on occupational stress and disease, there are several other measures of psychosocial risk whose impact we believe may be more effectively understood with the use of these methods. For example, there is a large body of evidence linking personality factors, such as hostility and the Type A behavior pattern, with increased risk for cardiovascular disease (Rozanski et al., 1999). Individuals who score higher on standard measures of hostility are hypothesized to exhibit more frequent social conflicts with others, and they are expected to show larger physiological changes during social stress as well

(Miller, Smith, Turner, et al., 1996), both of these effects acting individually or synergistically to enhance disease risk. Although several ambulatory monitoring studies have presented evidence consistent with these hypotheses (e.g., Brondolo, Rieppi, Erickson, et al., 2003), there have been no published reports, to date, linking the hypothesized daily-life effects of hostility with cardiovascular disease. Use of the methods described here should allow us to examine the mechanisms linking personality factors with cardiovascular disease.

Social support is another psychosocial variable that has been widely linked with health outcomes; numerous epidemiological studies have shown that individuals who are socially isolated or have fewer social supports may be at increased risk for cardiovascular and all-cause mortality (Rozanski et al., 1999). We have shown that EMA methods may be particularly well suited for examining social interactions in the natural environment and their physiological effects. For example, our previous work suggests that social interactions with one's spouse or significant other during daily life may be associated with momentary reductions in blood pressure relative to being alone or in interaction with others (Gump, Polk, Kamarck, & Shiffman, 2001). What remains is to examine whether and how these effects may mediate the impact of the social environment on disease progression. Once again, the methods described here should allow investigators to begin to address such questions in a sophisticated manner.

Finally, in addition to measures of occupational stress, personality, and the social environment, a fourth class of psychosocial measures, assessed in the psychophysiology laboratory, has been proposed as a marker of individual difference in disease vulnerability. An emerging body of animal and human epidemiological evidence suggests that those showing exaggerated cardiovascular reactivity to psychological stress or challenge may be greater risk for the development of coronary heart disease or hypertension (Treiber, Kamarck, Schneiderman, et al., 2003). Such findings are usually based on measures of reactivity derived in response to standardized challenges administered in a laboratory setting (Kamarck & Lovallo, 2003). The hypothesized effects of exaggerated reactivity, however, are usually proposed to accumulate over the course of daily living. In a recently published report using the same sample described in this chapter, we showed that individuals who show exaggerated blood pressure responses in the laboratory tend to show larger blood pressure changes, by ABP measures, during situations rated as high in task demand or low in decisional control (Kamarck, Schwartz, Janicki, et al., 2003). What remains to be demonstrated is the extent to which such changes, observed during daily life using EMA methods, may mediate or moderate the effects of laboratory reactivity on disease progression.

In the future, additional methodological advances not employed here could enhance the use of EMA methods for assessing the biological pathways linking psychosocial factors with disease. In the current study, we used an interval sampling method, and because our self-report and biological assessment devices were not explicitly linked, we could not alter our sampling in one domain (biology or behavior) to capture the determinants of acute events unfolding in the other. In future work, the use of event-related data collection strategies that link self-report and biological assessments in real time might provide us with a better understanding of some of the acute psychological processes that may underlie discrete biological events of significance for health risk. Such a system would be useful, for example, in identifying daily life correlates of acute myocardial ischemia (transient problems with oxygen delivery to the heart) in cardiac patients (Gullette, Blumenthal, Babyak, et al., 1997). Methods for facilitating real-time pattern recognition and communication between monitoring devices will require further development toward this end.

A large body of research in cardiovascular behavioral medicine has been based on the premise that alterations in autonomic nervous system responding may mediate, in part, the effects of psychosocial factors on cardiovascular risk (Manuck, Marsland, Kaplan, & Williams, 1995). The effects of such processes in humans have usually been inferred from standardized interviews, questionnaires, or laboratory simulations. In contrast, the behavioral and biological characteristics of daily life that may contribute to disease risk have remained largely unexplored. This study illustrates how EMA methods may help us take an important step in this direction, assisting, at the same time, in testing some of the major models linking psychosocial factors with health and disease.

References

Belkic, K., Landsbergis, P., Schnall, P., Baker, D., Theorell, T., Siegrist, J., Peter, R., & Karasek, R. (2000). Psychosocial factors: Review of the empirical data among men. In P. L. Schnall, K. Belkic, P. Landsbergis, & D. Baker (Eds.), *Occupational medicine: The workplace and cardiovascular disease. State of the Art Reviews, 15*, 24–49.

Bosma, H., Marmot, M. G., & Hemingway, H., et al. (1997). Low job control and risk of coronary heart disease in Whitehall II (prospective cohort) study. *British Medical Journal, 314*, 558–565.

Brisson, C. (2000). Women, work, and CVD. In P. L. Schnall, K. Belkic, P. Landsbergis, & D. Baker (Eds.), *Occupational medicine: The workplace and cardiovascular disease. State of the Art Reviews, 15*, 49–57.

Brondolo, E., Rieppi, R., Erickson, S. A., Bagiella, E., Shapiro, P. A., McKinley, P., & Sloan, R. P. (2003). Hostility, interpersonal interactions, and ambulatory blood pressure. *Psychosomatic Medicine, 65*, 1003–1011.

Devereux, R. B., Waber, B., & Roman, M. J. (1992). Conclusions on the measurement of arterial wall thickness: Anatomic, physiologic and methodologic considerations. *Journal of Hypertension — Supplement, 10*, S119–121.

Fehrenbacher, M. C., & Hummel, A. A. (1996). Evaluation of the mass balance model used by the Environmental Protection Agency for estimating inhalation exposure to new chemical substances. *American Industrial Hygiene Association Journal, 57*, 526–536.

Fossum, E., Hoieggen, A., Moan, A., Rostrup, M., & Kjeldsen, S. E. (2000). The cardiovascular metabolic syndrome. In P. L. Schnall, K. Belkic, P. Landsbergis, & D. Baker (Eds.), *Occupational medicine: The workplace and cardiovascular disease. State of the Art Reviews, 15*, 146–162.

Goodie, J. L., & Kamarck, T. W. (1996). Use of the Accutracker DX to assess behavioral influences on ambulatory cardiovascular activity: A preliminary investigation. *Blood Pressure Monitoring, 1*, 135–140.

Gullette, E. C. D., Blumenthal, J. A., Babyak, M., Jiang, W., Waugh, R. A., Frid, D. J., O'Coner, C. M., Morris, J. J., & Krantz, D. S. (1997). Effects of mental stress on myocardial ischemia during daily life. *Journal of American Medical Association, 277*, 1521–1526.

Gump, B. B., Polk, D. E., Kamarck, T. W., & Shiffman, S. (2001). Partner interactions are associated with reduced blood pressure in the natural environment: Ambulatory monitoring evidence from a healthy, multiethnic adult sample. *Psychosomatic Medicine, 63*, 423–433.

Hackshaw, A. K., Law, M. R., & Wald, N. J. (1997). The accumulated evidence on lung cancer and environmental tobacco smoke. *British Medical Journal, 315*, 980–988.

Hemingway, H., & Marmot, M. (1999). Psychosocial factors in the aetiology and prognosis of coronary heart disease: Systematic review of prospective cohort studies. *British Medical Journal, 318*, 1460–1467.

Kamarck, T. W., Janicki, D. L., Shiffman, S., Polk, D. E., Muldoon, M. F., Liebenauer, L. L., & Schwartz, J. E. (2002). Psychosocial demand and ambulatory blood pressure: A field assessment approach. *Physiology and Behavior, 77*, 699–704.

Kamarck, T. W., & Lovallo, W. (2003). Cardiovascular reactivity to psychological challenge: Conceptual and measurement considerations. *Psychosomatic Medicine, 65*, 9–21.

Kamarck, T. W., Muldoon, M. F., Shiffman, S., Sutton-Tyrrell, K., Gwaltney, D., & Janicki, D. L. (2004). Experiences of Demand and Control in daily life as correlates of subclinical carotid atherosclerosis in a healthy older sample. *Health Psychology, 23*, 24–32.

Kamarck, T. W., Shiffman, S., Smithline, L., Goodie, J., Thompson, H., Ktuarte, P. H., Jong, J., Pro, V., Paty, J., Kassel, J., Gnys, M., & Perz, W. (1998). The Diary of Ambulatory Behavioral States: A new approach to the assessment of ambulatory cardiovascular activity. In D. Krantz & A. Baum (Eds.), *Perspectives in behavioral medicine: technology and methodology in behavioral medicine* (pp. 161–193). Hillsdale, NJ: Lawrence Erlbaum.

Kamarck, T. W., Schwartz, J. E., Janicki, D. L., Shiffman, S., & Raynor, D. A. (2003). Correspondence between laboratory and ambulatory measures of cardiovascular reactivity: A multilevel modeling approach. *Psychophysiology, 40*, 675–683.

Karasek, R. A. (1979). Job demands, job decision latitude, and mental strain: Implications for job redesign. *Administrative Science Quarterly, 24*, 285–308.

Karasek, R., Baker, D., Marxer, F., Ahlbom, A., & Theorell, T. (1981). Job decision latitude, job demands, and cardiovascular disease: A prospective study of Swedish men. *American Journal of Public Health, 71*, 694–705.

Labarthe, D. R. (1998). Advancement of epidemiologic research for the prevention of cardiovascular diseases. In D. R. Labarthe, *Epidemiology and prevention of cardiovascular disease: A global challenge* (pp. 649–662). Gaithersburg, MD: Aspen Publishers.

Landsbergis, P., Theorell, T., Schwartz, J., Greiner, B. A., & Krause, N. (2000). Measurement of psychosocial workplace exposure variables. In In P. L. Schnall, K. Belkic, P. Landsbergis, & D. Baker (Eds.), *Occupational medicine: The workplace and cardiovascular disease. State of the Art Reviews, 15*, 163–188.

MacKinnon, D. P., Lockwood, C. M., Hoffman, J. M., West, S. G., & Sheets, V. (2002). A comparison of methods to test the significance of the mediated effect. *Psychological Methods, 7*, 83–104.

Manuck, S. B., Marsland, A. L., Kaplan, J. R., & Williams, J. K. (1995). The pathogenicity of behavior and its neuroendocrine mediation: An example from coronary artery disease. *Psychosomatic Medicine, 57*, 275–283.

Miller, T. Q., Smith, T. W., Turner, C. W., Guijarro, M. L., & Hallet, A. J. (1996). A meta-analytic review of research on hostility and physical health. *Psychological Bulletin, 119*, 322–348.

O'Brien, E., Coats, A., Owens, P., Petrie, J., Padfield, P. L., Littler, W. A., de Swiet, M., & Mee, F. (2000). Use and interpretation of ambulatory blood pressure monitoring: Recommendations of the British Hypertension Society. *British Medical Journal, 320,* 1128–1134.

O'Leary, D., Polak, J. F., Kronmal, R. A., Manolio, T., Burke, G., & Woltson, S. (1999). Carotid-artery intima and media thickness as a predictor for myocardial infarction and stroke in older adults. *New England Journal of Medicine, 340,* 14–22.

Pickering, T. G., & Kario, K. (2001). Nocturnal non-dipping: What does it augur? *Current Opinion in Nephrology and Hypertension, 10,* 611–616.

Pignoli, P., Tremoli, E., Poli, A., Oreste, P., & Raoletti, R. (1986). Intimal plus medial thickness of the arterial wall: A direct measurement with ultrasound imaging. *Circulation, 74,* 1399–1406.

Rozanski, A., Blumenthal, J. A., & Kaplan, J. (1999). Impact of psychological factors on the pathogenesis of cardiovascular disease and implications for therapy. *Circulation, 99,* 2192–2217.

Schnall, P. L., Schwartz, J. E., Landsbergis, P. A., Warren, K., & Pickering, T. G. (1992). Relation between job strain, alcohol, and ambulatory blood pressure. *Hypertension, 19,* 488–494.

Schnall, P. L., Schwartz, J. E., Landsbergis, P. A., Warren, K., & Pickering, T. G. (1998). A longitudinal study of job strain and ambulatory blood pressure: Results from a three-year follow-up. *Psychosomatic Medicine, 60,* 697–706.

Schwartz, J. E., & Stone, A. A. (1998). Strategies for analyzing ecological momentary assessment data. *Health Psychology, 17,* 6–16.

Stone, A. A., Shiffman, S., Schwartz, J. E., Broderick, J. E., & Hufford, M. R. (2002). Patient non-compliance with paper diaries. *British Medical Journal, 324,* 1193–194.

Stone, A. A., Turkkan, J. S., Bacharch, C. A., Jobe, J., Kurtzman, H. S., & Cain, V. S. (1999). *The science of self-report: Implications for research and practice.* Mahwah, NJ: Lawrence Erlbaum.

Theorell, T., Perski, A., Akerstedt, T., Sigala, F., Ahlberg-Hulen, G., Svensson, J., & Eneroth, P. (1988). Changes in job strain in relation to changes in physiological state: A longitudinal study. *Scandinavian Journal of Work and Environmental Health, 14,* 189–196.

Treiber, F. A., Kamarck, T., Schneiderman, N., Sheffield, D., Kapuku, G., & Taylor, T. (2003). Cardiovascular reactivity and development of preclinical and clinical disease states. *Psychosomatic Medicine, 65,* 46-62.

Wong, M., Edelstein, J., Wollman, J., & Bond, M. G. (1993). Ultrasonic-pathological comparison of the human arterial wall. *Arteriosclerosis and Thrombosis, 13,* 482–486.

PART III

FUTURE DEVELOPMENTS IN REAL-TIME DATA CAPTURE

15

Momentary Health Interventions: Where Are We and Where Are We Going?

Brian L. Carter, Susan X Day, Paul M. Cinciripini, and David W. Wetter

Recent advances in communications and computer technology give health professionals several powerful new tools that can dramatically increase the effectiveness of health interventions. In contrast to health interventions that take place within the professional setting, the key to momentary health interventions is their ability to capture and influence critical moments as they happen in the patient's everyday life. For example, Newman, Consoli, and Taylor (1999) used a palmtop computer to assist in the treatment of generalized anxiety disorder (GAD). Patients carried a portable computer designed to deliver a standard cognitive-behavioral therapy for GAD. The computer-assisted treatment was shown to be effective. The success of this treatment was likely due in part to the fact that patients could use the device in their everyday environment when they felt anxious instead of traveling to the professionals' site.

This chapter reviews momentary health interventions, the technologies being used, the theoretical underpinnings of momentary health interventions, some of the interventions currently being employed, potential disadvantages, and ethical dilemmas of these approaches and what the future may hold for momentary health interventions.

Technological Overview

Technologies proving most useful for momentary health interventions include, not surprisingly, those used by people in their everyday lives: cellular phones, personal digital assistants (PDAs), computers, and the Internet.

Cell phones (and land-based phones), in their most basic utility, enable people to find (or send) information on demand. In terms of momentary health interventions, an important tool is the interactive voice response (IVR) phone system. These days it is virtually impossible to call an airline or credit card company without being engaged by an IVR system. Typically, a recorded voice gives you a series of menu options, asks you to respond by pressing a key on your phone or using voice recognition, and directs your call accordingly. With the IVR's ability to place calls as well as receive them, health professionals are using IVRs to provide tailored information to patients and to collect health information from the patient (see Corkrey & Parkinson, 2002, and Lee, Friedman, Cukor, & Ahern, 2003, for an overview of IVR systems).

Computers are beginning to rival telephones in everyday communication use. In 2001 there were estimated to be more than 100 million Internet users in the United States (U.S. General Accounting Office, February 2001). As a result, never in history has so much information been so readily available to so many people. The Internet offers health professionals a way to provide, on demand, health information and interventions to anyone with Internet access.

The PDA is another widely used device that can identify or influence important moments in a person's everyday environment. These devices are essentially miniature computers that can perform a variety of functions, from managing appointments to running software programs. The most basic PDA model weighs just a few ounces, fits easily into a trouser pocket or purse, and costs approximately $100. With PDAs, health professionals now have the ability to put reams of health information and tailored interventions in a patient's pocket.

Levels of Complexity in Momentary Health Interventions

One way to categorize various approaches to momentary health interventions is based on level of complexity—that is, how complex the relationship is between the intervention and the user. For simplicity's sake, the technological devices mentioned above are referred to as *tools*. A low level of intervention is informational, in which the user looks up a topic and receives preexisting information. The Internet and IVRs represent much of this level, which formerly was occupied by reference books.

At a more interactive level of intervention, both the user and the tool are changed. The tool records input (e.g., behaviors) from the user and may solicit responses, such as requesting information from the user at random times of the day. The tool stores and organizes the information the user enters and can display it on demand. This level also may provide preexisting, unchanging information, such as educational and inspirational messages.

An integrated level of intervention can have both of the above functions but also interprets the user's input and tailors its responses to the user's past performance. At this level of complexity, the tool interacts most personally with the user. For example, it may detect something amiss about the user's ordinary pattern of entries and poll the user with a series of questions about the anomaly, questions based on its knowledge of this individual. At the highest level of complexity, the tool may deliver a tailored intervention for the user to follow, based on current

Table 15-1. Levels of intervention

	Level 1: Simple	Level 2: Interactive	Level 3: Integrative
How does user interact with tool?	User requests information	User requests information, enters data	User requests information, enters data
How does tool interact with user?	Gives prepared material	Gives material, initiates contact, compiles and presents user input	Gives material, initiates contact, compiles and presents, uses algorithms to interpret data individually
Are there momentary assessments (collection of user responses)?	No	Yes	Yes, both pre-programmed and learned from user's past performance
Are there momentary interventions (provision of services)?	Depends on person's use of the material	Intervention through providing organized data as feedback	Intervention specific to the moment and tailored to user

and past input. This input may also include information about the context of the user's environment, so the intervention will be practical for the setting.

Table 15-1 presents this categorization system graphically. We use levels of intervention to organize most of our discussion in this chapter, since several different tools may function at each level of intervention.

Like most classification systems, this one appears more categorical than the situation is in reality; many of the momentary health interventions occur along a continuum ranging from Level 1 to Level 3. For example, at Level 1 a user might request information over a cell phone but also discuss the situation with a nurse, who might provide more than prepackaged material in the interaction by giving support and encouragement.

Using New Technologies as Educational and Training Tools

In its simplest use, the Internet, IVR system, or PDA can serve as a library, providing health information, training materials, and support for a variety of health-related concerns. Nguyen and colleagues (Nguyen, Carrieri-Kohlman, Rankin, et al., 2004) recently reviewed 17 studies that provided health professional-facilitated Internet-based health education interventions covering a wide range of medical conditions from AIDS to obesity. These interventions typically provided some or all of the following: health and self-care information, decision support, problem-solving strategies, or social support. In general, user satisfaction with these programs was positive, and their findings suggest that medical outcomes can be improved using this approach.

Mundt, Kaplan, and Greist (2001) used an IVR system to provide education and access to resources related to dementia. During the 1-month study, 193 calls were made to the toll-free system, averaging 9.5 minutes. Although only 19 of the callers consented to provide feedback on the system (most callers simply hung up when they obtained the desired information), 13 of these 19 callers rated the system as "very helpful" and indicated the information was "easy to find." Mundt and colleagues concluded that such an IVR system could prove effective for the elderly, rural populations, and people of lower socioeconomic status who may not have computers or access to the Internet.

A PDA, properly programmed, can also perform many of these same functions. A diabetic patient can carry a PDA that contains hundreds of pages of useful information about diabetes: sugar content of foods, meal plans, the importance of weight loss, and so on. A diabetic patient in the supermarket may be unsure whether a particular food item poses a threat to health. A PDA with a *Find* command and built-in hot links will provide the answer quickly. A PDA may also contain written health interventions, to be referred to as needed. For example, a cancer patient with frequent pain can request instructions on deep breathing from a PDA in the situation in which it is most needed.

Programmed instruction is an educational technique that can be exploited by PDAs, IVRs, and Internet websites, increasing the interaction between the user and the technology. Programmed instruction is also known as computer-assisted instruction (CAI). Since its beginnings in the 1950s (e.g., Skinner, 1954), boosted by the development of software that provided unique responses based on user input, programmed instruction has focused on improving the design of educational materials by providing individualized instruction to students. For example, many of today's CAI programs function as virtual instructors. They guide a student through a set of material by providing instantaneous feedback on student responses: analyzing student mistakes, making suggestions on which material should be reviewed more carefully, skipping over material already learned, and praising correct responses. Although historically there has been controversy concerning the effectiveness of CAI, Fletcher-Flinn and Gravatt (1995) conducted a meta-analysis of 120 studies that compared CAI to traditional instruction and found that CAI significantly improved test scores. In terms of momentary health interventions, when familiarity with a body of knowledge is required for a more effective health intervention, CAI may help augment the basic information provided to the patient.

Using New Technologies to Monitor Behavior

Assessment and monitoring of behavior in real time are covered in depth in other chapters in this volume. A brief summary is provided here demonstrating how this level of intervention helps set the foundation for more complex momentary health interventions. In terms of providing accurate feedback on behavior and eventually providing tailored interventions based on the behavior recorded, effective and accurate means of recording the behavior of interest are paramount. However, separate methodological issues arise when simply assessing behavior for basic scientific research compared to behavior assessments as part of a momentary health intervention. For example, does a person who joins a study solely for compensation behave differently from a person who joins a study expecting personal health benefits? We know that the demand characteristics of an experiment (e.g., the nature of the reward) can affect participants' behavior (Orne, 1962).

Reactivity of measurement, the principle that being asked to record behaviors can alter the frequency of behaviors being recorded (Romancyzk, 1974), has different implications for basic research assessments versus assessments as part of a momentary health intervention. Reactivity of measurement is undesirable in basic research assessments but can be a positive aspect of momentary health interventions because behavior change is often a central goal of the intervention. This principle is discussed in more detail in the next section of this chapter. The present discussion is not meant to be exhaustive concerning the methodological issues of basic research using real-time assessments versus those collected as part of a momentary health intervention, but to highlight subtle distinctions of quality, error, and purpose that exist between these two forms of assessment.

Using New Technologies to Provide Feedback on Behavior

Behavioral self-monitoring has been employed for several decades both as a means of studying behavior and as a component of therapeutic interventions. Behavioral recordkeeping increases the patient's awareness of the frequency, patterns, and circumstances attendant to a target behavior. Moreover, the simple act of keeping a behavioral record tends to increase desirable behaviors and decrease negative behaviors (Kazdin, 1974). Most likely, this effect is due to the inherent feedback provided by recordkeeping. A person who records his or her weight daily can easily see the progress or lack thereof. People asked to tally their unhealthy behaviors (e.g., smoking, drinking, or overeating) may decrease the undesired behavior rather than watch their failures go on the record. PDAs, IVRs, and Web-based interventions have not only made this task easier and more reliable (in part by prompting the user for timely input), but they also offer the advantages of computer power to customize, consolidate, and analyze the behavioral input and provide feedback to the user.

Basen-Engquist and colleagues, in an intervention for breast cancer patients with fatigue, use PDAs to enhance adherence to a walking program. Participants can set goals, schedule walks, and receive feedback on how they are doing. From the device-initiated side, the application prompts walks and records data on the length and intensity of walks. Before and after the walk, the user enters data on fatigue, pain, and mood, which is formatted into graphs and charts for feedback to the user.

Cunningham, Humphreys, and Koski-Jännes (2000) used an Internet-based pilot program to assess problem drinking and provide individualized feedback. Participants entered the website and were assessed for baseline drinking habits with a 21-item questionnaire. They were then provided a personalized drinking profile that included comparisons of the participant's drinking level to national norms. Although this was a pilot study that did not assess drinking behavior in real time and did not offer any specific intervention, the authors noted other research that suggests that this type of feedback can promote changes in drinking behavior. With a PDA or cell phone, this approach could be expanded to monitor participants' drinking patterns in real time and, based on these patterns, offer tailored interventions.

Using New Technology to Provide Intervention Delivery

At the most sophisticated level, PDAs, IVRs, and Internet programs can deliver momentary health interventions with the aid of complex computer algorithms that incorporate some or all aspects of education, training, monitoring, and feedback previously discussed. In contrast to the type of program that simply tracks behavior (e.g., calorie intake) and plots the data on a graph for the user to reinforce progress, the most sophisticated programs use the monitoring information to design customized interventions based on these data.

To cite a simple example where a program tracks diet, the device is already tracking food intake, but it could also look for patterns of consumption and make recommendations for future meals. If, for example, the patient's profile indicates potential problems with diverticulitis, the program could notice a steady decline in dietary fiber in content of the food recorded. In this case, a recommendation could appear suggesting that, over the next few meals, the patient increase fiber intake. It could even suggest a number of recipes or meal plans to choose from.

In programs that seek to ameliorate psychological disorders, in addition to using monitoring and feedback, most of the technologies mentioned earlier can help guide the individual through a specific treatment plan. For example, computer-assisted treatments for anxiety disorders exist, and recent research suggests this treatment can be extended into the patient's daily environment. Kenardy and colleagues (Kenardy, Dow, Johnston, et al., 2003) provided cognitive-behavioral therapy (CBT) for 186 patients with panic disorder. Some patients received CBT provided entirely by a therapist, while others received a combination of therapist- and computer-assisted CBT. Patients in the computer-assisted group used, in their own environment, a palmtop computer that prompted them five times a day to practice components of CBT. The computer contained modules on self-talk, breathing control, and situational and interceptive exposure. Results indicated that the computer-assisted CBT reduced panic symptoms as well as traditional CBT treatments.

Przeworski and Newman (2004) used a palmtop computer to assist in the delivery of CBT for social phobia. During a baseline period, participants were instructed to carry the palmtop with them at all times. Four times daily the palmtop sounded an alarm and prompted the participant to record current levels of anxiety, highest level of anxiety experienced during the past hour, and percentage of time spent worrying during the past hour. During the treatment phase the computer continued to prompt the participant for anxiety-related symptoms, but also provided relaxation training, imagery exercises, and exercises in cognitive reframing (e.g., *"Are there alternative explanations for that person's behavior?"*). In a case study illustration, the authors reported that the computer-assisted therapy was effective at reducing anxiety symptoms, was well tolerated by the patient (80% compliance with computer-generated homework), and was frequently used by the patient (90 times during the first 2 weeks of treatment). In follow-up interviews, the researchers found that once the computer was taken away, the participant had retained the training from the computer and had not become dependent on it.

Cinciripini and colleagues are using PDAs to administer a smoking cessation treatment involving scheduled smoking (Cinciripini, Lapitsky, Seay, et al., 1995). This approach aims primarily to control the timing of smoking for a predetermined period before the quit date. Individuals are prompted to smoke by the PDA only at specific times during the day (based solely on the passage of time between cigarettes), and without regard for the social, behavioral, and psychological cues that normally accompany smoking behavior. The program progressively increases the interval between cigarettes, leading up to the quit date. The strength of association between smoking and the smoking cues that normally trigger smoking may be reduced by this process. As a result, the power of former smoking cues is weakened. Example PDA screen shots appear in Figure 15-1.

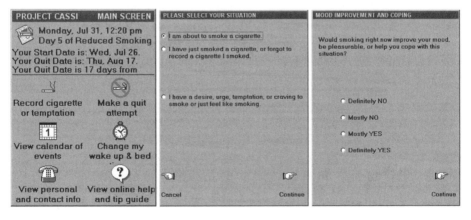

Figure 15-1 Example screen shots from Cinciripini and colleagues' smoking cessation treatment program.

In the first phase, to establish baseline smoking patterns, participants carry a PDA and are asked to record every cigarette they smoke. In the second phase, the computer program generates a 21-day individualized smoking schedule based on the baseline smoking frequency. During this phase participants are instructed to smoke only when prompted by the computer. Using a predetermined algorithm, the program reduces the number of cigarettes allowed per day and increases the interval between cigarettes so that only three or four cigarettes are consumed the day before the quit date. Participants carry the palmtop computer and are instructed to smoke only during the first 5 minutes of each specified smoking interval. They are not allowed to accumulate missed cigarettes for later use. The PDA also prompts the user for random, smoking-specific, and global assessments of mood. It has an on-line user guide, built-in functions to accommodate an early quit attempt (before the quit date), and a re-initiating of the schedule in case of relapse. A sample schedule is presented in Table 15-2.

In the third phase, the participant has reached his or her quit date but still continues to carry the PDA. During this time, random prompts from the PDA assess mood, craving, and other withdrawal symptoms. The PDA also has a library of information on coping with stress and cravings and tips to avoid risky situations that increase the likelihood of relapse. Participants are instructed to record any cigarettes they smoke after their quit date. If a participant relapses, the PDA encourages him or her to make another quit attempt, offering the opportunity to set another quit date (within a specified time period). The PDA then generates a new reduced smoking schedule leading up to the new quit date.

Cinciripini and colleagues' study is based on principles drawn from classical and operant conditioning. The thrust of the treatment is designed to attenuate the incentive value of environmental cues associated with cigarette smoking during the prequit period by inserting a number of unreinforced trials, and to increase the smokers' tolerance for longer periods of nicotine withdrawal. Weakening the

Table 15–2. Example of reduced smoking schedule

		Scheduled smoking data		
Baseline data		Days of schedule	Cigarettes/ day	Intercigarette interval (minutes)
Total cigarettes/day	35	1–3	30	30
Wake time	6:30 AM	4–6	25	45
First cigarette	7:15 AM	7–9	19	45
Sleep time	11:30 PM	10–12	14	60
Total time awake	16:15	13–15	11	75
Start date	12/5/97	16–17	7	120
Quit date	12/26/97	18–20	4	195

incentive value of smoking cues and increasing the tolerability of nicotine withdrawal should, in theory, make smokers less prone to relapse when they encounter smoking cues during a quit attempt and should help them experience longer periods of abstinence.

The applications previously discussed, using new technologies as educational tools, to monitor behavior, to provide feedback, and to deliver sophisticated health interventions, provide the framework for the current capabilities of momentary health interventions. These technological tools have evolved into increasingly more sophisticated and versatile devices able to perform complex tasks in the service of a widening variety of health and psychological problems.

Basic research using devices to collect real-time data is a rapidly growing enterprise that will eventually lay the foundation for a number of effective momentary health interventions spanning the fields of health and psychology. These approaches have been used to investigate pain in women with fibromyalgia (Affleck, Tennen, Zautra, et al., 2001); mood states associated with asthma (Affleck, Apter, Tennen, et al., 2000); the comfort level with obstetric patients' use of PDA-assisted self-interviews (Bernhardt, Strecher, Bishop, et al., 2001); psychosocial variables in hypoglycemic awareness (Broers, Van Vliet, Everaerd, et al., 2002); alcohol use in problem and moderate drinkers (Carney, Tennen, Affleck, et al., 1998); time management skills in individuals with mental retardation (Davies, Stock, & Wehmeyer, 2002); auras in migraine headaches (Honkoop, Sorbi, Godaert, & Spierings, 1999); chronic pain (Jamison, Raymond, Levine, et al., 2001); treatment of generalized anxiety disorder (Newman et al., 1999); and computer-assisted insulin therapy for diabetics (Schrezenmeir, Dirting, & Papazov, 2002). At this point, it is reasonable to predict that a great deal of this research will eventually translate into practical momentary health interventions for treating these disorders.

Theoretical Implications of Momentary Health Interventions

Four theoretical aspects of momentary health interventions are worthy of discussion. First, the design of momentary health interventions should include considerations of human factors psychology, communication theory, and theories related to learning and memory. Second, momentary health interventions themselves should be based on solid theoretical foundations. Third, momentary health interventions can test theoretical constructs by the unique way they collect information. And fourth, the information collected with momentary health interventions can, in turn, lead to the refinement of existing theory.

Human factors psychology, the study of the interaction between humans and machines, is an important basic consideration in the design of momentary health interventions. For example, PDA interventions with an elderly population could be compromised by sensory deficits associated with aging. PDAs have small screens, small print, and small buttons, are typically operated with a thin stylus, and have alarms that may not be loud enough for the hearing-impaired.

Furthermore, momentary health interventions that impart information should be designed with communication theories in mind. For example, how efficiently people process information, at least in part, is dependent on their "need for cognition" (see Cacioppo, Petty, Feinstein, & Jarvis, 1996, for review). Other barriers to effective interventions are discussed elsewhere in this volume.

Well-designed momentary health interventions should be grounded in theories that apply to the particular problem of interest. In general, many PDA user-initiated or computer-instigated interventions are based on CBT, with instantiations such as feedback, reinforcement, and contingency management (Skinner, 1974) and cognitive appraisal and self-monitoring (Beck, Rush, Shaw, & Emery, 1979). From a cognitive-behavioral perspective, giving feedback to someone on his or her behavior, such as a graph or frequency chart on a PDA or website, is not simply information. Instead, under the proper conditions it acts as a motivating influence by representing future outcomes symbolically and thus influencing immediate choices of action (Bandura, 1974). The proper conditions for this type of learning, Bandura (1986) argued, include:

- An attention to the feedback pattern or information
- The ability to remember it
- Some motivation to learn from it
- Belief that you are capable of learning from it (self-efficacy)
- Some reason to believe you will benefit from learning it (outcome expectations)

Psychotherapists work diligently to establish these conditions in conventional behavior modification plans. The hand-held or computerized device can enhance each of the five conditions listed above. The device can solicit attention during each day, can act as a memory aid, and can provide motivational information (including self-monitoring records, as explained above). A sense of mastery over the program and choice over its use bolsters self-efficacy and outcome expectations. Research on perceived control supports this last assertion: when people believe that they hold responsibility over their behavioral program and that their cooperation is voluntary, learning and motivation are increased and resistance is decreased (Deci & Ryan, 1987; Ryan & Deci, 2000).

The critical element provided by the momentary methods discussed here is the "momentariness" itself. Most life decisions and emotions happen in the moment, and most therapists are not present for them. Yet the more closely in time a learning opportunity is associated with a behavior, the more effective it is as a reinforcer or motivator (Watson & Tharp, 1997). To make the most of the motivating and incentive value of self-monitoring, for example, the recording task should ask for "high attention to one's actions and the disruption of ongoing activity" (Kanfer & Gaelick-Buys, 1991, p. 333). The reason is that the behavior being monitored probably became automatized, and any additional conscious attention to it is illuminating. Breaking the automaticity of unwanted actions is a basic of behavior change. Kanfer and Gaelick-Buys also point out the utility of premonitoring—for example, keeping a record of an urge to smoke, in which case a programmed device can provide support and exhortation on the spot. Owning a computerized record of conquered urges adds the aspect of reinforcement to such a technique. The above discussion is provided to emphasize that the use of momentary techniques is not syncretic but has a strong theoretical background in cognitive-behavioral learning.

Another theoretical consideration is that real-time data capture techniques provide a unique opportunity to test existing theories as they apply to real-world situations. In terms of momentary health interventions, a number of psychological theories of human behavior (e.g., self-efficacy, motivation, stages of change) have been postulated in an attempt to account for various health-related behaviors, and many assessments have been created to measure these attributes. These attributes are typically measured in the laboratory or clinic. However, a new ex-smoker can score high on a scale of self-efficacy to resist smoking, but relapse only hours after leaving the clinic. An overweight person can be assessed as having a strong motivation to lose weight but show up for the next visit a few pounds heavier. A person interested in beginning an exercise program may be assessed at Prochaska and DiClemente's (2002) Preparation Stage but never seem to advance to the Action Stage. One explanation for these types of setbacks is that people tend to make decisions that are more changeable than unchangeable and are poor predictors of how they will feel about the result of the decisions they make (Gilbert & Ebert, 2002). It is also possible that levels of self-efficacy and motivation, or stages of change, are not static constructs, but in fact wax and wane throughout the day depending on events experienced by the person. Momentary health interventions designed to assess fluctuations in these attributes in the real world can help answer this question. Interventions can conceivably be timed to arrive during periods conducive to behavior change.

Finally, the momentary health assessments received from the field have the potential to alter or augment existing theories. For example, Shiffman and colleagues were among the first to use PDAs extensively to examine variables related to cigarette smoking within the smoker's everyday environment (Shiffman, Paty, Gnys, et al., 1996). Their work demonstrated the PDA's utility in monitoring smoking behavior, as well as a number of other variables (e.g., mood, alcohol consumption) associated with smoking. A strong association between smoking and negative mood is well established in the clinical literature and in a number of research studies using retrospective self-reports (e.g., Gilbert, Sharpe, Ramanaiah, et al., 2000). In other words, when smokers are asked retrospectively about emotional antecedents to particular instances of smoking, they strongly endorse negative mood. However, Shiffman and colleagues, using PDAs to collect smokers' mood ratings in real time, found no difference in level of negative mood before smoking compared to random times (Shiffman, Gwaltney, Balabanis, et al., 2002). This research is helping reshape basic psychological and emotional assumptions underlying smoking behavior and is providing critical insight into what is actually happening with smokers in their natural environment.

Potential Disadvantages of Momentary Health Interventions

Questions often arise about the effects of technology upon the traditional social networks of family, friends, and workmates in face-to-face lives. Arguments have been made on both sides—that computerization has frayed the social fabric of everyday life, or that it has reduced isolation and built relationships for many people. From our point of view, the huge number of highly active online support groups is persuasive evidence that individuals who may feel isolated use the Internet to connect to others, receive social support, and learn new ways of handling problems. Research has frequently investigated the use of online support groups and typically found benefits for participants (Grohol, 2004). This phenomenon suggests that people are able to maintain psychological contact even when no face-to-face contact exists. In fact, people's imaginative ability to populate any space with the emotional features of human interaction is formidable and evidenced by several everyday situations in which we become attached and respond to characters, objects, and machines we know to be inert (Day, 1999; Lombard & Ditton, 1997). It is possible that the immediacy of the PDA-delivered intervention offers a similar feeling of connection with the therapist, and importantly offers a modicum of control over one's environment, a key factor in promoting behavior change.

From an intervention point of view, this question is important because the variable most predictive of good outcome in psychological treatments is the therapeutic alliance (Orlinsky, Ronnestad, & Willutzki, 2004), which is the quality of the personal relationship between therapist and client that allows them to function as a team with goals, and the positive affective aspect of the same relationship that allows the client to feel valued and liked. Whether this alliance can be built over technology has been a topic of psychological research. Cook and Doyle (2002), comparing face-to-face to online therapy, and Day and Schneider (2002), comparing face-to-face, videoconferencing, and audio-only therapy, found that the level of therapeutic alliance over all the modes was equivalent. In fact, Day and Schneider found that clients participated more during sessions in the distance (technology) modes than in the face-to-face mode. This suggests that interventions delivered through the Internet, cell phone, or PDA have the potential to develop an effective therapeutic alliance and help improve momentary health interventions.

There exists a digital divide in the United States, in which the wealthy and urban enjoy greater access to the Internet than the poor and rural. Lee (2000) reported that, in 1999, households with incomes of $75,000 and up were nine times more likely to have a computer at home than people at the lowest income levels, and even the urban poor were more likely to have computer access than the rural poor. However, there is evidence that the digital divide is narrowing (U.S. General Accounting Office, 2001) and that computer literacy and access to technology are increasing (Schwartz, 2003).

The design and implementation of momentary health interventions, as with any new computer-generated intervention, present some formidable challenges.

These include time, cost, and functionality. Programming time is expensive (over $100 an hour) and must be amply budgeted for design, testing, and debugging costs. Even the simplest of approaches can be costly, and with each increasing level of sophistication, more things can go wrong. That should not be a deterrent to designing a state-of-the-science intervention, but as the algorithms and branching logic become more complex for delivering content, controlling interactivity, and conducting assessments, it takes not only more time to program but also more time to test, and there is more opportunity for unanticipated conflicts in the computer code. Having said that, our recommendation is, if one has the funds, to plan the intervention components and the supporting programming in as flexible a way as possible. Anticipate future needs that go beyond the original planning. Allow for changes in the timing, frequency, and other sampling characteristics of the assessments, and build a module that provides options. If done well, new sampling events and content can be easily added, deleted, and changed so that during the pilot testing of the program, the researcher can adjust the program to obtain the best possible utility. In addition, allow for certain aspects of the program to be turned on or off at the researcher's discretion. This provides an opportunity to differentially manipulate independent variables (e.g., the presence or absence of a schedule) but under one program roof so that only one set of code needs to be maintained rather than several. Allow for use of external databases that provide some of the rules of the program so they can be easily switched out. Communication with the desktop for maintaining the assessment database can be accomplished in many ways (e.g., Web-based, direct cabling, wireless). Consider which one makes the most sense in the current computing environment.

Ethical Considerations of Momentary Health Interventions

Standard ethical care for patients applies in using new technological interventions: we must inspect our informed consent procedures to be sure that they include the special situations that might occur. For instance, privacy and confidentiality may be compromised in the age of hackers, missent e-mails, and family or workmate access to the same phones, computers, and PDAs. Meanwhile, health professionals need to learn about the latest encryption procedures and put them into effect, in efforts to act ethically. Childress and Asamen (1998) offered guidelines for therapeutic use of the Internet, and Reips (2002) and Smith and Leigh (1997) offered principles and methodologies for ethically gathering data from participants through computer-mediated means. In the case of PDAs, researchers may want to consider password protection for a patient's data entries. Technological failure is always a real possibility and may be especially daunting for the patient, who could feel abandoned and disillusioned. It is crucial to plan for the contingencies of breakdown and loss of devices, software, connections, batteries, and electricity. These contingencies should be discussed with patients and put into writing. A telephone hotline backup is desirable and should be considered where possible and appropriate.

Training for patients in using the technology can be seen as an ethical issue involving the general concern for the client's best interests. Running a series of pilot trials with nonexperts may reveal problems in using the tools that clinicians cannot predict. A detailed protocol for training patients, assessing their competence, and occasionally checking on their competence should be part of any program. When collecting intake material, data on amount of previous experience with the tool (e.g., e-mail, computer chat, PDA, videoconference) should be gathered, so that later we can see whether this experience affects patient outcome.

Because momentary health interventions hold so much promise for services to people who have traditionally been ill served by the conventional repeated-office-visit mode, intervention plans should address the digital divide where it exists and should not become part of a history of stratification of health and educational services. This ethical effort includes actively reaching out to include historically underserved populations, even to the point of providing technological tools to participants. This could be done by equipping local community centers, schools, and places of worship with the necessary equipment, perhaps by partnering with industry to provide low-cost devices.

The Future of Momentary Health Interventions

Three trends in electronics and computer technology can provide a sense for the innovations that lie ahead for momentary health intervention. First are the exponential increases in computer speed and memory storage, with a parallel decrease in the cost and size of electronic devices. Second is the massive proliferation of wireless communications, principally cell phones. Third is the trend of increasing connectivity between other electronic devices and computers—that is, due to the decreasing device size, components of different electronic devices with separate functions are being combined with computers into single devices.

Computer scientists and engineers, as they have since the late 1960s, continue to debate the impending death of Moore's Law (Moore, 1965), the proposition that the number of components (transistors) per integrated circuit (microchip) will double every 18 months while the price of these circuits falls inversely. However, most scientists today expect it to hold true for at least another 10 to 15 years (Tuomi, 2002). What this trend means in terms of momentary health interventions is that future PDA devices used to provide these interventions will be more powerful, hold more information, process information at higher speeds, and become smaller, while having the ability to accomplish even more increasingly sophisticated, complex, and multiple tasks.

Fortune magazine (Lewis, 2004) referred to South Korea as a "Broadband Wonderland" that puts Americans' Internet access "to shame." In South Korea, 75 percent of households have high-speed, always-on digital communications, compared to only 20 percent in the United States. The difference between these two countries is magnified by the difference in bandwidth. On the information superhighway, where cars represent packets of information, bandwidth is essentially the number of lanes on that highway: more lanes, more information, and greater speed. In the United States, our bandwidth is 2 megabits per second, good enough to download music. In South Korea, the bandwidth is 20 megabits per second, good enough to download high-definition television. By 2012 the South Koreans are expecting to have a bandwidth of 100 megabits per second.

Although there are no existing applications that require that much speed and capacity, researchers expect that services and applications will be created eventually to take advantage of it. Even with their present bandwidth, South Koreans enjoy unparalleled cell phone capabilities. The *Fortune* article lists 18 separate functions, including access to the Internet, e-mail, trading stocks, shopping, remote control of home appliances, videoconferencing, linking to video security cameras, sending and receiving photos, and watching television. If the United States can eventually catch up to South Korea in this technology, the implications for momentary health interventions are enormous.

Consider the momentary health interventions previously discussed. With the addition of a smart cell phone, along with a 100-megabit-per-second bandwidth, these interventions would have all the same capabilities they currently have, but the power to do much more. In terms of providing information as part of a health intervention, patients could access video streams that could cover any number of topics: smoking cessation tips, stress coping strategies, relaxation training, and so on. Patients could access, on demand, an actual or virtual therapist (over video) for an individual counseling session to address a critical situation that is occurring in real time. The option to videoconference means that patients could have nearly continuous access to support groups. Patients could send reports of their behavior to a health professional instantly and receive interventions, based on these reports, almost as quickly. The ability to combine one of these smart cell phones with other devices could enhance momentary health interventions even more.

Combining wireless technology with computers is just one example of the concept of disparate device connectivity. Other examples of device connectivity currently available are combination cell phones and PDAs. Although these devices have obvious advantages for the average consumer (one device takes the place of two), other examples of device connectivity are more dubious in terms of practical advantages. More recently, the cell phone has been combined with the digital camera. With this device, one can aim the cell phone camera, snap a picture, and send the photo over wireless technology to another user (who must have a display on his or her cell phone capable of viewing it). While the average consumer might have trouble justifying the purchase of such a device, it may have significant potential as a research and intervention tool, especially if combined with a PDA. For example, using a diet intervention, someday one may only need the PDA to snap a picture of a plate of food to record an accurate calorie count of a meal. As more and more electronic devices employ microchip technology, they are following the computer trend of becoming smaller, faster, and more powerful.

Perhaps one of the most uniquely useful of these devices is physiological monitoring equipment. Tracking and recording heart rate, blood pressure, temperature, skin conductance, and respiration in real time have important implications for a number of health-related interventions. Several companies are developing real-time data capture of physiological data. For example, Hewlett Packard (Cambridge Research Laboratory) has recently presented the BioStream system (Bar-Or, Goddeau, Healey, et al., 2004), which offers real-time ambulatory monitoring of electrocardiogram, body temperature, respiration, blood pressure, oxygen levels, and glucose levels over wireless technology to central computers monitored by trained technicians. TeleVital (San Jose, CA) (see http://www.televital.com) offers a similar system that monitors cardiovascular functioning over the Internet. This system allows physicians to monitor a patient's physical condition and perform diagnostic procedures in real time, potentially alerting the patient when asymptomatic problems arise.

The trend in electronics and computers suggests that devices like these someday could be miniaturized and combined with PDAs or cell phones. Other PDA combination devices may measure pain, assess cognitive functioning, measure blood gas, track REM sleep activity, test the air for pollen or other irritants, assess a patient's exposure to stressful noise, or measure a patient's overall activity level. Once these assessments are processed by a health professional, appropriate interventions could be delivered in real time with the same technology.

In summary, future advances in electronics and computer technology, combined with existing technology, portend greater and greater application, utility, and power as applied to the advancement of momentary health interventions. The use of this technology to dramatically improve health, ease suffering, and perhaps someday cure disease sounds like science fiction, but given the trends in electronics and computing, there is no reason to doubt that these approaches will march in pace with other dramatic health care advances that seem to be just around the corner.

References

Affleck, G., Tennen, H., Zautra, A., Urrows, S., Abeles M., & Karoly, P. (2001). Women's pursuit of personal goals in daily life with fibromyalgia: a value-expectancy analysis. *Journal of Consulting and Clinical Psychology, 69*, 587–96.

Affleck, G., Apter, A., Tennen, H., Reisine, S., Barrows, E., Willard, A., Unger, J., & ZuWallack, R. (2000). Mood states associated with transitory changes in asthma symptoms and peak expiratory flow. *Psychosomatic Medicine, 62*, 61–68.

Bandura, A. (1974). Behavior theory and the models of man. *American Psychologist, 29*, 859–869.

Bandura, A. (1986). *Social Foundations of thought and action.* Englewood Cliffs, NJ: Prentice Hall.

Bar-Or, A., Goddeau, D., Healey, J., Kontothanassis, L., Logan, B., Nelson, A., & Van Thong, J. M. (2004, September). *BioStream: A system architecture for real-time processing of physiological signals.* Paper presented at the IEEE Engineering in Medicine and Biology Society Conference, San Francisco, CA.

Beck, A. T., Rush, A. J., Shaw, B. F., & Emery, G. (1979). *Cognitive therapy of depression.* New York: Guilford.

Bernhardt, J. M., Strecher, V. J., Bishop, K. R., Potts, P., Madison, E. M., & Thorp, J. (2001). Handheld computer-assisted self-interviews: User comfort level and preferences. *American Journal of Health Behaviors, 25*, 557–563.

Broers, S., Van Vliet, K. P., Everaerd, W., Le Cessie, S., & Radder, J. K. (2002). Modest contribution of psychosocial variables to hypoglycaemic awareness in Type 1 diabetes. *Journal of Psychosomatic Research, 52*, 97–106.

Cacioppo, J. T., Petty, R. E., Feinstein, J. E., & Jarvis, W. B. G. (1996). Dispositional differences in cognitive motivation: The life and times of individuals varying in need for cognition. *Psychological Bulletin, 119*, 197–253.

Carney, M. A., Tennen, H., Affleck, G., Del Boca, F. K., & Kranzler, H. R. (1998). Levels and patterns of alcohol consumption using timeline follow-back, daily diaries and real-time "electronic interviews." *Journal of Studies on Alcohol, 59*, 447–54.

Childress, C. A., & Asamen, J. K. (1998). The emerging relationship of psychology and the Internet: Proposed guidelines for conducting Internet intervention research. *Ethics and Behavior, 8*, 19–35.

Cinciripini, P. M., Lapitsky, L., Seay, S., Wallfisch, A., Kitchens, K., & Van Vunakis, H. (1995). The effects of smoking schedules on cessation outcome: Can we improve on common methods of gradual and abrupt nicotine withdrawal? *Journal of Consulting & Clinical Psychology, 63*, 388–99.

Cook, J. E., & Doyle, C. (2002). Working alliance in online therapy as compared to face-to-face therapy: Preliminary results. *CyberPsychology and Behavior, 5*, 95–105.

Corkrey, R., & Parkinson, L. (2002). Interactive voice response: Review of studies 1989–2000. *Behavior Research Methods, Instruments, and Computers, 34*, 342–353.

Cunningham, J. A., Humphreys, K., & Koski-Jännes, A. (2000). Providing personalized assessment feedback for problem drinking on the internet: A pilot project. *Journal of Studies on Alcohol, 61*, 794–798.

Davies, D. K., Stock, S. E., & Wehmeyer, M. L. (2002). Enhancing independent time-management skills of individuals with mental retardation using a Palmtop personal computer. *Mental Retardation, 40*, 358–65.

Day, S. X. (1999). Psychotherapy using distance technology: A comparison of face-to-face, video, and audio treatments. *Dissertation Abstracts International, 60*(11), 5768B.

Day, S. X., & Schneider, P. (2002). Psychotherapy using distance technology: A comparison of face-to-face, video, and audio treatment. *Journal of Counseling Psychology, 49*, 499–503.

Deci, E. L., & Ryan, R. M. (1987). The support of autonomy and the control of behavior. *Journal of Personality and Social Psychology, 53*, 1024–1037.

Fletcher-Flinn, C. M., & Gravatt, B. (1995). The efficacy of computer assisted instruction (CAI): A meta-analysis. *Journal of Educational Computing Research, 12*, 219–242.

Gilbert, D. G., Sharpe, J. P., Ramanaiah, N. V., Detwiler, F. R., & Anderson, A. E. (2000). Development of a situation × trait adaptive response (STAR) model-based smoking motivation questionnaire. *Personality and Individual Differences, 29*, 65–84.

Gilbert, D. T., & Ebert, J. E. J. (2002). Decisions and revisions: The affective forecasting of changeable outcomes. *Journal of Personality and Social Psychology, 82*, 503–514.

Grohol, J. M. (2004). *The insider's guide to mental health resources online.* New York: Guilford Press.

Honkoop, P. C., Sorbi, M. J., Godaert, G. L., & Spierings, E. L. (1999). High-density assessment of the IHS classification criteria for migraine without aura: A prospective study. *Cephalalgia, 19*, 201–206.

Jamison, R. N., Raymond, S. A., Levine, J. G., Slawsby, E. A., Nedeljkovic, S. S., & Katz, N. P. (2001). Electronic diaries for monitoring chronic pain: 1-year validation study. *Pain, 91*, 277–285.

Kanfer, F. H., & Gaelick-Buys, L. (1991). Self-management methods. In F. H. Kanfer & A. P. Goldstein (Eds.), *Helping people change* (4th ed., pp. 305–360). New York: Pergamon.

Kazdin, A. E. (1974). Self-monitoring and behavior change. In M. J. Mahoney & C. E. Thoresen (Eds.), *Self-control: Power to the person* (pp. 218–246). Monterey, CA: Brooks/Cole.

Kenardy, J. A., Dow, M. G. T., Johnston, D. W., Newman, M. G., Thomson, A., & Taylor, C. B. (2003). A comparison of delivery methods of cognitive behavioral therapy for panic disorder: An international multicenter trial. *Journal of Consulting and Clinical Psychology, 71*, 1068–1075.

Lee, C. C. (2000). Cybercounseling and empowerment: Bridging the digital divide. In J. W. Bloom & G. R. Walz (Eds.), *Cybercounseling and cyberlearning: Strategies and resources for the millennium* (pp. 85–93). Alexandria, VA: American Counseling Association.

Lee, H., Friedman, M. E., Cukor, P., & Ahern, D. (2003). Interactive Voice Response System (IVRS) in health care services. *Nursing Outlook, 51*, 277–283.

Lewis, P. (2004, September 20). Broadband Wonderland. *Fortune, 105*(6), 191–198.

Lombard, M., & Ditton, T. (1997). At the heart of it all: The concept of telepresence. *Journal of Computer-Mediated Communication, 3*, Retrieved October 19, 2004 from http://www.ascusc.org/jcmc/vol3/issue2.

Moore, G. E. (1965). Cramming more components onto integrated circuits. *Electronics, 38*, n.p.

Mundt, J. C., Kaplan, D. A., & Greist, J. H. (2001). Meeting the need for public education about dementia. *Alzheimer Disease and Associated Disorders, 51*, 26–30.

Newman, M. G., Consoli, A. J., & Taylor, C. B. (1999). A palmtop computer program for the treatment of generalized anxiety disorder. *Behavior Modification, 23*, 597–619.

Nguyen, H. Q., Carrieri-Kohlman, V., Rankin, S. H., Slaughter, R., & Stulbarg, M. S. (2004). Internet-based patient education and support interventions: A review of evaluation studies and directions for future research. *Computers in Biology and Medicine, 34*, 95–112.

Orlinsky, D. E., Ronnestad, M. H., & Willutzki, U. (2004). Fifty years of psychotherapy process-outcome research: Continuity and change. In M. J. Lambert (Ed.), *Bergin and Garfield's handbook of psychotherapy and behavior change* (5th ed., pp. 307–389). New York: Wiley.

Orne, M. T. (1962). On the social psychology of the psychological experiment: With particular reference to demand characteristics and their implications. *American Psychologist, 17*, 776–783.

Prochaska, J. O., & DiClemente, C. C. (2002). Transtheoretical therapy. In F. W. Kaslow & J. Lebow (Eds.), *Comprehensive handbook of psychotherapy. Vol. 4: Integrative/Eclectic* (pp. 165–183). New York: Wiley.

Przeworski, A., & Newman, M. G. (2004). Palmtop computer-assisted group therapy for social phobia. *Journal of Clinical Psychology, 60*, 179–188.

Reips, U. (2002). Internet-based psychological experimenting: Five dos and five don'ts. *Social Science Computer Review, 20*, 241–249.

Romancyzk, R. G. (1974). Self-monitoring in the treatment of obesity: Parameters of reactivity. *Behavior Therapy, 5*, 531–540.

Ryan, R. M., & Deci, E. L. (2000) Self-determination theory and the facilitation of intrinsic motivation, social development, and well-being. *American Psychologist, 55*, 68–78.

Schrezenmeir, J., Dirting, K., & Papazov, P. (2002). Controlled multicenter study on the effect of computer assistance in intensive insulin therapy of type 1 diabetics. *Computer Methods and Programs in Biomedicine, 69*, 97–114.

Schwartz, W. (2003). *After-school and community technology education programs for low-income families.* (Report No. EDO-UD-03-2). New York: Institute for Urban and Minority Education. ERIC Document Reproduction Service No. ED478098.

Shiffman, S., Gwaltney, C. J., Balabanis, M. H., Liu, K. S., Paty, J. A., Kassel, J. D., Hickcox, M., & Gnys, M. (2002). Immediate antecedents of cigarette smoking: An analysis from ecological momentary assessment. *Journal of Abnormal Psychology, 111*, 531–545.

Shiffman, S., Paty, J. A., Gnys, M., Kassel, J. D., & Hickcox, M. (1996). First lapses to smoking: Within-subjects analysis of real time reports. *Journal of Consulting and Clinical Psychology, 64*, 366–379.

Skinner, B. F. (1954). The science of learning and the art of teaching. *Harvard Educational Review, 24*, 86–97.

Skinner, B. F. (1974). *About behaviorism.* New York: Vintage.

Smith, M. A., & Leigh, B. (1997). Virtual subjects: Using the Internet as an alternative source of subjects and research environment. *Behavior Research Methods, Instruments, and Computers, 29*, 496–505.

Tuomi, I. (2002). The lives and death of Moore's Law. *First Monday, 7.* Retrieved May 4, 2004, from www.firstmonday.org.

U.S. General Accounting Office. (2001). Telecommunications: Characteristics and choices of Internet users. Retrieved October 18, 2004, from http://www.gao.gov/new.items/d01345.pdf.

Watson, D. L., & Tharp, R. G. (1997). *Self-directed behavior: Self-modification for personal adjustment* (7th ed.). Pacific Grove, CA: Brooks-Cole.

16

Technological Innovations Enabling Automatic, Context-Sensitive Ecological Momentary Assessment

Stephen S. Intille

Health-related behavior, subjective states, cognitions, and interpersonal experiences are inextricably linked to context. Context includes information about location, time, past activities, interaction with other people and objects, and mental, physiological, and emotional states. Most real-time data collection methodologies require that subjects self-report information about contextual influences, notwithstanding the difficulty they have identifying the contextual factors that are influencing their behavior and subjective states. Often these assessment methodologies ask subjects to report on their activities or thoughts long after the actual events, thereby relying on retrospective recall and introducing memory biases. The "gold standard" alternative to these self-report instruments is direct observation. Direct observation in a laboratory setting, however, artificially constrains behavior. Direct observation is also typically too costly and invasive for long-term, large-sample-size studies of people in their natural environments.

Technological innovations are creating new opportunities to capture accurate, real-time data with minimal intrusiveness using techniques such as electronic Ecological Momentary Assessment (EMA). Other chapters in this collection discuss the benefits, challenges, and versatility of electronic EMA as it is being used in current research. This chapter, however, looks toward the future.

New technologies will enable two significant extensions to current EMA methodologies. First, most EMA studies to date have used intermittent collection of self-report data. New technologies will enable EMA studies that combine continuous data collection of subject activities and physiological states with intermittent self-report data collection. Second, new technologies will enable EMA studies where a computer automatically triggers context-sensitive intermittent self-reports based upon analysis of the continuous data stream. Intermittent self-reports can be tied to the observation of particular activities or states that are specified by the researcher but automatically detected by the computer.

The ability of a computer to continuously analyze sensor data to determine when and how to prompt a subject in response to that subject's activities is a significant extension of the EMA methodology, referred to here as context-sensitive EMA, or CS-EMA (Intille, Rondoni, Kukla, et al., 2003).[1]

The CS-EMA methodology for information acquisition is dependent upon the development of CS-EMA instruments that use sensors to measure and record contextual information such as a subject's location, movement, and physiological states. The sensor data is processed in real time so that the CS-EMA instrument can automatically respond to subject behavior with context-sensitive and tailored self-report queries. A diverse set of CS-EMA devices is possible, each exploiting different sensors, context inference algorithms, and output devices. The query can be triggered via physiological sensors, social interactions, or image processing. Self-reports can be obtained at the moment of interest, or data can be collected to help remind the subject of the key activity of interest and a report can be collected later. In all cases, however, the computer triggers some type of real-time data collection based upon processing a single or set of incoming data streams for a particular event. Each of these variations is considered to be an example of a CS-EMA in the remainder of this chapter.

CS-EMA is a methodological extension to EMA that cannot be achieved without computer instruments that perform the automatic context processing. CS-EMA may therefore require the development of new data analysis techniques because the triggering of self-report prompts (and the way prompted questions are structured) is dependent upon algorithms that automatically process continuous data streams to infer key moments in time that are of interest to the researcher. CS-EMA instruments must exploit advanced technologies, but within 10 years most of the input and output capabilities required will be built into common consumer electronic devices, thereby making CS-EMA instruments economical to deploy for large-sample-size research.

The Gold Standard Technology: Paper

Paper is a versatile and robust technology for gathering and conveying information and therefore provides a useful comparison point against which to assess new alternatives. Paper has many desirable attributes that, until recently, have been difficult for any other technology that supports real-time data collection to match. Paper is extremely lightweight and compact and has a flexible form factor (i.e., physical style that can be easily changed). It is inconspicuous when stored and used, inexpensive, and easy to replicate and modify without special expertise. Paper is familiar to people and easy for most to use, and it allows for easy correction if participants make a mistake during a particular recording session or at a later time. It also allows for subject adaptation when a subject wishes to express an idea the researcher may not have anticipated. Finally, paper has been validated: although the content on the paper may be debated, the use of paper as the medium through which information is collected is rarely questioned.

Paper as a real-time data collection technology does have some fundamental limitations because it is a static, not proactive medium that cannot tailor content to a subject's behavior, subjective states, or interpersonal experiences. Paper is also easy to forget and usually requires manual data entry and coding of information written on it. Paper has no automatic time-stamping of entries, and paper cannot be easily used to ensure that questions are answered in a particular order. Although paper can be combined with other technologies so that subjects can report different types of data, paper does not support the passive acquisition of multimodal data, and paper cannot automatically tailor data acquisition to the context.

The Emergence of Computerized EMA/ESM Tools

The fundamental problem with paper as a technology for real-time data collection is that it is a static medium that has no capability to be proactive. Paper is used in two ways: retrospectively or non-retrospectively. Retrospective instruments using paper require that a person be able to remember information and record that information at the end of each day, week, or some other time interval. Retrospective recall of mundane, regular, or frequent activity, however, is known to be unreliable (Gorin & Stone, 2001). Non-retrospective paper instruments, known as diaries, ask subjects to record information at the time of the activity of interest. Non-retrospective instruments limit recall bias and therefore should be better at reliably capturing the influence of contextual factors on behavior, subject states, cognitions, and interpersonal experiences. A recent study by Stone and colleagues, however, indicated that although subjects reported high compliance with a paper diary instrument, actual compliance was low; "hoarding," where subjects faked diary entries using retrospective recall, was common (Stone, Shiffman, Schwartz, et al., 2002).

One way to improve paper is to combine it with the use of an electronic beeper to trigger use of the paper technology (Csikszentmihalyi & Larson, 1987). Although such auditory signaling improves subject compliance, the result is "still unsatisfactory" (Broderick, Schwartz, Shiffman, et al., 2003). A better solution is to entirely replace the paper technology with an electronic device that can prompt for data entry and also time-stamp entries so that hoarding is not possible (Stone et al., 2002). When electronic devices are used as the medium for conveying and gathering information, diary compliance can be improved (Hyland, Kenyon, Allen, & Howarth, 1993; Stone et al., 2002). An additional benefit is that electronic entry devices can reduce researchers' data entry time and the likelihood of encoding errors.

Electronic EMA (Stone & Shiffman, 1994), also known as electronic experience sampling (Barrett & Barrett, 2001), is a technique where a small mobile computer such as a personal digital assistant (PDA) is programmed to prompt a subject with an audio or visual reminder on a schedule determined by the researcher. The other chapters in this collection describe how the electronic sampling methodology is being applied in health-related research fields. As more electronic sampling studies are conducted, recommendations for new experimental methods (Larson & Delespaul, 1990) and statistical models for data analysis (Schwartz & Stone, 1998) are being proposed. Electronic sampling does introduce some new potential problems, such as heightened reactivity, where the sampling may influence the measurement. Recent results, however, indicate that the magnitude of reactivity to electronic sampling may be smaller than previously thought (Hufford, Shields, Shiffman, et al., 2002). The cost of the enabling technologies is also a problem that is slowing widespread adoption of the technique.

The New Opportunity: Context-Sensitive Data Collection and Intervention

Most electronic sampling for real-time data collection in use today simply replaces the paper medium with an electronic device. The diary assessment content is adjusted for display on small screens, and responses are changed to allow for stylus or touch-screen input. The computer operates as an input, output, and time-stamping storage mechanism. These typical electronic EMA devices may improve the quality of data collected from paper instruments, but most are not yet fully exploiting the capabilities of the electronic devices. New technologies will support three key advances:

- **Continuous and passive collection of multimodal data.** New instruments will use emerging electronic devices to comfortably, continuously, and passively collect data. Sensors worn on the body and placed in the environment will record information about a subject's location, physiological states, and activities without requiring proactive self-report.
- **Context-sensitive prompting at appropriate times and places.** Emerging electronic devices will make context-sensitive prompting possible, where questions are automatically triggered based on the subject's behavior, location, physiological states, past responses, and/or activities.
- **Data collection tailored to the individual and to the situation.** Emerging electronic devices will allow an unprecedented amount of longitudinal data to be collected and stored locally on the sampling device. Algorithms that analyze this data will be able to tailor questions based upon a subject's prior behavior or reported subjective states, cognitions, or interpersonal experiences.

Each of these opportunities is described in the sections that follow.

An Example: Technology to Support CS-EMA

Technological innovations will support CS-EMA instruments that automatically compute an appropriate time and place to collect data based on a subject's past and current activity and then tailor the questions asked to the situation (Intille, Rondoni, Kukla, et al., 2003). Later in this chapter the full potential of CS-EMA is discussed, based on technologies likely to emerge in the next 10 years. However, current technologies can be used to create CS-EMA instruments.

First-generation software developed at MIT using present-day mobile computing devices is being used to test the capabilities of the CS-EMA methodology. Software written for PocketPC (Microsoft, Seattle, WA) PDA devices implements the basic functionality commonly found in commercial (e.g., DiaryPRO [invivo-data, Pittsburgh, PA]) and open-source (Barrett & Barrett, 2001; Brodsky, Consolvo, & Walker, 2002; Rafaeli, 2003; Weiss & Beal, 2003) EMA programs. The MIT software, referred to here as CAES, includes options for (1) chaining complex sequences of questions based on particular question responses, (2) multiple-choice and multiple-response questions, (3) flexible question recurrence patterns (by weeks, days, hours, minutes), and (4) bounded randomization (min/max time to next query). The researcher "programs" a diary assessment strategy by entering the questions in a comma-delimited file.

The most important aspect of the MIT CAES software is that it can record and respond to sensor data, such as a subject's position (from Global Positioning System [GPS]), the subject's posture (from accelerometers), and the subject's heart rate (from a wireless chest strap monitor). Typically a researcher using EMA has three options: (1) sampling on a time-based, regular-interval schedule, such as every 30 minutes, (2) sampling on a time-based variable random schedule, such as on average once every 30 minutes or sometime randomly within every 2-hour window, and (3) event-based sampling in response to subject initiative, where the subject is told to make a data entry whenever performing a particular activity (Stone & Shiffman, 1994). Devices with sensors allow a fourth option: triggering self-report based on sensor readings of the context. With such a device, contextual factors such as a subject's location, physical activity, proximity to others, or physiological state can trigger self-report assessments. Further, the assessments can be tailored to the context that has been detected from sensors. Any contextual situation that the device can automatically detect can be used to trigger, tailor, or trigger **and** tailor a self-report.

The MIT CAES software has been developed in a modular fashion that allows new context-sensing sensors and software to be plugged in. These sensors permit researchers to use context-sensitive sampling where questions are asked only when a subject does a specific thing. For example, in one study CAES software was used to implement a CS-EMA protocol where a subject was prompted to respond based upon changes in heart rate. Heart rate was monitored using a wireless chest strap that sent data to a receiver attached to a PDA (Rondoni, 2003). In another study, CAES software was used to implement a CS-EMA protocol where a subject was prompted based on changes in posture. Posture was detected by a CAES software module that analyzed data sent to a receiver plugged into the PDA from two wireless accelerometers worn on the body (Ho & Intille, 2005). In a pilot study, the CAES software has been used to implement a CS-EMA protocol where self-reports are triggered when someone is near a

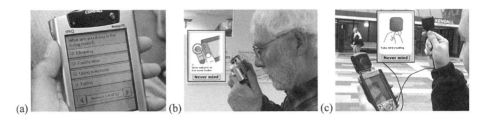

Figure 16-1. Screen shots of MIT CAES software.

particular part of the community, as determined by a GPS receiver plugged into the PDA and a GIS database.

In each of these experiments, the CS-EMA methodology was run using CAES software on a PDA. The researcher scheduled questions to occur during the time or just after the activities of most interest occurred, thereby minimizing the interruption burden of the EMA technique on a subject while maximizing the amount of data acquired about the target behavior. Figure 16-1 shows screen shots of the MIT CAES software.

Table 16-1 lists the properties of paper and current mobile computing devices (e.g., PDAs) that enable real-time data collection. The delivery technology dramatically affects the implementation of EMA. For instance, most current EMA options are implemented on PDA devices. PDAs are getting smaller, lighter, less expensive, and more convenient to use each year, but paper can still be carried much more inconspicuously and comfortably. PDAs offer the significant advantage of audio prompting with time-stamped and time-sensitive electronic data entry, but the prompting can become irritating for the participant in longer experiments or for those with aggressive prompting schedules. The interruption burden of traditional electronic sampling is one of its primary drawbacks.

By using new technology to prompt subjects only during activities of interest, CS-EMA may increase the volume and quality of data acquired about the target behaviors while minimizing the burden of sampling for the subject. CS-EMA, however, requires that subjects use computing devices that can receive data from sensors. Many sensors today are bulky, uncomfortable, and expensive, but this situation is about to change.

Driving Trends

There are four trends that will facilitate the creation of new instruments to support CS-EMA: miniaturization, plummeting costs, ubiquitous wireless networks, and accurate activity recognition algorithms.

Table 16-1. Properties of paper when used for a diary assessment, current PDAs when used for EMA, current PDAs with sensors when used for CS-EMA today, and mobile devices with sensors (in 10 years) when used for CS-EMA

Property	Paper for diary	PDA for EMA (today)	PDA with sensors for CS-EMA (today)	Mobile device with sensors (in 10 years) for CS-EMA
Lightweight	✓	✓-	✓-	✓
Compact	✓	✓-	✓-	✓
Inconspicuous	✓	✓-		✓
Inexpensive	✓			✓
Flexible physical form factor	✓			✓
Easy to replicate (technology readily available)	✓			✓
Easy to modify assessment strategies	✓			?
No special expertise required to implement	✓			?
Familiar to subject	✓	✓-		✓
Subject can adapt if desired	✓			
Validated	✓	✓		?
Not easy to forget/leave behind		✓-	✓	✓
Low interruption burden				
Proactive reminders to enter self-reports		✓	✓	✓
Automatic data entry		✓	✓	✓
Automatic time stamps		✓	✓	✓
Questions can be asked sequentially based on prior responses		✓	✓	✓
Multimodal continuous data collection			✓-	✓
Auto tailor prompts and questions to context			✓-	✓

A "✓" indicates the author believes the technique satisfies the property, with "✓- indicating the property is satisfied but to a somewhat lesser degree. A "?" indicates that the author is uncertain.

Device and Sensor Miniaturization

The computer industry has a phenomenal history of miniaturizing technologies— a trend expected to continue. Many of the portable phones, PDAs, and music players on the market today are actually 400-MHz+ computers with the capability to store gigabytes of information and transmit and receive data wirelessly. They can operate for a full day on a single night's charge. For output, these devices have bright, color video displays and audio. For input, the devices have touch screens, buttons, keyboards, handwriting recognition, and audio. These tiny computers can fit in a pocket, and they have enough speed and memory to collect, store, and process data from multiple sensors on wireless networks. The devices are essentially wearable computers, computing devices with small and ergonomic physical styles that permit users to comfortably wear or carry them at all times (Starner, 2002). The devices can perform nonstop data collection, processing, and archiving—functionality that could be exploited to create a device to implement CS-EMA protocols.

Miniaturization of wireless sensor technologies is also ongoing. Small, low-power sensors that can be worn on the body or placed in the environment are in development in labs today. Sophisticated sensors are already migrating into common consumer devices. New watches, for example, are capable of displaying and collecting information from wireless sensors worn on other parts of the body, such as a chest strap heart rate monitor (FitSense Technology, Southborough, MA). New mobile phones, PDAs, and watches have sensors such as GPS-based position locators, voice recognizers, fingerprint recognizers, and cameras. In labs, prototypes of jewelry that measure blood pressure volume, galvanic skin response, blood oxygen levels, and hand gestures have been created (Asada, Shaltis, Reisner, et al., 2003; Gandy, Starner, Auxier, & Ashbrook, 2000).

Plummeting Costs

Both the size and the cost of these devices are decreasing, even as their capabilities increase. Two barriers to widespread use of CS-EMA are the cost of the hardware required to collect and analyze sensor data in real time and the cost of developing, customizing, and maintaining the technology.

Intel, a manufacturer of computer, networking, and communications products, predicts that Moore's Law (Moore, 1965)—a doubling of computer power every 2 to 3 years—will hold for another decade. Therefore, the functionality-to-price ratio of mobile computing devices that can be used for computerized sampling will continue to improve. Within 10 years, mobile devices such as phones will have the computational, memory, and networking capacities of today's desktop computers but with "anytime, anywhere" access. These devices will have sensors such as miniature cameras, microphones, GPS, and accelerometers built in. They will have local area networking capabilities such as Bluetooth so that they can collect data such as heart rate and motion measurement devices from sensors or "sensor jewelry" worn on the body. Most significantly for researchers, many of the devices will be available "free" with the purchase of cellular phone contracts. As the technology matures, researchers will be able to exploit powerful computing infrastructures that have been purchased by people for their own entertainment, communication, and personal health care needs (Intille, Larson, & Kukla, 2002).

The cost of the technology will be spread across the consumer base. For example, the FCC has mandated that all new mobile phones must have GPS position-finding capability that can pinpoint the phone's position within 300 feet (Federal Communications Commission, 2004). Phone manufacturers are competing with each other to keep the cost of this technology, initially estimated to be $15 to $20 a phone, as low as possible. The ability to track a person in his or her community has benefits in nearly every subfield of preventive health research, and the capability to determine this information will exist in nearly all mobile phones in use by 2010.

The more significant barrier to the adoption of technology able to implement CS-EMA protocols may be the cost of developing, customizing, and maintaining the technology. Every study is different. Therefore, these costs will not drop unless tools are created that allow researchers to generate custom-designed EMA applications. Fortunately, the programming environments for mobile computing devices are improving. For example, many new mobile phones and PDAs can be programmed using platform-independent languages such as Java. Creating flexible tools for researchers so they can take advantage of CS-EMA and other new opportunities is a worthy and necessary goal toward achieving the vision of the ultimate mobile computing technology for running CS-EMA protocols described later in this paper.

Wireless Networks

The third force driving the adoption of CS-EMA will be "anytime, anywhere" wireless network capabilities. Three types of wireless networks will play a role. Wide-area wireless networks such as those used by the mobile phone carriers (e.g., GSM) can be used to send data long distances intermittently. High-speed local area wireless networks (e.g., 802.11b, or WiFi) that are common in workplaces and homes can be used for fast, low-cost transfer of video, audio, and other high-bandwidth data streams. On-body personal wireless networks such as Bluetooth can collect data from miniature, wearable on-body sensors. When combined, these three networks create new real-time data collection and analysis possibilities. For example, one lab prototype used a wireless heart rate chest strap monitor to send data via a personal wireless network to a receiver connected to a common mobile phone; the mobile phone sent the data via the wide-area network to a computer that processed the signal in real time and sent messages about heart condition back to the phone (Qi, 2003).

Activity Recognition Algorithms

The fourth trend that will lead to the development of new technologies that can support CS-EMA protocols is the creation and validation of accurate algorithms that use sensor data to automatically detect information, such as the subject's activity, about the subject's context.

The next three sections further discuss the three areas of innovation created by these technology trends: (1) continuous and passive collection of multimodal data, (2) context-sensitive prompting at appropriate times and places, and (3) data collection tailored to the individual and the situation.

Continuous and Passive Collection of Multimodal Data

Technological innovations will create new opportunities for continuous and passive collection of different types of data from people as they engage in free-living behavior. Manual data recording of certain data types, such as physiological states, is known to be difficult and error-prone (Hollenberg, Pirraglia, Williams-Russo, et al., 1997). Further, the more data that are being collected, the more burdensome and less practical self-report data collection becomes. The sensors for passive, multimodal data collection can be classified into two types: those worn or carried on the body and those placed in the environment.

Sensors Worn on the Body

Sensors worn by a person may passively collect data on three contextual factors: the person's motion, physiological states, and the state of the surrounding environment.

MOTION SENSORS

The actigraph may be the most widely used passive sensing device in use for studies of free-living subjects. An actigraph consists of one to three accelerometers in a watch-like casing that can be worn for long periods and used to estimate gross motion and energy expenditure (Melanson & Freedson, 1995). The actigraph has proven itself to be a useful tool to validate other instruments that measure physical activity (Welk, 2002). Unfortunately, commercial actigraphs do not permit data to be output in real time to a mobile computing device. They also do not sample motion data at sufficiently high rates so that the output from the devices can be used to detect specific activities.

New "real-time" actigraph extensions are being developed in laboratories. Figure 162 shows some "mobile MITes" (MIT environmental sensors): three-axis wireless accelerometers developed at MIT that transmit data to a PDA. Multiple mobile MITes can be worn simultaneously on different parts of the body. The PDA can either save the raw data for later analysis as a traditional actigraph does or process the multiple streams of acceleration data in real time to automatically infer ambulatory activities (e.g., walking, cycling) and the posture (standing, sitting, lying down) of the person. These motion states can be detected reliably in real time from raw accelerometer data, particularly when one accelerometer is placed on the upper body and one on the lower body and correlations between the two are detected (e.g., see Bao & Intille, 2004). Software on the PDA can then respond to the person's physical activity with a targeted question during or just after the behavior of interest. The MITes are designed to operate for a full waking day on a single coin cell battery. Participants can wear them continuously if they make one battery change each morning—a burden, but not an unacceptable one for many studies.

In Figure 16-2, mobile MITes transmit three-axis acceleration data in real time to a nearby PDA with a special sleeve that contains the receiver. The PDA can process the data to detect activities in real-time activity to support CS-EMA. MITes can be quickly installed in homes or other environments to detect use of specific devices and to trigger a context-sensitive self-report. The data, which are used to answer context-specific questions, can be transmitted to a PDA carried by the subject.

Some wireless motion sensors have already been commercialized. A wireless FootPod pedometer from FitSense can occasionally send distance traveled and speed data to a mobile computing device, such as a PDA or watch (FitSense Technology, Southborough, MA). The device is easy to use and easy to wear and can even transmit data to some Motorola mobile phones.

Accelerometers are not the only mechanisms that can measure body motion. Gyroscopes can also provide information about body motion, and they are small enough to include on the board shown in Figure 16-2. Gyroscopes, particularly when combined with accelerometers, could provide software running on a PDA or telephone with the relative orientation of the subject's limbs. Gyroscopes or accelerometers placed on both sides of a joint can detect the approximate joint angle. In laboratories, researchers are experimenting with up to 30 accelerometers placed simultaneously on a single person to determine the best number and placement for recognition of particular activities (Kern, Schiele, & Schmidt, 2003; Van Laerhoven, Schmidt, & Gellersen, 2002). Activity detection from these devices could enable CS-EMA protocols with activity-triggered self-reports.

PHYSIOLOGICAL SENSORS

Dramatic improvements in the size, performance, and comfort of on-body physiological sensors for ambulatory monitoring are being made in laboratories, and

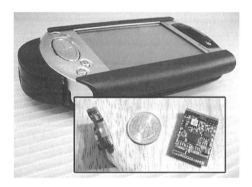

Figure 16-2. Mobile MITes.

these advances are migrating to consumer devices. The HealthWear armband is worn on the upper arm and continuously collects data on arm movement, skin temperature, heart rate, and galvanic skin response (BodyMedia, Pittsburgh, PA). The LifeShirt is a washable shirt that contains embedded sensors that monitor physiological states such as heart rate, blood pressure, and respiration (VivoMetrics, Princeton, NJ). Although these devices cannot send data in real time to a CS-EMA device, emerging technologies will provide new opportunities for context-sensitive sampling that is triggered by physiological state. For instance, heart rate can be measured with a commercial wireless heart rate chest strap (Polar Electro Oy, Kempele, Finland) (Goodie, Larkin, & Schauss, 2000). Monitoring can take place in real time from a PDA when the appropriate receiver is attached (Rondoni, 2003). Systems that are more comfortable to wear for extended periods are in development. For instance, the SmartShirt is a prototype shirt that sends EKG, heart rate, respiration, temperature, and pulse oximetry data wirelessly to a receiver (Sensatex, Bethesda, MD).

Other sensors enable similar physiological triggering. Galvanic skin response measures perspiration, which is known to correlate with stress. The galvanic skin response can be passively measured using a modified biker's glove (Healey & Picard, 1998). Blood pressure can be measured with an arm or finger cuff that automatically inflates at researcher-specified intervals of time (Kario, Yasui, & Yokoi, 2003). Finger touch can be measured without encumbering the fingertip using a tiny sensor that measures color change in the fingernail (Mascaro & Asada, 2004). A small finger ring can measure blood oxygen levels and wirelessly transmit the signal to a mobile computing device (Asada et al., 2003). "Sensor pills" (Given Imaging, Yoqneam, Israel) that are swallowed can transmit data wirelessly to an on-body receiver, measuring the body's internal state (Mow, Lo, Targan, et al., 2004).

Real-time analysis of multiple data streams from diverse sensor types will create the most powerful context detectors. For example, suppose a researcher wishes to use CS-EMA to trigger subject self-reports only during situations when the subject is undergoing psychological stress. A psychological stress detection algorithm could monitor three sensors for the following states: high heart rate, high galvanic skin response, and low body motion (to rule out excessive physical activity). Only when all three conditions are met (or just after they subside) would the subject receive the stress diary assessment.

Unfortunately, some ambulatory monitoring devices are intrusive and not easy to wear. Blood pressure measurement, for instance, will startle the person because a cuff must inflate, causing interruption and discomfort. Commercialization of the technologies, however, is bringing miniaturization (Bonato, 2003). Most of these sensor devices will soon be wireless and available in physical styles that permit them to be worn by participants inconspicuously, under clothing, for days or weeks at a time without discomfort (Pentland, 1996). Some of these sensors provide continuous streams of data (e.g., motion sensors on the body). Others provide intermittent signals because of the invasive nature of the sensing itself (e.g., blood pressure).

WEARABLE SENSORS THAT MEASURE THE ENVIRONMENT

Wearable sensors can measure not only motion or physiological states but also properties of the environment. For example, small ultra-violet photodiodes attached to a wireless transmitter worn on the wrist or neck can be used to send exposure data to software running on a PDA, allowing for sun-exposure context-sensitive queries. GPS systems in phones or PDAs can be used to identify a person's position outside, and software with a GIS database can trigger context-sensitive questions tailored to the subject's movement and the type of environment he or she is in (e.g. park, business district, or near a particular retail establishment).

Another property of the environment is sound, and mobile computing devices now contain sufficient amounts of storage to continuously record audio data. Mehl and colleagues have created the electronically activated recorder (EAR) (Mehl, Pennebaker, Crow, Dabbs, & Price, 2001). Subjects wear the EAR for 2–4 days during which time it records 30s samples of audio once every 12 minutes. The audio is then manually transcribed for analysis. Although the EAR records to tape, new versions of EAR-like devices that use digital devices could not only save the data but process the audio stream in real-time for important keywords or background sounds. If particular words or sounds are spotted, context-sensitive self-report diary assessments could be automatically triggered. In one study, researchers have used automatic speech recognition to determine how and when multiple subjects that work in the same physical environment are interacting with one another (Eagle & Pentland, 2003).

Beepers have been given to family members and simultaneously activated to signal multiple family members to make simultaneous entries on paper diaries (Larson and Richards, 1994). Radio frequency tags worn by subjects can *automatically* detect who is in a particular part of a space and when those people may be interacting with one another. Similarly, the networking capabilities of some mobile computing devices (e.g. Bluetooth) can be used to automatically determine when two people carrying the devices are within a short distance of one another.

Finally, video cameras can now be incorporated into phones or other mobile computing devices to create time-lapse video snapshots of what a person sees. A prototype extension for the MIT CS-EMA software has been used to capture such a record. The subject carries a PDA with a camera plug-in in the front shirt pocket. The device takes one (low-quality) time-stamped picture every 30 seconds that shows roughly what the subject sees. The image stream allows a researcher to more accurately reconstruct the subject's behavior, subjective states, cognitions, and interpersonal experiences throughout the day. The CS-EMA software can also prompt subjects to take pictures of certain objects in the environment. For example, subjects can be asked to take pictures of everything they eat—a new technique in nutrition research (Wang, Kogashiwa, Ohta, & Kira, 2002).

Environmental Sensors (Placed by the Researcher)

In addition to asking participants to wear sensors, other sensors can be installed in their environment. These sensors are also undergoing miniaturization and therefore are becoming less of a burden for participants to endure and for researchers to install. Ubiquitous sensor placement is made possible by reduction in sensor size and lengthening of battery life. Work is underway in laboratories to create wireless environmental sensors that are less than a cubic millimeter in size (Kahn, Katz, & Pister, 1999).

Sensors placed on objects in the environment provide information about what people in that environment are doing. If the sensors can wirelessly transmit information to a mobile computer, automatic detection of everyday activities can trigger context-sensitive sampling. For example, at MIT we are conducting experiments where MITes (and their earlier versions) are installed in participants' homes. The sensors are attached to any object that the person may manipulate: doors, cabinets, light switches, dials, appliances, and even large containers such as Tupperware (Intille, Munguia Tapia, Rondoni, et al., 2003). The sensors measure when the objects are moved.

Figure 16-3 shows some early versions of MITes that used magnetic contact switches "installed" in one participant's home. The sensors were literally taped to objects in the home and then used to collect data for 2 weeks. New wireless MITes dramatically cut installation time by using accelerometers instead of contact switches. Algorithms have been developed that use the data from the sensors to automatically detect some activities of daily living using statistical models (Munguia Tapia, Intille, & Larson, 2004).

Other researchers are implementing similar activity-detection algorithms that use different types of environmental sensors. For example, Philipose and colleagues have created a bracelet with an embedded radiofrequency identification tag (RFID) reader. When a subject wears the bracelet and inexpensive RFID stickers are placed on objects in the subject's home, a computer system can detect when the subject touches each of the tagged objects. Algorithms that recognize everyday activities (e.g., making tea) can then be detected automatically, in real time (Philipose, Fishkin, Fox, et al., 2003). In combination with software on a PDA, such systems could be used for studies where the subject's behavior is monitored for specific eating patterns and then context-sensitive questions are asked during or after particular target behaviors.

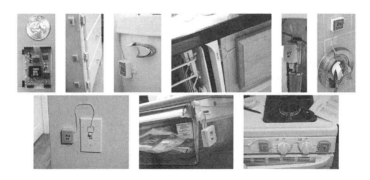

Figure 16-3. Early versions of MITes.

Other sensors such as microphones or video cameras can easily be placed throughout an environment for research studies. For instance, automatic computer vision analysis of video streams from inexpensive webcams attached to laptops can be used to detect when a person is in a particular room and can transmit his or her location to a PDA running assessment software. The software can implement a CS-EMA protocol that asks for self-reports depending upon how people move about the environment. Air quality properties such as carbon monoxide and dioxide levels, temperature, and even particulate levels can be measured with sensors and used as CS-EMA triggers.

Not all environmental monitoring must lead to CS-EMA-triggered interruptions for the participant. For example, image data can be used as a memory trigger rather than a self-report trigger to minimize the interruption burden of sampling. We call this technique image-based EMA. In a prototype implemented at MIT, a computer monitors a video stream for motion events. When significant motion is detected, a sample is triggered. However, instead of interrupting the subject with a prompt, a static image of the environment and the person is taken, time-stamped, and stored. Later, at a convenient time, such as when riding the bus, waiting in line, or just being idle, the participant can use a PDA device to answer questions. The image-based EMA program displays previously captured images and then presents the researcher's question. In many cases, the image will trigger the subject's memory, helping him or her provide more accurate answers to the assessment questions by providing visual contextual cues about that particular moment in time (Intille, Kukla, & Ma, 2002).

Environmental Sensors Already in Place

Although in many studies investigators may wish to have participants wear sensors or may place them in their living environments, researchers may also be able to exploit the proliferation of sensors in devices and environments. Working with public institutions or corporations, researchers may obtain access to valuable data sources. With appropriate conversion software, it may be possible to send the data via wireless networks to a device enabling CS-EMA protocols. For example, suppose a researcher wanted to explore the relationship between sedentary behavior and television viewing. TiVo (TiVo, Alviso, CA) or another digital recorder company might provide the researcher access to real-time data on the current television station settings. These data could be combined with data from wireless accelerometers worn by participants in the home and enable real-time context-sensitive questioning that is tailored to how people are moving and what content they are watching.

Similarly, suppose a researcher is interested in studying the relationship between sedentary behavior, driving, and the built environment. An automobile manufacturer may be able to provide real-time data from the vehicle itself, and more vehicles have built-in GPS. A PDA will be able to collect data from wireless accelerometers worn by the person, a GPS system in the car, and GIS information obtained over the Internet to implement a CS-EMA protocol where questions are triggered based on driving and walking behavior.

Obtaining access to data sources from companies or governments can be challenging because these organizations often wish to protect the privacy of their patrons, as well as their trade secrets. Furthermore, implementing the technology required to get access to the data in real time to enable CS-EMA may not always be possible without substantial investment in technology middleware. However, as devices such as home theater systems and automobiles improve, the technologies they use to communicate with other electronic devices are likely to improve, making possible novel data transfer for real-time health assessment research.

Other existing data sources installed in the environment that might interest health researchers are public surveillance cameras, satellite imagery, usage data from home appliances such as stovetops, and radiofrequency tollbooth payment trackers.

In summary, researchers using real-time data collection have new tools at their disposal for passively collecting multimodal data in real time and, most significantly, triggering additional data collection based on automatic, real-time processing of the incoming data streams.

Context-Sensitive Prompting at Appropriate Times and Places

The key technological innovation enabling the CS-EMA methodology is the automatic detection of context. In the simplest case, questions can be triggered in response to a single, prespecified sensor reading—for example, heart rate jumps above a subject-specific threshold. Alternatively, the computer combines many sensor readings simultaneously to infer more complex subject states using pattern recognition algorithms. However a trigger is detected, the key insight is that a subject's context and activities can be used to determine when and where self-report data are collected. Mobile computing devices, including mobile phones, are now sufficiently powerful to perform this "just-in-time" questioning (Intille, 2002).

Conveying Information at the Appropriate Place

Telephones have been used for many years to deliver and collect health information from people in their home settings (Friedman, 1998). More than 95 percent of U.S. homes have telephone service (U.S. Census Bureau, 1990). Although the telephone is a ubiquitously available technology, as a technology for real-time data collection it has two serious limitations. First, it is fixed in the home and most people spend a significant amount of time in other settings. Second, the telephone, without additional technologies, has no information available about when it is opportune to prompt for information. Finally, the technology required to use the traditional phone system to proactively call people is costly and complex to maintain.

By comparison, new mobile computing devices are making "anyplace" communication possible at a very low cost. Mobile phones are exploding in usage, and many people carry them everywhere they go. There is almost one mobile phone for every two people in the United States (*Trends in Telephone Service,* 2003). The percentage of mobile phone owners will grow because many people are replacing wired telephones with wireless service (Horrigan, 2003). By 2002 in Finland (which the U.S. tends to follow in technology adoption), 86 percent of the male population and 78 percent of the female population over age 10 had a mobile phone (Statistics Finland, 2003). As these devices are further miniaturized and more sensing capability is incorporated into them, they can be exploited by health researchers to get information to or acquire information from subjects (Collins, Kashdan, & Gollnisch, 2003). New phones will have built-in GPS positioning that will automatically provide position information when outdoors. Wireless networking capability may soon provide information about location when the devices are inside buildings (Bahl & Padmanabhan, 2000).

Other emerging technologies will make it easier to get messages to a subject at the appropriate place. Bluetooth headsets such as the FreeSpeak (JABRA Corporation, Ballerup, Denmark) can wirelessly transmit a private audio message to a person's ear from a mobile computing device. Heads-up display devices such as the SV-6 PC Viewer (MicroOptical Corporation, Westwood, MA) that attach to the ear or glasses and provide a video display to a person as he or she moves about the environment are also dropping in price. Even interactive voice response systems in vehicles, such as OnStar (General Motors, Detroit, MI), could be used to collect data from subjects.

Looking 10 to 15 years into the future, new low-cost display devices for homes and workplaces may transform typical home environments into spaces where information can be presented not only in the right room but also on the most appropriate object, such as furniture, walls, floors, overlaying a picture, or placed on a particular device such as an outlet.

Figure 16-4 shows a prototype living room at MIT. In the corner is an Everywhere Displays Projector (EDP) (Pinhanez, 2001) consisting of a computer

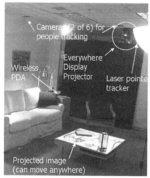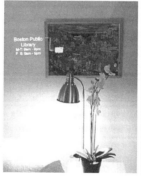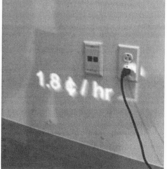

Figure 16-4. Prototype living room with an Everywhere Displays Projector in one cabinet; it can display information on most surfaces in a typical-size room.

projector, a computer-controlled mirror, and a standard desktop computer. After calibrating the device, the computer can use a perspective transformation to warp an image so that, when it is projected onto objects in the environment, it retains its correct size and shape. If the computer is also connected to a computer-controlled camera, it can detect the laser dot and allow the laser pointer to be used to "click" on the image, no matter where it is projecting (Intille, Lee, & Pinhanez, 2003). Such advances in computer hardware and the widespread adoption of consumer technologies for communication and entertainment will create new opportunities to display messages at the appropriate place, possibly allowing prompting strategies that grab a person's attention without audio interruption.

Detecting an Appropriate Time

A greater challenge than presenting or requesting information at the right place may be to develop algorithms that can use sensors to determine an appropriate time.

DETECTING THE ACTIVITIES THAT MATTER

Entire fields in engineering are devoted to developing algorithms that can collect noisy sensor readings and infer a person's activity or context. Recent advances in pattern recognition algorithm development and improvements in processor speed have led to systems that can robustly infer events from noisy sensor data. The most promising techniques typically use a supervised learning algorithm, where a set of labeled examples is used to create exemplar models of each target class and then new examples are classified based on similarity functions with the targets (Witten & Frank, 1999).

Using pattern recognition, raw sensor data can be converted into more meaningful labels. For example, data on limb motion collected from accelerometers worn on multiple body parts can be used to automatically determine which of a list of known activities such as "walking," "cycling," "scrubbing," "working at a computer," and "vacuuming" a person may be performing (Bao & Intille, 2004). One of the key challenges for health researchers is to learn how to exploit these pattern recognition algorithms. The algorithms are statistical—they output only a statistical likelihood that an activity is observed given the observed data. Therefore, when developing CS-EMA sampling protocols and performing data analysis, researchers need to account for both the variability among subjects and the uncertainty in the triggering algorithms. The data analysis methods needed to analyze data collected with CS-EMA tools demand future research.

MINIMIZING INTERRUPTION BURDEN

In most electronic sampling studies, the researcher assumes that, given a full day and random sampling, the sampling will eventually capture a sufficient number of events of interest. However, a well-known limitation of EMA is the burden the technique places on the participant. One way to reduce the burden is to keep the measures brief to avoid subject fatigue (Stone & Shiffman, 1994). This strategy, however, may not be sufficient for long-term sampling studies or for studies where the events of interest are short in duration.

The CS-EMA methodology may provide a solution by limiting sampling to the moments of greatest interest to the researcher. A variation on this approach is to also use context-sensitive computing to determine good (or poor) times to interrupt if a specific activity of interest cannot be detected. Because of the proliferation of electronic devices vying for the user's attention, the detection of good times to interrupt using sensors is becoming an active topic of research for computer scientists (Horvitz & Apacible, 2003). Ironically, EMA is a technique being used to conduct these studies. In one study conducted in the workplace setting, researchers found that a few sensors that detect use of the phone, if anyone is talking, or other indicators of conversation could be better than 75 percent effective at predicting interruptability in the office (Hudson, Fogarty, Atkeson, et al., 2003). Another study found that information proactively presented at physical activity transitions (e.g., a transition from sitting to walking) rather than at random times has a higher perceived value (Ho & Intille, 2005). Future versions of CS-EMA might use such sensors to reduce the burden of sampling by triggering prompts during automatically detected activities or during activity transitions when participants are likely to be most receptive to an interruption.

Exploiting the Network

Even with a variety of sensor inputs available, automatic detection of subject activity is challenging for many activities of interest. For example, although galvanic skin response and other physiological measures can provide some information about emotional state, reliable detection of most emotions is still an active research problem (Picard, 2003). Similarly, automatic detection of certain activities or parameters of those activities (*"he's cooking lazily," "she's being passive-aggressive"*) may be far beyond current capabilities of machine perception. In these cases, a researcher interested in using CS-EMA may need to fall back on other EMA designs.

An alternative is to exploit the ubiquitous networking capability of emerging computing devices. For example, suppose two people living in the same home are participating in a study. Instead of sampling the target individual, if PDA software detects that the two people are near one another, the software might silently prompt the second individual (perhaps using vibration) and present questions about the state of the first. The software can attempt to exploit human intelligence of other people as triggers for sampling the subject of greatest interest. Moreover, answers from the second individual might change the sequence of questions asked of the first. Although this network-triggered CS-EMA protocol could occur in a home, it might also occur in a workplace or other environment where large groups of people work and where not all the people participating know each other well.

Text messaging using the network could also trigger data collection among groups. Text messages have already been used as economical interventions for diabetes for children (Franklin, Waller, Pagliari, & Greene, 2003), asthma management (Neville, Greene, McLeod, et al., 2002), and bulimia research (Bauer, Percevic, Okon, et al., 2003). Clever use of simultaneous communication between groups of subjects could heighten the sense of perceived value of the experience for subjects by exploiting social norms. For instance, if subjects in a study are receiving prompts at the same time, a real-time update about who has answered the queries might be a useful tool to increase compliance.

Data Collection Tailored to the Individual and to the Situation

The CS-EMA methodology as described thus far involves continuous collection and analysis of data that are used to prompt self-report at appropriate times and places. However, emerging computer technologies will also facilitate opportunities for personalized tailoring based on an individual's past behavior, subjective states, cognitions, and interpersonal experiences.

User-Specific Devices

The mobile computing technologies that will enable the next generation of CS-EMA instruments will be highly personal devices. Already mobile phone users are beginning to use their phones to store detailed personal information and files. As the interfaces between the phones and desktop computers are improved in the next 5 years, phones will become the primary mechanism by which people carry and exchange data. For heavier computer users, phones are likely to contain information about personal contacts, meetings, and movement patterns around the community (from GPS). It is not unreasonable to expect the mobile devices to also contain large amounts of health data. As the physiological and motion sensors reach comfortable sizes, first athletes and then the general public will begin to use them for personal health monitoring.

Longitudinal Data Storage—Lifelong Records

A trend toward personalizing mobile computing devices will take place at the same time as another important technological innovation: "free memory." Storage devices the size of a quarter can now store gigabytes of information, and the cost of memory has plummeted. For all practical purposes, within 10 years digital memory storage capacity will no longer be a consideration for most typical data collection tasks, even those that take place on mobile computing devices. "Free memory" and personalized devices will mean that people will never need to delete the digital data they collect. Suppose a mobile phone user has a wireless pedometer that saves walking data and GPS position data on the phone. That person could easily save a lifetime of walking data on a single phone and never have a reason to delete it. In fact, as discussed in the next section, the phone might collect a longitudinal record of nearly everything the person sees, hears, and does.

Looking to the Future: CS-EMA+10

In the next 10 years, new technologies will enable CS-EMA protocols to be widely deployed for health research. How will the properties of new CS-EMA instruments compare with the current dominant technology of paper? Consider what an instrument that implements a CS-EMA protocol might be like 10 years from now (CS-EMA+10), after mobile computing, wireless sensors, ubiquitous networks, and "free memory" have permeated the marketplace.

A device implementing a CS-EMA protocol for studying how, when, and where people engage in physical activity might operate as follows. The device would consist of software that runs on all major mobile phones. Ten years from now, well over 150 million mobile phones will be in use daily in the United States. People who wish to become research subjects will obtain the software using the touch screen on the phone to access the project website and download and run the program.

The typical phone will be a powerful, miniature computer with a 0.5- to 1-terabyte storage card; it will easily synchronize with a computer via low-power wireless networks. Some people will use phones with a pocket-sized physical shape and style; others will have phones with watch or armband physical styles. Nearly all phones will have color screens with touch-input displays.

Each phone will have a local body network used to collect data from built in and add-on sensor devices. Pedometers and some physiological monitors (e.g., heart rate) may be common. These devices will always be activated and collecting data, most likely so phone users can monitor their own health. Researchers using phones for CS-EMA protocols may distribute additional sensors to subjects as well, and the sensors will use the local body network to transmit data to sampling software running on the phone. For physical activity measurement, the sensors will consist of miniature accelerometers embedded in comfortable elastic wrist and ankle bands and a wireless heart rate chest patch. Subjects may wear them for months, charging their batteries at night. Two to five accelerometer bands may be worn on different parts of the limbs. Additional data will be collected on the subject's position from the phone's built-in GPS or indoor tracking system using the local network inside buildings. The researchers may ask subjects to place a few hundred sensors like MITes around their home to improve recognition of certain types of activities and detect events such as eating, opening the refrigerator, cooking, exercising, sleeping, and socializing.

The software for monitoring physical activity will save and then immediately process the incoming signals. The accelerometers will send three-axis accelerometer data to the phone at 20 Hz. The phone will continuously process the sensor data and use statistical learning algorithms to automatically detect certain physical activities specified by the researcher. The algorithms will recognize many activities with 80 to 90 percent accuracy (Bao & Intille, 2004). Using more sensors will typically improve recognition performance. Heart rate in combination with the accelerometer data will determine what activity is being performed and with what intensity.

When a target physical activity is detected, such as "walking," "cycling," "scrubbing," or "vacuuming," the phone will prompt the subject and present context-specific (multiple-choice) questions that the researcher has constructed. The questions may change based on the subject's prior activity, including pedometer data collected 2 years ago but saved on the subject's phone. Subjects will use the phone's touch screen to answer the questions after receiving an audio prompt.

As it gathers the self-report data, the CS-EMA+10 device can create a "digital diary" of the subject's activity by recording what a user sees and hears (Clarkson, 2002; Gemmell, Bell, Lueder, et al., 2002). The researcher can use this diary to interpret surprising results. The value of such an experiential memory device was realized as early as 1945, but only recently have improvements in the size and cost of technology made the vision achievable (Bush, 1945; Gemmell et al., 2002).

The phone will collect all of the following information: a continuous video stream (from an embedded camera), a continuous audio stream of everything the subject hears and says (from the phone's microphone), a continuous accelerometer data stream of the subject's limb motion, a continuous data stream of physiological parameters such as heart rate, a continuous data stream of subject's location in the community, and other miscellaneous data about how the subject is feeling as reported by the user occasionally via a mobile computing device user interface. When compressed, a year of data can be stored with less than 1 terabyte of memory. By 2007, 1 TB of memory may retail for approximately $300 (Gemmell et al., 2002).

In some situations the software running on the telephone may change the question that is asked based on an automatically detected deviation from past baseline performance. For example, a person may be reminded of previous answers from the previous days, weeks, or years (e.g., *Yesterday at this time you felt tired. Do you feel more or less tired right now?* or *You've done this activity at about the same time every day for the last month. Why do you think that is the case?*). The device can go one step further, however, and use image-based EMA to show the subject video or play the subject audio from periods of time in the past. The computer might play a video clip of an activity that occurred 2 months ago and ask the subject to compare the current situation to the past event.

People using the telephone software might participate in CS-EMA studies for years if researchers ensure that the context-sensitive interruptions do not become a burden. Participation would require no more than telling the telephone how many questions a week are tolerable and letting the program automatically run in the background. In some studies, participants using devices running CS-EMA protocols may start to view themselves less as "subjects" and more as "active volunteers." The software could be structured so that some studies are experienced as long-term participatory conversations rather than impersonal and untailored question-and-answer sessions.

All the technologies that are needed to make this scenario a reality exist today and prototypes are being tested at MIT and elsewhere. As consumer technologies drop in size and price, such instruments could be deployed on very large scales with millions of telephone users. Open research questions include how to analyze the huge amount of data that such a tool would produce and how to provide researchers with the tools they need to develop context-sensitive sampling protocols without requiring expertise in the sensor technologies.

Privacy, Ethical, and Practical Considerations

As with any research study, the use of CS-EMA protocols, particularly those deployed with tools available 10 years from now, requires that informed consent be obtained from subjects. The investigators must ensure that participants understand what data are being collected, what the data could be used to infer, and how they can opt out of data being collected at particular times. Investigators must take the most care when sensors are being used to continuously collect data without the direct input of participants, because they may not realize how much data a consumer device such as a mobile phone could (or already does) collect. They may also forget that data are being collected when no proactive action is required.

A device implementing a CS-EMA protocol may be capable of recording a person's location, activities, interactions with other people, physiological states, and psychological states. Such descriptive data sets may make it increasingly likely that EMA data collected in one study can be retroactively reused for a different purpose in another study at a later date. However, the density and versatility of the datasets may also make it more likely that datasets will be of value to other parties, such as the government or family members interested in the behavior of particular subjects. The probative power of the data sets may necessitate improved procedures for masking subject identity. This is especially true because the data sets may contain audio and video samples that can be used to identify the participant, and current technologies do not allow researchers to automatically anonymize those data sources without obscuring much potentially relevant data.

The EMA technology that is continuously monitoring raises several other concerns that need to be addressed. One is that investigators may wish to request data collected by consumer devices used by participants prior to their enrollment in the study. A standard mobile phone, for instance, may store detailed information on the person's prior whereabouts, social connections, and physiological state—perhaps from the last several years. A participant may wish to provide only the relevant longitudinal data to the researcher, but in practice it will be more difficult to recall and flag data that he or she does not wish the researcher to see. The participant may therefore turn over the data without fully comprehending the amount of information it contains.

Another concern raised by EMA continuous monitoring is that some sensors may unintentionally capture data on nonconsenting people who interact with the subject. In situations where data about interaction with others are collected, it may not be possible for the investigator to obtain informed consent from all people with whom the subjects interact, either before or after the study. Such data could be removed once it is identified, but marking instances for deletion may require seeing of the data.

Finally, EMA continuous monitoring may capture data from the participant that is unrelated to the core study goals but that requires a response by the investigator. For example, while analyzing heart-rate–prompted questions, the investigators may discover heart arrhythmias. Should the researcher communicate this information to the subject? Alternatively, the investigators may determine that the subject engaged in an illegal activity. Do they report this information to the authorities? Subjects may also mistakenly feel that they are being monitored in real time and adjust their behavior accordingly. A researcher would not want a subject to defer medical care because he or she mistakenly felt that the system monitoring heart rate would trigger a warning if a serious heart problem was observed.

In addition to privacy and ethical concerns, future CS-EMA studies offer some practical challenges. A device running a CS-EMA protocol on a future computing device could generate orders of magnitude more data than current studies. New tools will be needed to manage these datasets and allow researchers to easily manipulate multimodal data sources with sampling rates that vary from days to milliseconds. Although many studies will be possible using standard telephones and commercial sensors such as electronic pedometers, in other cases a substantial infrastructure investment may required to collect the data desired (e.g., television content from a proprietary digital video recorder/tuner). Once again, special tools may be required for some studies that collect and process data. In most cases, the context detection algorithms will function as "black boxes." This may create some analysis challenges because the researcher may not have access to reliable data on the performance on the algorithms that are analyzing data to trigger self-reports.

Conclusions

Electronic sampling techniques, and particularly context-sensitive sampling techniques that use new sensor technologies, will create exciting new opportunities for health researchers interested in studying behavior, subjective states, cognitions, and interpersonal experiences of free-living subjects in natural settings. The CS-EMA methodology is likely to provide value for any health-related research where behavior and context are intertwined. For example, one can imagine studies such as the following:

- A study using CS-EMA to gather data on the links between television viewing, eating behaviors, and sedentary behaviors. Sensors worn on the body, placed in the kitchen, and placed on the television trigger questions when people are sedentary, snacking, and/or watching particular types of television shows.

- A study on ultraviolet exposure where questions about sun exposure are triggered only when a subject has been getting unusually high UV exposure for at least 15 minutes.
- A study on walking behavior and the built environment, where subjects are asked specific questions based on their typical walking behavior, current walking speed and duration, and type of space they are currently in.
- A study on the impact of social contact on perceptions of psychological well-being, where a group of friends or coworkers are prompted to describe how they feel just after an encounter with one another. Audio snippets from the conversations could be saved and analyzed by the researchers.

Table 16-1 (presented earlier in the discussion of emerging technologies) compares four technologies for real-time assessment: paper used for a diary, PDA software used for computerized EMA, PDA devices with context-sensitive software and sensors used for CS-EMA, and mobile devices 10 years from now used for CS-EMA+10. The table, which is speculative and makes gross simplifications, nonetheless suggests that researchers interested in studying free-living subjects may have a powerful new assessment instrument at their disposal as the technology that enables widespread adoption of CS-EMA matures. This new tool may be characterized by the following:

- A CS-EMA+10 device will be as lightweight and compact as the typical mobile phone, which most people will carry everywhere they go. The CS-EMA+10 device will be as inconspicuous as the mobile phone, which will have permeated society.
- A CS-EMA+10 device will be inexpensive to deploy for research. Consumers will absorb the cost of the mobile computer and sensor technology for personal entertainment and communication purposes. Hundreds of millions of people will own sufficiently powerful mobile computers, permitting instruments to be deployed in studies with extremely large sample sizes.
- A CS-EMA+10 device will not have a flexible physical form factor but it will have a comfortable one. It will have flexible function; the researcher can structure the way that information is presented to the subject to achieve a particular end.
- Many versions of CS-EMA+10 devices will be easy to replicate and modify without special expertise because tools will be developed so researchers can set up context-sensitive protocols. The investment in such tools will be justified by the enormous sample sizes that can be obtained for tools that are widely deployed.
- The CS-EMA+10 technology will operate on mobile computing devices that are familiar to subjects and easy for most people to use.

- The CS-EMA+10 technology can be developed so that participants can correct and adapt their entries—for example, by leaving audio notes for the researcher to explain their answers.
- The CS-EMA+10 tool may still raise questions about validation, reactivity, and selection bias, as does current electronic EMA.
- Although CS-EMA+10 instruments will be easy to carry everywhere, they will not be easy to forget because they will proactively prompt for information and the technology will be the subject's primary phone.
- Most data collected via CS-EMA+10 tools will not require costly, time-consuming, and error-prone manual data entry and coding.
- CS-EMA+10 technology will have automatic time stamping of entries, prohibiting hoarding. It will also allow the researcher to ensure that questions are answered in a particular order.
- The CS-EMA+10 device will allow acquisition of both self-report data and passive acquisition of multimodal data.
- In ways not possible via any other instrument, the CS-EMA+10 device will permit researchers to automatically tailor data acquisition to the context.

Finally, although this chapter is about the use of new technologies for real-time, context-sensitive assessment, the same technologies could be powerfully deployed for just-in-time intervention (Intille, 2004). A computing device can automatically determine when and how to present information to motivate behavior, attitude, or belief changes at "teachable" moments. Evaluation of such technologies is likely to require the use of the CS-EMA protocols.

ACKNOWLEDGMENTS

Dr. Intille is supported, in part, by National Science Foundation ITR grant #0112900 and the House_n Consortium. He thanks Jennifer Beaudin for comments on a draft of this paper. Emmanuel Munguia Tapia designed the wireless sensors shown in Figure 16-2. John Rondoni implemented the first version of the MIT PDA software for CS-EMA.

Note

1. In past work, this extension to the EMA methodology has been called context-aware experience sampling, or CAES (CAES, 2003; Intille, Rondoni, Kukla, et al., 2003). Context-aware is a term commonly used by ubiquitous computing researchers to indicate systems that automatically detect and respond to context.

References

Asada, H. H., Shaltis, P., Reisner, A., Rhee, S., & Hutchinson, R. C. (2003). Mobile monitoring with wearable photoplethysmographic biosensors. *IEEE Engineering in Medicine and Biology Magazine, 22*(3), 28–40.

Bahl, P., & Padmanabhan, V. N. (2000). RADAR: An in-building RF-based user location and tracking system. In *Proceedings of IEEE Infocom 2000* (Vol. 2, pp. 775–784). IEEE Press.

Bao, L., & Intille, S. S. (2004). Activity recognition from user-annotated acceleration data. In A. Ferscha & F. Mattern (Eds.), *Proceedings of PERVASIVE 2004* (Vol. LNCS 3001, pp. 1–17). Berlin Heidelberg: Springer-Verlag.

Barrett, L. F., & Barrett, D. J. (2001). An introduction to computerized experience sampling in psychology. *Social Science Computer Review, 19*(2), 175–185.

Bauer, S., Percevic, R., Okon, E., Meermann, R., & Kordy, H. (2003). Use of text messaging in the aftercare of patients with bulimia nervosa. *European Eating Disorders Review, 11,* 279–290.

Bonato, P. (2003). Wearable sensors/systems and their impact on biomedical engineering. *IEEE Engineering in Medicine and Biology Magazine, 22*(3), 18–20.

Broderick, J. E., Schwartz, J. E., Shiffman, S., Hufford, M. R., & Stone, A. A. (2003). Signaling does not adequately improve diary compliance. *Annals of Behavioral Medicine, 26*(2), 139–148.

Brodsky, M. Z., Consolvo, S., & Walker, M. (2002). *IESP Software.* Retrieved April 15, 2004, from http://seattleweb.intel-research.net/projects/ESM/iESP.html

Bush, V. (1945, July). As we may think. *The Atlantic Monthly, 176,* 101–108.

CAES. (2003). *Context-Aware Experience Sampling Website.* Retrieved January 15, 2003, from http://web.media.mit.edu/~intille/caes

Clarkson, B. P. (2002). *Life patterns: Structure from wearable sensors.* Unpublished Ph.D. thesis, Massachusetts Institute of Technology, Cambridge, MA.

Collins, R. L., Kashdan, T. B., & Gollnisch, G. (2003). The feasibility of using cellular phones to collect ecological momentary assessment data: Application to alcohol consumption. *Experimental and Clinical Psychopharmacology, 11*(1), 73–78.

Csikszentmihalyi, M., & Larson, R. (1987). Validity and reliability of the Experience-Sampling Method. *The Journal of Nervous and Mental Disease, 175*(9), 526–536.

Eagle, N., & Pentland, A. (2003). Social network computing. In A. K. Day, A. Schmidt, & J. F. McCarthy (Eds.), *Proceedings of the International Conference on Ubiquitous Computing* (Vol. LNCS 2864, pp. 289–296). Berlin, Heidelberg: Springer-Verlag.

Federal Communications Commission. *Enhanced 911.* Retrieved May 31, 2004, from http://www/fcc/gov/911/enhanced

Franklin, V., Waller, A., Pagliari, C., & Greene, S. (2003). "Sweet Talk:" Text messaging support for intensive insulin therapy for young people with diabetes. *Diabetes Technology and Therapeutics, 5*(6), 991–996.

Friedman, R. H. (1998). Automated telephone conversations to assess health behavior and deliver behavioral interventions. *Journal of Medical Systems, 22*(2), 95–102.

Gandy, M., Starner, T., Auxier, J., & Ashbrook, D. (2000). The Gesture Pendant: A self-illuminating, wearable, infrared computer vision system for home automation control and medical monitoring. In *Proceedings of the Fourth International Symposium on Wearable Computers (ISWC'00)* (pp. 87–102). IEEE Press.

Gemmell, J., Bell, G., Lueder, R., Drucker, S., & Wong, C. (2002). MyLifeBits: Fulfilling the Memex vision. In *Proceedings of ACM Multimedia '02* (pp. 235–238). New York: ACM Press.

Goodie, J. L., Larkin, K. T., & Schauss, S. (2000). Validation of Polar heart rate monitor. *Journal of Psychophysiology, 14*(3), 159–164.

Gorin, A. A., & Stone, A. A. (2001). Recall biases and cognitive errors in retrospective self reports: A call for momentary assessments. In A. Baum, T. Revenson, & J. Singer (Eds.), *Handbook of health psychology* (pp. 405–413). Mahwah, NJ: Erlbaum.

Healey, J., & Picard, R. (1998). StartleCam: A cybernetic wearable camera. In *Proceedings of the Second International Symposium on Wearable Computers* (pp. 42–49). IEEE Press.

Ho, J., & Intille, S. S. (2005). Using context-aware computing to reduce the perceived burden of interruptions from mobile devices. In *Proceedings of the Conference on Human
Factors and Computing* (pp. 909–918). New York: ACM Press.

Hollenberg, J. P., Pirraglia, P. A., Williams-Russo, P., Hartman, G. S., Gold, J. P., Yao, F. S.,
& Thomas, S. J. (1997). Computerized data collection in the operating room during
coronary artery bypass surgery: A comparison to the hand-written anesthesia record.
Journal of Cardiothoracic and Vascular Anesthesia, 11(5), 545–551.

Horrigan, J. B. (2003). *Consumption of information goods and services in the United States.*
Washington, DC: Pew Internet and American Life Project.

Horvitz, E., & Apacible, J. (2003). Learning and reasoning about interruption. In *Proceedings
of the 5th International Conference on Multimodal Interfaces* (pp. 20–27). New York:
ACM Press.

Hudson, S. E., Fogarty, J., Atkeson, C. G., Avrahami, D., Forlizzi, J., Kiesler, S., Lee, J. C., &
Yang, J. (2003). Predicting human interruptability with sensors: A Wizard of Oz feasi-
bility study. In *Proceedings of the Conference on Human Factors and Computing* (pp. 257–264).
New York: ACM Press.

Hufford, M. R., Shields, A. L., Shiffman, S., Paty, J., & Balabanis, M. (2002). Reactivity to
ecological momentary assessment: An example using undergraduate problem
drinkers. *Psychology of Addictive Behaviors: Journal of the Society of Psychologists in Addictive
Behaviors, 16*(3), 205–211.

Hyland, M. E., Kenyon, C. A., Allen, R., & Howarth, P. (1993). Diary keeping in asthma:
Comparison of written and electronic methods. *British Medical Journal, 306*(6876),
487–489.

Intille, S. S. (April/June, 2002). Designing a home of the future. *IEEE Pervasive Computing,*
80–86.

Intille, S. S. (2004). A new research challenge: persuasive technology to motivate healthy
aging. *Transactions on Information Technology in Biomedicine, 8*(3), 235–237.

Intille, S. S., Kukla, C., & Ma, X. (2002). Eliciting user preferences using image-based
experience sampling and reflection. In *Proceedings of the CHI '02 Extended Abstracts on
Human Factors in Computing Systems Human Interface Short Abstracts* (pp. 738–739).
New York: ACM Press.

Intille, S. S., Larson, K., & Kukla, C. (2002). Just-in-time context-sensitive questioning for
preventative health care. In *Proceedings of the AAAI 2002 Workshop on Automation as
Caregiver: The Role of Intelligent Technology in Elder Care.* Menlo Park, CA: AAAI Press.

Intille, S. S., Lee, V., & Pinhanez, C. (2003). Ubiquitous computing in the living room:
Concept sketches and an implementation of a persistent user interface. In *Adjunct
Proceedings of the Ubicomp 2003 Video Program* (pp. 265–266).

Intille, S. S., Munguia Tapia, E., Rondoni, J., Beaudin, J., Kukla, C., Agarwal, S., et al.
(2003). Tools for studying behavior and technology in natural settings. In A. K. Dey,
A. Schmidt, & J. F. McCarthy (Eds.), *Proceedings of UbiComp 2003: Ubiquitous Computing,*
(Vol. LNCS 2864, pp. 157–174). Berlin, Heidelberg: Springer.

Intille, S. S., Rondoni, J., Kukla, C., Anacona, I., & Bao, L. (2003). A context-aware experience sampling tool. In *Proceedings of the Conference on Human Factors in Computing
Systems: Extended Abstracts* (pp. 972–973). New York: ACM Press.

Kahn, J. M., Katz, R. H., & Pister, K. S. J. (1999). Mobile networking for "Smart Dust." In
*Proceedings of the 5th Annual ACM/IEEE International Conference on Mobile Computing and
Networking* (pp. 271–278). New York: ACM Press.

Kario, K., Yasui, N., & Yokoi, H. (2003). Ambulatory blood pressure monitoring for cardiovascular medicine. *IEEE Engineering in Medicine and Biology Magazine, 22*(3), 81–88.

Kern, N., Schiele, B., & Schmidt, A. (2003). Multi-sensor activity context detection for wearable computing. In *European Symposium on Ambient Intelligence (EUSAI)* (Vol. LNCS 2875, pp. 220–232). Heidelberg: Springer-Verlag.

Larson, R., & Richards, M. (1994). *Divergent realities: The emotional lives of mothers, fathers, and adolescents.* New York: Basic Books.

Larson, R., & Delespaul, P. (1990). Analyzing experience sampling data: A guidebook for the perplexed. In M. deVries (Ed.), *The experience of psychopathology: Investigating mental disorders in their natural settings* (pp. 58–78). Cambridge, UK: Cambridge University Press.

Mascaro, S. A., & Asada, H. H. (2004). Measurement of finger posture and three-axis fingertip touch force using fingernail sensors. *IEEE Transactions on Robotics and Automation, 20*(1), 26–35.

Mehl, M. R., Pennebaker, J. W., Crow, M. D., Dabbs, J., & Price, J. H. (2001). The Electronically Activated Recorder (EAR): A device for sampling naturalistic daily activities and conversations. *Behavior Research Methods, Instruments, and Computers, 33*(4), 7.

Melanson, Jr., E. L. & Freedson, P. S. (1995). Validity of the Computer Science and Applications, Inc. (CSA) activity monitor. *Medicine and Science in Sports and Exercise, 27*(6), 934–940.

Moore, G. E. (1965). Cramming more components onto integrated circuits. *Electronics, 38*(8).

Mow, W. S., Lo, S. K., Targan, S. R., Dubinsky, M. C., Treyzon, L., Abreu-Martin, M. T., & Papadakis, K. A. (2004). Initial experience with wireless capsule enteroscopy in the diagnosis and management of inflammatory bowel disease. *Clinical Gastroenterology and Hepatology, 2*(1), 31–40.

Munguia Tapia, E., Intille, S. S., & Larson, K. (2004). Activity recognition in the home setting using simple and ubiquitous sensors. In A. Ferscha & F. Mattern (Eds.), *Proceedings of PERVASIVE 2004* (Vol. LNCS 3001, pp. 158–175). Berlin, Heidelberg: Springer-Verlag.

Neville, R., Greene, A., McLeod, J., Tracy, A., & Surie, J. (2002). Mobile phone text messaging can help young people manage asthma. *British Medical Journal, 325*(7364), 600.

Pentland, A. (1996). Smart clothes. *Scientific American, 274*(4), 73.

Philipose, M., Fishkin, K. P., Fox, D., Kautz, H., Patterson, D., & Perkowitz., M. (2003). Guide: Towards understanding daily life via auto-identification and statistical analysis. In *Ubihealth 2003: The 2nd International Workshop on Ubiquitous Computing for Pervasive Healthcare Applications.*

Picard, R. W. (2003). Affective computing: Challenges. *International Journal of Human-Computer Studies, 59*(1–2), 55–64.

Pinhanez, C. (2001). The Everywhere Displays Projector: A device to create ubiquitous graphical interfaces. In G. D. Abowd, B. Brumitt, & S. A. N. Shafer (Eds.), *Proceedings of the Conference on Ubiquitous Computing* (pp. 315–331). Berlin, Heidelberg: Springer-Verlag.

Qi, Y. (2003). iDen Heart Rate Demo. Cambridge, MA: Personal communication.

Rafaeli, E. (2003). *The Personality, Motivation, and Cognition (PMC) Diary (Version 2. 0).* Retrieved October 1, 2004, from http://www.personality-project.org/pmc/diary.html

Rondoni, J. (2003). *A Context-Aware Application for Experience Sampling and Machine Learning.* Unpublished M.Eng. Thesis, Massachusetts Institute of Technology, Cambridge, MA.

Schwartz, J. E., & Stone, A. A. (1998). Strategies for analyzing ecological momentary assessment data. *Health Psychology, 17*(1), 6–16.

Starner, T. E. (2002). Wearable computers: no longer science fiction. *IEEE Pervasive Computing, 1*(1), 86–88.

Statistics Finland. (2003). *The Evolution of the Information Society.* Retrieved August 15, 2004, from http://www.stat.fi/index_en.html

Stone, A. A., & Shiffman, S. (1994). Ecological momentary assessment (EMA) in behavioral medicine. *Annals of Behavioral Medicine, 16*(3), 199–202.

Stone, A. A., Shiffman, S., Schwartz, J. E., Broderick, J. E., & Hufford, M. R. (2002). Patient non-compliance with paper diaries. *British Medical Journal, 324*(7347), 1193–1194.

Trends in Telephone Service. (2003). Retrieved April 15, 2004, from http://www.fcc.gov/Bureaus/Common_Carrier/Reports/FCC-State_Link/IAD/trend803.pdf

U.S. Census Bureau. (1990). *Historical census of housing tables telephones.* Retrieved April 15, 2004, from http://www.census. gov/hhes/www/housing/census/historic/phone. html

Van Laerhoven, K., Schmidt, A., & Gellersen, H. W. (2002). Multi-sensor context aware clothing. In *Proceedings of the 6th IEEE International Symposium on Wearable Computers* (pp. 49–56). IEEE Press.

Wang, D. H., Kogashiwa, M., Ohta, S., & Kira, S. (2002). Validity and reliability of a dietary assessment method: The application of a digital camera with a mobile phone card attachment. *Journal of Nutritional Science and Vitaminology, 48*(6), 498–504.

Weiss, H., & Beal, D. (2003). *PMAT: Purdue Momentary Assessment Tool.* Retrieved October 1, 2004, from http://www.mfri.purdue.edu/pages/PMAT/

Welk, G. J. (2002). Use of accelerometry-based activity monitors to assess physical activity. In G. J. Welk (Ed.), *Physical activity assessments for health-related research* (pp. 125–142). Illinois: Human Kinetics Publishers, Inc.

Witten, I. H., & Frank, E. (1999). *Data mining: Practical machine learning tools and techniques with Java implementations.* San Francisco: Morgan Kaufmann.

17

Statistical Issues in Intensive Longitudinal Data Analysis

Theodore A. Walls, Bettina B. Höppner, and
Matthew S. Goodwin

Innovation in scientific data collection involving new kinds of protocols has proceeded at a breakneck pace over the past 10 years. Starting from a tradition of diary studies (Almeida, 2005; Bolger, Rafaeli, & Davis, 2003), researchers have increasingly used emerging "smart" electronic devices to collect data reflecting experience over time in real-life contexts. Many scientific studies have emerged using these devices; for example, there are studies using beepers for diary data collection (Csikszentmihalyi & Larson, 1987), computerized ambulatory recording devices (e.g., Wilhelm, Roth, & Sackner, 2003), automated behavioral observational tools (e.g., Borrie, Jonsson, & Magnusson, 2002; Hirschhauser, Frigerio, Grammer, & Magnusson, 2002), and sensing devices in physical and architectural environments (Intille, Chapter 16, this volume). Consistently, in many areas of psychology and in behavioral medicine, studies using Ecological Momentary Assessment (EMA) techniques have become commonplace (Stone & Shiffman, 1994). At the same time, other technological advances, including developments in GPS and GIS technology, fMRI and PET imaging, road network analysis, Web interfaces for transactions, and many other technology-based data collection mechanisms have equipped researchers with tools to collect much more detailed and complex time-graded data than ever before.

These technological advances have given rise to a new class of multivariate, multiple-subject databases with many more time points than are typically found in behavioral science. This class of data is called intensive longitudinal data (ILD) (Walls & Schafer, 2006). Inherent to this new class of data are both challenges and opportunities. In this chapter, we describe the nature of some analytical opportunities that are inherent to ILD and review some statistical approaches that we believe researchers should consider for the analysis of these data.

The Nature of Intensive Longitudinal Data

The most defining characteristic of an intensive longitudinal database is the large number of occasions recorded per person or research unit of interest.

These databases typically consist of at least 20 and often 200 or more recorded occasions per unit or person. In the social sciences, the ability to collect data from this great number of occasions constitutes a revolutionary change. Since the beginning of social science itself, questions have most often been explored through labor-intensive and often high-delay survey and observational techniques that use few occasions of measurement. In the past, this limitation vastly curtailed scientists' ability to characterize processes of change as they unfold over time. With the advent of ILD, researchers can now more clearly investigate and delineate microgenetic patterns of change over time. This development has caused an explosion of interest in the types of data collection techniques that yield ILD, particularly within the prevention sciences that span several applied disciplines including psychology, medicine, and education.

In general, our goal is to identify analytical opportunities for ILD and to describe promising statistical methods that have been considered by methodologists working on these kinds of data. The remainder of this chapter is organized as follows. First, we briefly review each dimension of Cattell's (1957, 1982) "data box" (persons, occasions, and variables) and point out areas of opportunity that arise within each dimension in the case of ILD (Figure 17-1). We think that it is useful for researchers to think through their own databases on these dimensions. However, here we are using the data box mainly as an organizational framework to describe opportunities in the analysis of ILD. Second, we consider multilevel modeling, reviewing how this approach is used to model change, and explain the

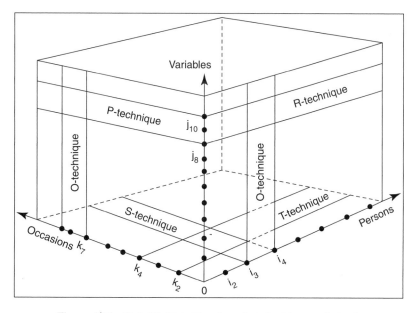

Figure 17-1. Cattell's Data Box (reprinted with permission).

heterogeneity on the persons (or units) dimension. Because this topic is undertaken carefully by Schwartz in this volume (Chapter 5), we limit the discussion to pointing out some key issues and possibilities in the case of ILD. Third, we consider some emerging methods that may help capitalize on the areas of opportunity that we have raised. These methods excel at handling the occasions dimension in ways that multilevel models do not. We are careful to note that the application of many of these methods to ILD is new and that not all of the strengths, weaknesses, and limitations in their application are known. We conclude with a discussion of open issues and likely next steps for modeling ILD in the future.

Dimensions and Opportunities of ILD Data

Cattell's data box consists of three axes or dimensions that contain units for persons, occasions (indicating a time dimension), and variables, respectively (see Figure 17-1). Each of these three dimensions can be sampled to a lesser or greater extent depending on the focus of the research study. Extensive sampling on a particular dimension typically indicates a substantive focus on that dimension. We consider some trends in sampling that have led to and continue to influence ILD modeling needs on each dimension.

The Persons Dimension

With regard to sampling on the persons dimension, consider the typical sample sizes found in different psychological studies. Sample sizes range from a minimum of 30 participants in experimental or pilot research studies, to 400 or more for sophisticated blocked designs, to thousands in population-level investigations. Sample sizes in intensive longitudinal studies are frequently low to moderate, although we might expect to see increased sizes as scientists use data collection mechanisms with broad access, such as Web interfaces; as familiarity with instrumentation on handheld devices becomes a societal norm; and as the need for more complex designs and population-level data increases.

Two special issues arise on the variables dimension in the case of ILD: classical heterogeneity and the possibility of accounting for time-graded heterogeneity.

Classical Heterogeneity

Psychological studies have increasingly attended to individual differences over the past few decades. This focus on heterogeneity among study participants has taken many forms, including extensive collection of demographic variables to use as controls, exploration of understudied populations, and the development of statistical models that describe both individual and group characteristics. For example, multilevel models separate individual-level and group-level stability and change effects and provide ways to explain differences in these effects among study participants. Many modeling frameworks can deal with aspects of heterogeneity as it has been thought of traditionally.

TIME-GRADED HETEROGENEITY

As a function of the large number of occasions in ILD, a new kind of heterogeneity has emerged: time-graded heterogeneity. Given at least a moderate number of individuals, aggregate patterns of change may be detectable across all participants or study units. At the same time, (a) participants may be tracked as members of specific a priori defined groups or (b) patterns may emerge for clusters of participants over time. Both of these possibilities involve a heterogeneity of participants that evolves over time. In the former case of a priori defined groups, several plausible pre- and post-intervention (interruption) patterns can be reviewed in Velicer and Fava (2004) and Shadish, Cook, and Campbell (2002). As a conceptual example, Shiffman and colleagues (Shiffman, Gwaltney, Balabanis, et al., 2002) tracked smokers' reports of feelings before and after they quit to shed light on smoking cessation. Such a design may enable the researchers to discriminate patterns for groups for which an approach to quitting is more or less successful. Note that a multilevel model, can easily address this need through the use of dummy-coded predictors for groups and pre- and post-intervention time periods. Similarly, researchers may be interested in the relative efficacy of a diversity of approaches to quitting and may want to compare trajectories within and across conditions.

In the latter case, emergent characteristics of participants may be reflected in patterns of responses over time that suggest group membership. Moreover, individuals may move from one group into another or may form new groups over the series. These emergent patterns would be undetectable using current typical multilevel analyses. Various strategies for determining clusters of individuals who share commonalities along an ILD series are needed but are near the outset of development. Methods that attend to the presence of possible latent classes and transitions, such as those found in stage-sequential models, may become relevant (Collins & Wugalter, 1992; Vermunt, Langenheine & Böckenholt, 1999). New methods that attend to continuous change patterns and movement among groups are also beginning to emerge and could possibly be extended to apply to ILD situations (Muthén, 2001; Nagin, 1999).

The Time Dimension

With regard to sampling from the time dimension, we have seen studies with thousands of occasions of measurement in laboratory-based studies, such as those using MRI or PET technologies (e.g., Waldorp, 2004). However, most longitudinal studies in areas of psychology that have traditionally attended to change include substantially fewer occasions of measurement, typically not more than 20 (Jones, 1991). Although there are some exceptions in studies examining the full life course in which occasions rise to approximately 30, such as the Elder (1985, 1999) and Thomas and Chess (1977) studies, changes in the protocols over distinct human developmental periods and differential tracking of cohorts often reduce the number of occasions available for consideration of the entire series within a single analysis. With the increased prevalence of intensive longitudinal databases, three issues have become prominent: a focus on time scale, spacing of measurement intervals, and time-graded covariates.

Focus on Time Scale

Measurement in a time scale that is appropriate to detect states of change in a given phenomenon must be defined during the research design phase. For example, if intimacy is composed of events of caring that emerge at the lowest level on an hourly basis, researchers typically attempt to measure these events on this time scale. It may be that the salience of time scale is not known a priori, resulting in the need to collect information at multiple time scales or to organize measurements taken at lower-level units of information into higher-level time blocks in some way. Work by Newell (1990) in cognitive science provides one rubric for considering time-scale issues by describing scales, time units, and levels of system for four hierarchical bands of cognitive scientific inquiry into human action: biological, cognitive, rational, and social. For example, cognitive and bio-logical bases of action are classed into units of less than a second.

Specific considerations for time scale in ILD resulting from EMA studies are outlined by Shiffman (Chapter 3, this volume); key issues revolve around a sample's intensity (e.g., how often it occurs when it's available for measurement), class (episodic vs. continuous), and the best method for establishing a recording interval (random, fixed, or some combination of the two). The goals of studies producing ILD involve determining what is happening over time. As such, the nature of the phenomena under study and the corresponding data structure need to be carefully considered in order to set the time scale in appropriate, real-istic, and meaningful units. These design decisions bear heavily upon design selection, protocol development, selection of statistical models, and model deployment. For example, the loess and point process models described in this section require the researchers to select a bandwidth at varying time scales in order to properly characterize data over a series.

Spacing of Measurement Intervals

Due to the high number of occasions measured per person or unit in ILD, time can be understood in an increasingly continuous fashion rather than through the use of broad categorical heuristics (e.g., pre- and post-intervention), as has been the case traditionally. The data collection devices used for ILD are fre-quently "smart," which means, among other things, that they can employ different time sampling strategies from individual to individual depending on the research question of interest and the phenomenon under study (see Chapter 3). Consequently, ILD may consist of complex temporal sampling, in which both the frequency and the spacing of measurements can vary (e.g., measured at all occasions or not; even or uneven spacing). Fortunately, most of the methods discussed in this chapter are flexible in handling interval spacing issues.

With the possibility of assessing patterns of change, researchers readily take interest in other factors that may influence or be influenced by their main variables of interest. For instance, cortisol levels in studies of stress may vary over time, potentially reflecting time-varying covariation with stress reports. A participant's gender, ethnicity, and other time-invariant variables may also define characteristics of change; most current modeling approaches can include time-invariant predictors. We also note that many intensive longitudinal databases include markers of both time-varying and time-invariant covariates and that assessing the effects of these predictors simultaneously can involve a good amount of iteration in the model building process.

The Variables Dimension

With regard to sampling from the variables dimension, the total number of constructs under consideration in studies producing ILD may actually be lower than in past studies. In past studies, researchers collected fewer occasions of measurement because of the high cost and burden to participants of collecting self-report data at many occasions. Instead, they often increased variable counts in protocols in order to gain more information about traits. Analysis of covariation usually followed from these studies. By contrast, studies producing ILD make within-person change analyses possible by increasing the number of units on the occasions dimension. Hence, there may be a trade-off of occasions for variables, of a sort, in moving to studies that collect ILD.

As the field progresses, studies that need to burden participants will probably find a threshold of protocol length and those that do not will likely be able to increase it. The number of variables may increase in the future as researchers develop ways to collect information from multiple devices, such as GPS, cellular networks, wearable computers and monitors, and so forth (Intille, Chapter 16, this volume; Nusser, Intille, & Maitra, 2006), because these devices do not add to participant burden.

Two special analytical opportunities arise on the variables dimension when ILD are under study: diverse underlying distributions of measured variables and issues of measurement equivalence.

Underlying Distributions of Measured Variables

The variables found in ILD may describe either more continuous experiences or discrete events or both. Examples of more continuous variables include psychological states reported on interval scales, such as mood or motivation. Discrete events include the event of having a drink, the event of one child hitting another, and so forth. The complexity that such a selection of variables introduces in ILD is that these variables, while sampled over the same period, can have different underlying distributions. For example, the normal (or Gaussian) distribution commonly assumed in social science research may work well for continuous experiences, but it reflects the distribution of discrete events improperly. These data are often measured in counts, which are best modeled using the Poisson distribution or other strategies for estimation of marked point processes. Intensive longitudinal databases often contain temporally complex data composed of normally distributed variables and other types of distributions simultaneously.

Measurement Equivalence

The perennial issue of measurement equivalence in longitudinal research involves the extent to which a construct measured by several items in one group or another or, more recently, at one time point or another, reflects comparable measurement characteristics. This issue fundamentally resides at the variables dimension, but it is particularly challenging in the longitudinal context (or occasions dimension) when variation among items or a set of items (e.g., factor scores) is used to reflect a construct's comparability from time point A to time point B. Extensive methodological consideration of this issue has been produced over the years (see, in particular, Baltes, Reese, & Nesselroade, 1988; Bartholomew, 1985; Meredith & Horn, 2001; Meredith & Tisak, 1990). The issue becomes even more challenging in intensive longitudinal data for at least two reasons. First, there are many more occasions that can differ due to chance alone, including changes in states or changes tied to longer periodicities, such as those typically thought of as traits in psychology. Second, new measurement issues emerge in ILD, such as participants centering on one score over time or responding to simultaneous periodic influences on more than one time scale (Fok & Ramsay, 2006). For example, Figure 17-2 illustrates a time series from an individual who appears to have centered on one score from an item over time. This kind of series reflects very little variation about its own mean over time, possibly suggesting a stable characteristic. However, this participant may have alternatively found a comfortable default score and varied from it only when life events dramatically altered his or her perceptions. Or, the apparent aberrations on a couple of days may suggest a daily or weekly pattern that can be detected only with an even longer series.

In general, a key question is whether to treat the scores about the mean as random error variance, measurement error, or meaningful temporal variation. Examination of the prevalence of such a situation across diary and EMA studies (both of which use self-report) has not yet been pursued formally. Consideration of measurement topics by Schwartz (Chapter 5, this volume) may be particularly useful in considering these issues.

These are some of the analytical opportunities on each dimension of intensive longitudinal databases that we face in developing appropriate statistical models. Taken together, they present a hearty challenge. However, few databases present

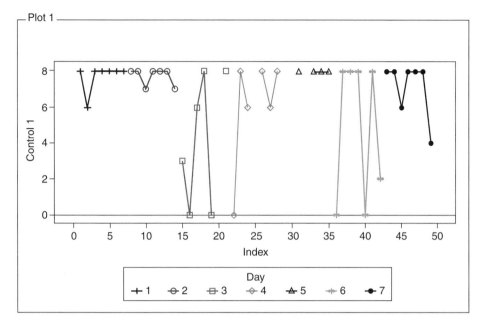

Figure 17-2. Time series centered on one score from an item over time.

all of these opportunities, and no current modeling framework can be used to address all of them at the same time. What is needed, then, are the means to select an appropriate method for a given study. Therefore, we proceed with our review of potentially useful models and strive to point out when a model excels in attending to some of the analytical opportunities highlighted in the last section.

The Prevailing Approach to ILD: Multilevel Modeling

Multilevel models enable researchers to model the heterogeneity of individual and group intercepts and growth curves. In general, multilevel models are elaborated forms of hierarchical linear regression. They have appeared in the statistical literature under a variety of terms, including "random effects model" (Laird & Ware, 1982); "general mixed linear model" (Goldstein, 1986); "random coefficient model" (de Leeuw & Kreft, 1986; Longford, 1993), "variance component model" and "hierarchical linear model" (Bryk & Raudenbush, 1992; Raudenbush & Bryk, 2002). More extensive pedagogical and conceptual discourse on multilevel modeling can be found in Fitzmaurice, Laird, and Ware (2004), Goldstein (2003), Hox (2002), Kreft and de Leeuw (1998), Raudenbush and Bryk (2002),

Snijders and Bosker (1999), and Singer and Willett (2003). Multilevel models have been at the forefront in addressing the emerging statistical modeling needs of social scientific researchers collecting diary and EMA data (Armeli, Tennen, & Todd, 2003; Laurenceau, Feldman Barrett, & Pietromonaco, 1998).

A brief contrast between traditional regression techniques and multilevel modeling highlights the advantage that multilevel modeling offers in dealing with heterogeneity. Traditional regression techniques, such as analysis of variance (ANOVA), rely on fixed group values for the intercept and slope of a given growth pattern over time. Thus, one set of values is used to characterize all individuals in a sample. In contrast, in multilevel modeling strategies, individual intercepts and slopes are calculated and their variances are assessed at the second or higher levels of the model. These models most often include fixed or time-varying covariates to predict the heterogeneity of the interindividual intercepts and slopes, thereby allowing each individual to be characterized by his or her own set of values.

Key Considerations in Using Multilevel Models

We now consider some key issues in multilevel modeling of ILD, point out advantages of some recently developed adaptations of the model for ILD, and raise some unanswered questions about heterogeneity that may be beyond the scope of multilevel models. In general, the multilevel modeling framework is very versatile and offers many advantages in modeling ILD. It deals well with the need to explain classical heterogeneity and it is flexible with respect to the handling of variable spacing of measurement intervals and time-varying/invariant covariates. However, much depends on the depth of knowledge and experience of the modeler. Those considering use of these models are well advised to undertake one of the many short courses currently available on the topic and to review specialized literature on models involving intensive longitudinal data (see Schwartz, Chapter 5, this volume, and Walls, Schwartz, & Jung, 2006). Other modeling strategies at times use some features of multilevel modeling and offer complementary opportunities for the analysis of ILD (e.g., Boker & Laurenceau, 2006; Rovine & Walls, 2006).

The first issue to consider in modeling growth curves of ILD with multilevel models is the need to determine whether the phenomenon reflects a temporal process at work within the series—that is, prevailing models focus on assessing whether the series reflects a stable mean or a gradual, long-term change over the entire series. If a temporal process does exist, without modification to the standard multilevel modeling procedures at the first level (using a linear or lower-order polynomial function to fit a line through the points for each individual), the model will discount meaningful temporal patterns and reflect them as random error. Because multilevel models pass quantities among "levels," inferences drawn at multiple levels of the model could be biased. Therefore, a standard multilevel model is appropriate only in the presumed absence of temporal influences within the series; that is, the temporal variation is seen as a nuisance parameter and the focus is on a longer-term trend. An example of such an appropriate situation could be a period of evenly increasing stress reported over a few weeks.

Second, consider a situation in which periodic daily measures of classroom functioning are randomly sampled over a set of different classes progressing over a moderate period of time. In this case, contextual variation tied to different subject matter and teachers may be so great that the assumption of within-subject serial dependence is unwarranted. In this hypothetical study, let us assume that only long-term change would be of interest and the many measurements are intended only to produce the best estimated individual intercepts over the series; that is, serial dependence is seen as unimportant. This would be a good circumstance in which to employ a marginal (growth) model in which estimation (via Generalized Estimating Equations [GEE]) depends only on the mean response and a vector of covariates (Walls, Schwartz, & Jung, 2006).

Third, assuming that the phenomenon under study does not include a complex temporal process, some typical considerations are made in conducting growth curve analyses with multilevel models. A range of error structures can be selected in most statistical software packages. Since the strength of relationships is generally expected to decline from occasion to occasion, modeling of the residual error structure is typically assumed to follow an autoregressive process, often a first-order AR process. However, in some cases, there may be sufficient knowledge of a phenomenon to know at which points over a series measurements are serially dependent or not. For example, studies of rapid eye movement (REM) may reflect little serial dependence at the outset of REM sleep and high serial dependence once a given depth of REM is achieved. Some alternative error structures have been considered for these kinds of databases and may be more appropriate for intensive longitudinal data (Diggle, 1998; Rovine & Molenaar, 1998; Schwartz, Chapter 5 in this volume).

Fourth, if a temporal process of some kind is anticipated, a different set of modeling options needs to be considered. If the process can be specified explicitly as a cyclical pattern of some kind, this pattern can be specified and the model can be estimated against it. One example of such an innovation involves the use of sinusoidal curves to model heart rate data (Schwartz, Chapter 5). In the presence of strong theory, many specific curves could be modeled in such a way. Another alternative to modeling temporal processes within a series involves the integration of time series techniques with multilevel modeling. For example, a given autoregressive process can be assumed (such as first order) and autoregressive parameters can be calculated for each case. In turn, these values can be modeled in a multilevel framework (Rovine & Walls, 2006; see also Timmerman & Kiers, 2003; van Buuren, 1997). More challenging scientific questions about temporal processes, such as when multiple processes reside at varying time scales, can be undertaken in other modeling frameworks, through the use of basis coefficients to reflect periodicities (Fok & Ramsay, 2006) and through the use of state space models (see general treatments in Fahrmeier & Tutz, 2001; Hershberger, Molenaar, & Corneal, 1996; and Jones, 1991). A data-smoothing approach called loess can also be integrated with multilevel modeling; the loess is discussed in greater detail later in this chapter.

Fifth, a possible limitation of using a multilevel model for ILD is that, over many participants' individual series, relatively flat slopes may reflect interindividual variability due to the large number of measurements being sensitive to contextual or other random influences over time. However, this is perhaps more aptly treated as an issue tied to study design and deployment origins, with data analytic implications for interpretation, than as a consideration fundamental to the multilevel model.

Finally, we note that although the multilevel model is perhaps the gold standard for dealing with classical heterogeneity, it does not track groups or clusters that emerge over time—that is, it cannot specify effects that involve time-graded heterogeneity. Other models that may approach this need are discussed later.

Models for the Occasions (Time) Dimension

In this section, we encourage analysts to consider four different models for handling ILD. Each model excels in different ways and each has its own inherent limitations. Near the beginning of each description, we point out some of the particular analytical opportunities that the model addresses well in the case of ILD.

Time Series Analysis

Many techniques are available for the study of time series (Box & Jenkins, 1976; Chatfield, 1996; Pena, Tiao, & Tsay, 2001), although these methods are used less frequently in the very areas of social science now producing ILD. Time series modeling is the best-known approach for studying temporal variation. These models frequently use autoregressive models and lagging techniques or moving averages to correct for local-in-time aberrations. The general strategy is to find the best-fitting autoregressive structure for a time series AR(1), AR(2), and so forth. The key principle in time series models is that one moment predicts for a subsequent moment, reflecting a lawfulness of the phenomenon over time. Another way of putting this is that one is looking for temporal regularities. For example, one might ask, does my motivation now relate to my subsequent motivation, or is my motivation "stable" or "erratic" over time? For a short primer on time series techniques and their relevance to diary data, see Velicer and Fava (2004).

Time series models excel in their focus on the occasions (time) dimension and have diverse and sophisticated capacities for detecting whether a process is in control. However, these models differ in the nature of their focus on time from many of the other models on the time dimension in that change trends over the series are not central; in fact, trends are often removed from series. Rather, the series are assessed for the presence of occasion-to-occasion prediction. Once these effects are assessed, time-varying covariance among series can be also explored. Time series measurements inherently assume that moment-to-moment regularity will be reflected in meaningful time-scale units; in fact, analysts routinely iterate among different levels of time aggregation (e.g., minutes, hours, days) in order to find the time scale at which the process can be identified.

The time series design also has great advantages in evaluating experimental designs involving many conditions. In this situation, it is possible to take advantage of randomization of subjects while simultaneously controlling for maturation (effectively, a multiple-group interrupted time series design). In this situation, it is possible to evaluate interesting questions such as whether a slope change before and after interruption is likely to occur in the outcome and whether groups differ in this slope change (Walls, 2003). All of the models discussed in this chapter could be adapted to evaluate such a design more effectively than is possible with currently prevailing methods.

In more sophisticated time series models, it is possible to pursue understanding of dynamic relationships—how one series may lead to another—where the information contained in the historical data of another series may allow understanding of dynamic processes if they are modeled jointly (Nesselroade & Molenaar, 2004). Multilevel versions of time series may allow interpretation of individual differences in these dynamic processes (within and between individuals) (Rovine & Walls, 2006). Relevant time series domain approaches using state-space modeling techniques have also been reviewed by Oud and Jansen (2000). Examples of these kinds of models tailored to ILD data can be found in Ho, Shumway, and Ombao (2006).

Locally Weighted Polynomial Regression (AKA Loess)

Another data analysis technique that excels in addressing the issue of time-scale selection in ILD is locally weighted polynomial regression, also known as loess. Loess is well suited to dealing with the selection of the appropriate time scale in understanding a given phenomenon over time and to properly modeling non-normally distributed observed variables. Loess is also flexible enough to allow time-varying covariates and irregular spacing of measured time intervals. Because this approach is not yet widely known, a brief primer is provided with attention to the opportunities in ILD modeling that it addresses well.

In looking at data series that stem from ILD, it readily becomes obvious that some ILD defy description by linear or other global (such as higher-order polynomial) functions. Consider, for instance, heart rate data collected through an ambulatory recording device for a person immediately after exercising on a stationary bike (Höppner, Goodwin, & Velicer, 2003). An example of such a series is shown in Figure 17-3. The ambulatory recording device recorded heart rate approximately every 0.5 seconds, and thus the resulting timeline for the participant's heart rate follows a highly sensitive, jagged and erratic trend. To understand this general underlying trend, a researcher may use some of the commonly available parametric statistical tools and describe these data through a global function. In Figure 17-3, two commonly used global functions, a linear and a quadratic trend, are fit to the heart rate data.

Both functions are a poor fit. The straight line (i.e., linear trend) captures the decrease in the person's overall heart rate as the study participant recovers from

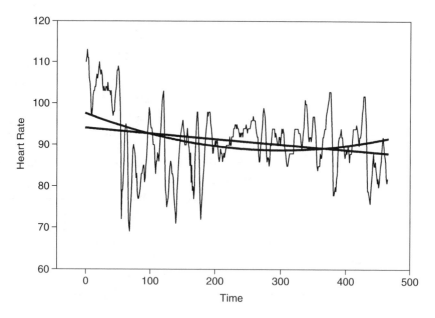

Figure 17-3. Global growth functions applied to heart rate data.

exercising, but it does not capture any of the different types of variation around the overall decreasing trend. For instance, the person's heart rate fluctuates considerably more at the beginning of the timeline than toward the end. Apart from invalidating the inferences drawn from a regular regression approach that assumes homogeneity of variance, it is also clear that much of the interesting part of the series is not captured through the linear trend. The curved line (i.e., the quadratic trend) also fails to describe the series well. Just as the straight line, the curved line misses much of the variation occurring in the data. Even worse, however, is the increasing trend that the curved line suggests toward the end of the timeline, which is at odds with the overall trend discernible in Figure 17-3.

This example illustrates that, at times, ILD cannot be well described using global functions, such as linear, polynomial, or even exponential functions, and thus cannot be easily modeled through the use of currently available parametric statistical tools. An alternative approach to dealing with such data is the use of locally weighted polynomial regression, or loess.

Loess was originally proposed by Cleveland (1979), and its application was demonstrated by Cleveland, Devlin, and Grosse (1988); Cleveland and Grosse (1991); and Cleveland, Grosse, and Shyu (1992). The name "loess" is based on the German word *Löss*, which is a deposit of fine clay or silt along a river valley. Because the *Löss* describes the surface of a river valley, Cleveland, Grosse, and Shyu (1992) used this word as a short name for locally weighted polynomial regression, a method for estimating a regression surface. Specifically, loess is a nonparametric method that estimates a regression surface without assuming an underlying global function.

The basic idea of loess is that while the data cannot be globally described through one function, it can be locally approximated, as illustrated in Figure 17-4.

To use this basic idea to estimate one locally defined underlying trend, three issues need to be considered: the weighting of the individual data points, the shape of the local functions, and the size of the local neighborhood used to estimate the local functions. Each of these three issues is considered in turn.

Weighting

Like classical regression tools, loess is based on the method of least squares. Specifically, loess uses weighted least squares in the estimation of the local functions. The weighting scheme gives the most weight to data points nearest the point of estimation and the least weight to data points furthest away. The idea is that data points that are close to each other are more likely to be related through a simple relationship than points that are further away.

Shape of Local Functions

The shapes of the functions used to locally describe the data are all of the polynomial family (i.e., no exponential or sigmoidal shapes). The idea is to approximate the data, and this approximation is useful only if it is simpler than the observed data. Hence, the loess method uses predominantly low-order polynomial functions to locally describe the data. Commonly, only first-order (linear) and second-order

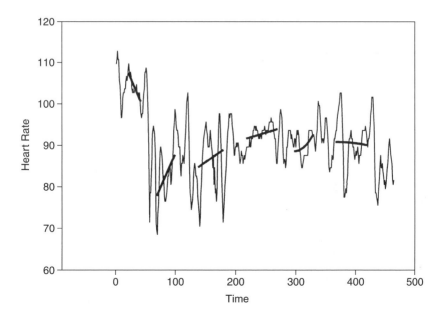

Figure 17-4. Locally fitted functions applied to heart rate data.

(quadratic) polynomial functions are used. Note that a zero-order polynomial function would turn the loess solution into a weighted moving average.

SIZE OF LOCAL NEIGHBORHOODS

The size of the local neighborhood is the number of data points used in each fitting of a localized function. All neighborhoods are of the same size and represent a specified proportion of the overall sample size. This specified proportion is called the "smoothing parameter" (also bandwidth), or q. Determining the appropriate size of the smoothing parameter is of critical importance as q defines how closely the estimated underlying trend follows the observed data. The larger the smoothing parameter, the more data points are used in the estimation of the localized functions. Accordingly, the localized functions become increasingly global as the smoothing parameter increases. Thus, as the smoothness of the estimated trend increases, the accuracy with which this trend describes the observed data decreases. The trade-off between accuracy and smoothness due to an increasingly large smoothing parameter is illustrated in Figures 17-5 through 17-7, which graph loess solutions for the heart rate data using smoothing parameters of 0.01, 0.05, and 0.25, respectively.

The selection of the size of the smoothing parameter may vary from application to application and can be selected based on a number of different approaches ranging from a priori selection to empirical estimation. The empirical estimation procedure is often used as a default in software packages, such as SAS PROC LOESS.

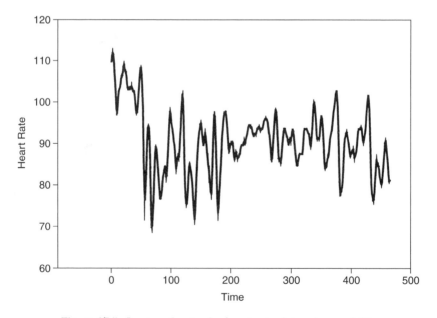

Figure 17-5. Loess estimates for heart rate data using q=0.01.

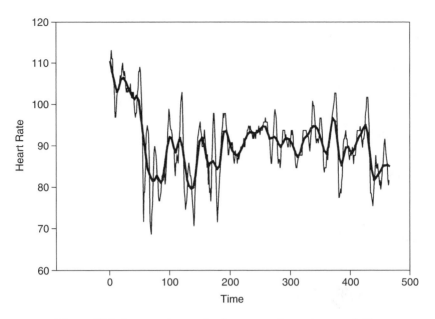

Figure 17-6. Loess estimates for heart rate data using q = 0.05.

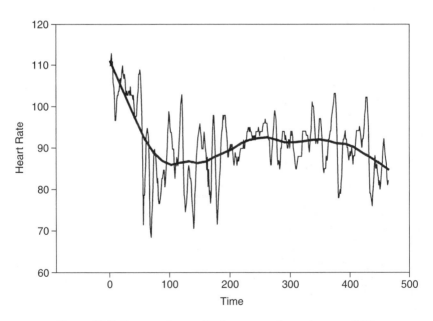

Figure 17-7. Loess estimates for heart rate data using q = 0.05.

After specification of the three factors discussed above, the loess solution for the ILD can be found. This solution provides an empirical estimate of the underlying, deterministic trend of the observed data. It can be used as a visual exploration of the data or to explore the behavior of the variable of interest over time, or it can be used as the dependent variable in further parametric tests. Furthermore, the loess method is not limited to one independent and one dependent variable at a time but can accommodate any number of independent and dependent variables. Some inferential testing tools are also available for the loess method, but their properties relating to temporally linked data are not well understood. More detailed descriptions of local polynomial regression can be found in Fox (2000) and Cohen, Cohen, West, and Aiken (2003), and an advanced application to ILD can be found in Li, Root, and Shiffman (2006).

Survival Analysis

Most researchers are familiar with survival-type models, which focus on the time to censoring for a given event, and there are well-known resources for deploying these models (Allison, 1995; Hosmer & Lemeshow, 1999). These texts cover a range of Cox regression, hazard, and survival models. In most of these models, events are typically assumed to be independent and the standard errors are adjusted for this assumption.

Survival analysis is a particularly useful method when the focus is on time. It also permits an estimation of the time it takes for a discrete or continuous event to occur and can use a diversity of underlying distributions to achieve this. Depending on the nature of the data to be analyzed and the research questions guiding the analysis, survival analysis can be used to characterize the distribution of time-to-event data, test for differences among groups of individuals (one facet of classical heterogeneity), and model the influences that covariates have on duration data using regression procedures (Hosmer & Lemeshow, 1999). Historically used for predicting death in medical and biological sciences, survival analysis is now widely used in the social, economic, and engineering sciences to determine the time it takes for an event to occur (Kalbfleisch & Prentice, 2002; Lawless, 2002; Lee & Wang, 2003).

However, there are several special issues in modeling of recurrent events in ILD. First, as was mentioned in the case of context of multilevel outcomes, event dependence over time needs to be modeled appropriately, in this case for binomial or multinomial response distributions—that is, once an event (dichotomous or polytomous) occurs, the probability of it occurring again may be higher or lower, and with many occasions of measurement the estimation of these probabilities becomes more complicated. Several modeling frameworks have attempted to address aspects of this issue, specifically frailty models (Sastry, 1997; Therneau & Grambsch, 2000), marginal models (Liang & Zeger, 1996), and competing risk models.

Second, there may be spells or episodes in which the events recur more regularly. Survival models may need to account for spells through specific adaptations.

This can be accomplished using multilevel models—for example, through concomitantly modeling spells (or states) and competing risks (Steele, Goldstein & Browne, 2004) or otherwise adjusting for these spells (Box-Steffensmeier & Zorn, 2002). Recently, multilevel versions of survival models have also emerged that facilitate ways to account for interindividual differences in the time to censoring and support the use of covariates to explain these differences (Barber, Murphy, Axinn, & Maples, 2000; Reardon, Brennan, & Buka, 2002). The standard approach to survival modeling may be adaptable to ILD; however, at this time such approaches are only beginning to emerge.

Third, sometimes interest lies not in the time to censoring of events or in predictions or recurrence of particular episodes, but in the intensity of events within a time increment (cf. earlier discussion of time scale). In these cases, when the focus of the analysis is on a series of successive events and the duration of time between them, event history modeling is useful (Lindsey, 1999). Event history modeling is a family of techniques including, but not limited to, the survival analysis approach and point process modeling (Allison, 1984; Blossfeld & Rohwer, 2002; Box-Steffensmeier & Jones, 2004). A brief discussion of point process modeling follows.

Point Process Models

Point process models are frequently used in the physical sciences to model various characteristics of recurrent events (Blossfeld & Rohwer, 2002); however, these models are relatively new to social science. Using a record of all previous times an event has occurred, spatial or temporal point process models (Diggle, 1983) can indicate the potential for and intensity of an event occurring in the near future (Lindsey, 1999). Rather than considering time to events, as is customarily done in survival analysis, temporal point processes can generate an "intensity function" that describes recurrent events as an average number of events per unit time. This complex response function can assist with time-scale selection because it reflects when an event will occur on a specified time scale, an advantage over survival analysis when more than time to censoring is of interest in the response. Advanced point process models can also be used to model time-varying covariates such as time-dependent patterns or periodicities (e.g., daily, weekly, or monthly changes) in a response since they focus on the moment an event occurs. For example, a point process model could account for a reduced rate of alcohol consumption in the late evening relative to the early evening by capturing the diurnal sleep–wake cycle. These models can also be used to model event dependence where one event increases or decreases the likelihood of a subsequent event occurring.

An example application of this technique applied to EMA data on smoking behavior can be reviewed in Rathbun, Shiffman, and Gwaltney (2006). This application is the first in social science and clearly illustrates the advantages of applying point process models to reflect the role that timing and other covariates have on an event's temporal occurrence. Future possibilities for this approach include the ability to estimate multilevel versions that reflect estimation of both discrete and continuous events simultaneously and that account for time-graded heterogeneity on the response.

Conclusions

A range of sophisticated modeling options exist for ILD and many are already in use, particularly multilevel modeling and survival modeling. Efforts to make these approaches more accessible to practitioners are underway and researchers can look forward to a wealth of new modeling strategies to emerge in peer-reviewed literature and edited volumes, including this volume and the Walls and Schafer volume (2006). Moreover, supporting software and manuals are likely to make it possible to deploy some of these approaches much more easily than in the past.

The greatest challenge arising from intensive longitudinal databases is the presence of large amounts of data on multiple dimensions. As discussed previously, the complexity is greatest when the focus is on the occasions dimension. Many methodologists are working to address the relative lack of available methods for drawing inferences based on all three dimensions in a single analysis or through a series of analyses (Moskowitz & Hershberger, 2002; Schwartz & Stone, 1998; Walls & Schafer, 2006). Additional analytical approaches that handle questions that describe and explain time-graded heterogeneity, systemic relations, and stability and change over time are needed. Perhaps statistical methods currently employed in other scientific disciplines such as economics, demography, or engineering can be used (e.g., Ramsay, 2006; von Bertalanffy, 1968).

An exciting possibility is that the availability of new methods for ILD may itself promote new and diverse kinds of scientific questions for inquiry into intensive longitudinal databases. Studies may also be specifically designed to take advantage of some of these models. Given these trends, we can look forward to a period of rapid scientific innovation among methodologists and investigators collecting ILD.

Finally, it may take time before some of these methods will be routinely used in the analysis of ILD. This is because much additional statistical evaluation of the consequences of using each of these methods for the analysis of ILD is still underway. It will also take time for the efforts of substantive researchers and editorial boards to bring examples of applications of these models to their scientific communities. We look forward to the exciting process of methodological innovation and dissemination that this progress will entail.

References

Allison, P. D. (1984). *Event history analysis, regression for longitudinal event data.* Beverly Hills, CA: Sage.

Allison, P. D. (1995). *Survival analysis using the SAS system: A practical guide.* Cary, NC: SAS Institute.

Almeida, D. M. (2005). Resilience and vulnerability to daily stressors assessed via diary methods. *Current Directions in Psychological Science, 14,* 64–68.

Armeli, S., Tennen, H., & Todd, M. (2003). A daily process examination of the stress-response dampening effects of alcohol consumption. *Psychology of Addictive Behaviors, 17*, 266–276.

Baltes, P. B., Reese, H. W., & Nesselroade, J. R. (1988). *Life-span developmental psychology: Introduction to research methods*. Hillsdale, NJ: Erlbaum.

Barber, J., Murphy, S., Axinn, W. G., & Maples, J. (2000). Discrete time multilevel survival analysis. *Sociological Methodology, 30*, 201–235.

Bartholomew, D. J. (1985). Foundations of factor analysis: Some practical implications. *British Journal of Mathematical and Statistical Psychology, 38*, 1–10.

Blossfeld, H. P., & Rohwer, G. (2002). *Techniques of event history modeling: New approaches to causal analysis* (2nd ed.). Mahwah, NJ: Lawrence Erlbaum.

Boker, S. M., & Laurenceau, J. P. (2006). Dynamical systems modeling: An application to the regulation of intimacy and disclosure in marriage. In T. A. Walls & J. L. Schafer (Eds.), *Models for Intensive Longitudinal Data*. (pp. 195–218) New York: Oxford.

Bolger, N., Rafaeli, E., & Davis, A. (2003). Diary methods: Capturing life as it is lived. *The Annual Review of Psychology, 54*, 579–616.

Borrie, A., Jonsson, G. K., & Magnusson, M. S. (2002). Temporal pattern analysis and its applicability in sport: An explanation and exemplar data. *Journal of Sports Sciences, 20*, 845–852.

Box, G. E. P., & Jenkins, G. M. (1976). *Time series analysis, forecasting and control*. San Francisco: Holden-Day.

Box-Steffensmeier, J. M., & Jones, B. S. (2004). *Event History Modeling: A guide for social scientists*. Cambridge: Cambridge University Press.

Box-Steffensmeier, J. M., & Zorn, C. J. W. (2002). Duration models for repeated events. *Journal of Politics, 46*, 1069–94.

Bryk, A. S., & Raudenbush, S. W. (1992). *Hierarchical linear models: Applications and data analysis methods*. Thousand Oaks, CA: Sage Publications, Inc.

Cattell, R. B. (1957). *Personality and motivation structure and measurement*. Yonkers, NY: World Book.

Cattell, R. B. (1982). The Data Box: Its ordering of total resources in terms of possible relational systems. In R. B. Cattell (Ed.), *Handbook of multivariate experimental psychology*. Chicago: Rand McNally.

Chatfield, C. (1996). *The analysis of time series: An introduction* (6th ed.). Boca Raton, FL: CRC Press.

Cleveland, W. S. (1979). Robust locally weighted regression and smoothing scatterplots. *Journal of the American Statistical Association, 74*, 829–836.

Cleveland, W. S., Devlin, S. J., & Grosse, E. (1988). Regression by local fitting. *Journal of Econometrics, 37*, 87–114.

Cleveland, W. S., & Grosse, E. (1991). Computational methods for local regression. *Statistics and Computing, 1*, 47–62.

Cleveland, W. S., Grosse, E., & Shyu, M. J (1992). Local regression models. In J. M. Chambers & T. Hastie (Eds.), *Statistical Models* (pp. 309–376). New York: Chapman and Hall.

Cohen, J., Cohen, P., West, S. G., & Aiken, L. S. (2003). *Applied multiple regression/correlation analysis for the behavioral sciences*. Mahwah, NJ: Erlbaum.

Collins, L. M., & Wugalter, S. E. (1992). Latent class models for stage-sequential dynamic latent variables. *Multivariate Behavioral Research, 27*, 131–157.

Csikszentmihalyi, M., & Larson, R. (1987). Validity and reliability of the experience—sampling method. *Journal of Nervous and Mental Disease, 175*, 509–513.

de Leeuw, J., & Kreft, I. (1986). Random coefficient models of multilevel analysis. *Journal of Educational Statistics, 11*, 57–85.

Diggle, P. J. (1983). *Statistical analysis of spatial point patterns.* New York: Academic Press.

Diggle, P. J. (1998). An approach to the analysis of repeated measurements. *Biometrics, 44,* 959–971.

Elder, G. H., Jr. (1985). *Life course dynamics: Trajectories and transitions* (pp. 1968–1980). Ithaca: Cornell University Press.

Elder, G. H., Jr. (1999). *Children of the Great Depression* (25th Anniversary Edition). Boulder, CO: Westview Press.

Fahrmeier, L., & Tutz, G. (2001). *Multivariate statistical modeling based in generalized linear models* (2nd ed.). New York: Springer.

Fitzmaurice, G. M., Laird, N. M., & Ware, J. H. (2004). *Applied longitudinal analysis.* New York: Wiley.

Fok, C. C., & Ramsay, J. O. (2006). Fitting curves with periodic and nonperiodic trends and their interactions with intensive longitudinal data. In T. A. Walls & J. L. Schafer (Eds.), *Models for intensive longitudinal data* (pp. 109–123). New York: Oxford University Press.

Fox, J. (2000). *Nonparametric regression: Smoothing scatterplots.* Thousand Oaks, CA: Sage.

Goldstein, H. (1986). Efficient statistical modeling of longitudinal data. *Annals of Human Biology, 13,* 129–141.

Goldstein, H. (2003). *Multilevel statistical models* (3rd ed.). New York: Oxford University Press.

Hershberger, S. L., Molenaar, P. C. M., & Corneal, S. E. (1996). A hierarchy of univariate and multivariate structural time series models. In G. A. Marcoulides & R. E. Schumacker (Eds.), *Advanced structural equation modeling: Issues and techniques* (pp. 159–194). Mahwah, NJ: Erlbaum.

Hirschhauser, K., Frigerio, D., Grammer, K., & Magnusson, M. S. (2002). Monthly patterns of testosterone and behavior in prospective fathers. *Hormones and Behavior, 42,* 172–181.

Ho, M., Shumway, R., & Ombao, H. (2006). The state-space approach to modeling dynamic processes. In T. A. Walls & J. L. Schafer (Eds.), *Models for intensive longitudinal data* (pp. 148–175). New York: Oxford University Press.

Höppner, B. B., Goodwin, M. S., & Velicer, W. F. (2003). *Pooled time series analysis: An applied example.* Paper presented at the 1st Annual Graduate Student Pre-conference of the Society for Multivariate Experimental Psychology, Keystone, CO.

Hosmer, D. W., & Lemeshow, S. (1999). *Applied survival analysis: Regression modeling of time to event data.* New York: Wiley.

Hox, J. J. (2002). *Multilevel analysis: Techniques and applications.* Mahwah, NJ: Erlbaum.

Jones, K. (1991). The application of time series methods to moderate-span longitudinal data. In L. M. Collins & J. L. Horn (Eds.), *Best methods for the analysis of change: Recent advances, unanswered questions, future directions* (pp. 75–87). Washington, DC: American Psychological Association.

Kalbfleisch, J. D., & Prentice, R. L. (2002). *The statistical analysis of failure time data* (2nd ed.). New York: Wiley.

Kreft, I. G. G., & de Leeuw, J. (1998). *Introducing multilevel modeling.* Thousand Oaks, CA: Sage.

Laird, N. M., & Ware, H. (1982). Random-effects models for longitudinal data. *Biometrics, 38,* 963–974.

Laurenceau, J.-P., Feldman Barrett, L., & Pietromonaco, P. R. (1998). Intimacy as an interpersonal process: The importance of self-disclosure, partner disclosure, and perceived responsiveness in interpersonal exchanges. *Journal of Personality and Social Psychology, 74,* 1238–1251.

Lawless, J. F. (2002). *Statistical models and methods for lifetime data* (2nd ed.). New York: Wiley.

Lee, E. T., & Wang, J. W. (2003). *Statistical methods for survival data analysis* (3rd ed.). New York: Wiley.

Li, R., Root, T. L., & Shiffman, S. (2006). A local linear estimation procedures for functional multilevel modeling. In T. A. Walls & J. L. Schafer (Eds.), *Models for intensive longitudinal data* (pp. 63–83). New York: Oxford University Press.

Liang, K. Y., & Zeger, S. L. (1996). Longitudinal data analysis using generalized estimating equations. *Biometrika, 73,* 13–22.

Lindsey, J. K. (1999). *Models for repeated measurements* (2nd ed.). New York: Oxford.

Longford. (1993). *Random coefficient models.* New York: Oxford University Press.

Meredith, W., & Horn, J. (2001). The role of factorial invariance in modeling growth and change. In Collins, L. M., & A. Sayer (Eds.), *New methods for the analysis of change* (pp. 204–240). Washington, DC: American Psychological Association.

Meredith, W., & Tisak, J. (1990). Latent curve analysis. *Psychometrika, 55,* 107–122.

Moskowitz, D. D., & Hershberger, S. L. (2002). *Modeling intraindividual variability with repeated measures data: Methods and applications.* Mahwah, NJ: Erlbaum.

Muthén, B. (2001). Latent variable mixture modeling. In G. A. Marcoulides & R. E. Schumacker (Eds.), *New developments and techniques in structural equation modeling* (pp. 1–33). Mahwah, NJ: LEA.

Nagin, D. S. (1999). Analyzing developmental trajectories: A semi-parametric, group-based approach. *Psychological Methods, 4,* 139–157.

Nesselroade, J. R., & Molenaar, P. C. M. (2004). Applying dynamic factor analysis in behavioral and social science research. In D. Kaplan (Ed.), *The Sage handbook of quantitative methodology for the social sciences.* Thousand Oaks, CA: Sage.

Newell, A. (1990). *Unified theories of cognition.* Cambridge, MA: Harvard University Press.

Nusser, S. Intille, S. S., & Maitra, R. (2006). The future of longitudinal measurement and analysis. In T. A. Walls & J. L. Schafer (Eds.), *Models for intensive longitudinal data* (pp. 254–278). New York: Oxford.

Oud, J. H. L. & Jansen, R. A. R. G. (2000). Continuous time state space modeling of panel data by means of SEM. *Psychometrika, 65,* 199–215.

Pena, D., Tiao, G. C., & Tsay, R. S. (Eds.) (2001). *A course in time series analysis.* New York: Wiley.

Ramsay, J. O. (2006). The control of input/output systems. In T. A. Walls & J. L. Schafer (Eds.), *Models for intensive longitudinal data* (pp. 176–194). New York: Oxford.

Rathbun, S. L., Shiffman, S., & Gwaltney, C. J. (2006). Point process models for even history data: Applications in behavioral science. In T. A. Walls & J. L. Schafer (Eds.), *Models for intensive longitudinal data* (pp. 219–253). New York: Oxford University Press.

Raudenbush, S. W., & Bryk, A. S. (2002). *Hierarchical linear models: Applications and data analysis methods.* Thousand Oaks, CA: Sage.

Reardon, S. F., Brennan, R. T., & Buka, S. L. (2002). Estimating multi-level discrete-time hazard models using cross-sectional data: Neighborhood effects on the onset of adolescent cigarette use. *Multivariate Behavioral Research, 37,* 297–330.

Rovine, M. J., & Molenaar, P. C. M. (1998). A LISREL model for the analysis of repeated measures with a patterned covariance matrix. *Structural Equation Modeling, 5,* 318–343.

Rovine, M. R., & Walls, T. A. (2006). A multilevel autoregressive model to describe interindividual differences in the stability of a process. In T. A. Walls & J. L. Schafer (Eds.), *Models for intensive longitudinal data* (pp. 124–147). New York: Oxford.

Sastry, N. (1997). A nested frailty model for survival data, with an application to the study of child survival in Northeast Brazil. *Journal of the American Statistical Association, 92,* 426–435.

Schwartz, J. E., & Stone, A. A. (1998). Strategies for analyzing ecological momentary assessment data. *Health Psychology, 17*(1), 6–16.

Shadish, W. R., Cook, T. D., & Campbell, D. T. (2002). *Experimental and quasi-experimental designs for generalized causal inference.* Boston: Houghton-Mifflin.

Shiffman, S., Gwaltney, C. J., Balabanis, M. H., Liu, K. S., Paty, J. A., Kassel, J. D., Hickcox, M., & Gnys, M. (2002). Immediate antecedents of cigarettes smoking: An analysis from ecological momentary assessment. *Journal of Abnormal Psychology, 111*, 531–545.

Singer, J. D., & Willett, J. (2003). *Applied longitudinal data analysis.* New York: Oxford.

Snijders, T. A. B., & Bosker, R. L. (1999). *Multilevel analysis: An introduction to basic and advanced multilevel modeling.* Thousand Oaks, CA: Sage.

Steele, F., Goldstein, H., & Browne, W. (2004). A general multistate competing risks model for event history data, with an application to a study of contraceptive use dynamics, *Statistical Modelling, 4*(2), 145–159.

Stone, A. A., & Shiffman, S. (1994). Ecological momentary assessment (EMA) in behavioral medicine [Special Issue]. *Annals of Behavioral Medicine, 16*, 199–202.

Therneau, T. M., & Grambsch, P. M. (2000). *Modeling survival data: Extending the Cox model.* New York: Springer.

Thomas, A., & Chess, S. (1977). *Temperament and development.* Oxford, England: Brunner/Mazel.

Timmerman, M. E., & Kiers, H. A. (2003). Four simultaneous component models for the analysis of multivariate time series for more than one subject to model intraindividual and interindividual differences. *Psychometrika, 68*, 105–121.

van Buuren, S. (1997). Fitting ARMA time series by structural equation models. *Psychometrika, 62*, 215–236.

Velicer, W., & Fava, J. L. (2004). Time series analysis. In J. A. Schinka & W. F. Velicer (Eds.) (I. B. Weiner, Editor-in-Chief), *Handbook of psychology: Research methods in psychology* (Vol. 2) (pp. 581–606). New York: Wiley.

Vermunt, J. K., Langeheine, R., & Böckenholt, U. (1999). Latent Markov models with time-constant and time varying covariates. *Journal of Educational and Behavioral Statistics, 24*, 178–205.

von Bertalanffy, L. (1968). *General system theory.* New York: George Brazilier, Inc.

Waldorp, L. (2004). *Statistical model identification in electromagnetic source analysis.* Doctoral Dissertation, University of Amsterdam. Defended April 27, 2004. PrintPartners Ipskamp. ISBN 90-9017817-1.

Walls, T. A. (2003, June). *Defining the developmental window and selecting measurement occasions in middle childhood intervention trials.* Poster session presented at the MacArthur Network Conference on Middle Childhood Development: Building Pathways to Success.

Walls, T. A., & Schafer, J. L. (2006). *Models for intensive longitudinal data.* New York: Oxford.

Walls, T. A., Schwartz, J. E., & Jung, H. (2006). Multilevel models and intensive longitudinal data. In T. A. Walls & J. L. Schafer (Eds.), *Models for intensive longitudinal data* (pp. 3–37). New York: Oxford.

Wilhelm, F. H., Roth, W. T., & Sackner, M. A. (2003). The lifeshirt: An advanced system for ambulatory measurement of respiratory and cardiac function. *Behavior Modification, 27*, 671–691.

18

Thoughts on the Present State of Real-Time Data Capture

Arthur A. Stone

The aim of this book is to present readers with an overview of the theory and technology available to researchers for capturing data from people as they go about their daily lives. Undoubtedly, a conference on real-time data held 10 years from now will include presentations of unimaginably sophisticated monitoring devices and, given advances in the field, will yield recommendations quite different than ones found in this volume. As more researchers from the behavioral sciences and from other scientific disciplines adopt real-time methods for their work, there will be a deepening of all aspects of the field—from data capture techniques through the analyses of the data. The chapter authors have argued persuasively that there are compelling reasons for collecting real-time data, including the importance of the data and the potential knowledge gained from the availability of repeated daily assessments to examine dynamic and complex processes.

In this concluding chapter, I reflect upon some of the themes and issues presented, adding my own perspective to the discussion, and touch upon several issues not previously discussed. I don't mean to suggest that this is a systematic review; rather, it is a more personal and idiosyncratic one based largely upon my own experiences as a researcher conducting momentary studies and digesting the work of other Ecological Momentary Assessment (EMA) researchers. Some of the comments also reflect the discussion periods that followed the formal presentations at the conference on which this book is based, and I thank the audience members for their thoughtful and challenging questions. Let me also establish a convention of using the terms "EMA" and "real-time data capture" interchangeably.

The Utility of Real-Time Data

The chapters in this book show that EMA data are useful for addressing a wide array of questions. A recent paper by Bolger, Davis, and Rafaeli (2003) outlines three typologies of estimates that can be addressed by real-time data. I present two of these categories as a jumping-off point for my comments.

First, EMA studies can generate reliable between-person estimates of a construct over some period of time. For example, if a researcher was interested in weekly pain intensity as an outcome measure in a clinical trial, then the EMA alternative to a single weekly recall at the end of the period would be to take the average of multiple momentary assessments.

An intriguing issue comes up when researchers discuss comparisons of recall measures versus summary measures based on EMA such as the average of all assessments. Some researchers may hold a naïve belief that because the EMA measure is more reliable and valid than a recall measure (I am making the assumption that the average EMA measure is more valid for this argument), it will necessarily perform better than less psychometrically sound measures, for example, as an outcome measure in a clinical trial. The key here is the word "perform," which might be interpreted in the following way: if a recall measure in a clinical trial yielded a treatment effect size of .2, for instance, then a more reliable and valid measure should produce an even larger effect size. Let's first consider the case where the recall measure used in a trial was valid, although not entirely reliable (say, due to some random measurement error). Because the measure was valid, the effect observed in the trial would therefore be valid. In this case, the implication of increasing reliability with real-time data would be to increase the study's statistical power. I believe that most researchers think that this would be a likely outcome of moving to real-time data capture.

In a second scenario, however, the catch is that a modestly valid recall measure could show a greater effect than a more valid diary measure, because the recall measure was biased in ways that accentuate treatment-versus-control-group differences (whereas the EMA measure did not). This could happen when patients know that they received an active medication (e.g., by noticing side effects or because a trial was not blinded) and also held the belief that the treatment should be effective. The expectation would be likely to color participants' reports of their retrospective pain and lead to apparently better improvement when compared to the EMA assessment of pain. This outcome is contrary to what the researchers were expecting when they moved to real-time data capture. In general, when the validity of a measure is improved, the association it has with other measures can change in unpredictable ways—and not simply "improve" the discrimination between groups.

A second class of associations discussed by Bolger and colleagues focuses on within-person estimates of variability and change. Repeated measurements of momentary phenomena present the opportunity to examine fluctuations of the measures in unique ways. Prior to real-time procedures, participants could be asked about their impression of how fluctuating, for example, their pain was over a day or week, but actual measurement of the variability was uncommon.

I think it is evident that, apart from very simple appraisals such as *"Pain was constant throughout the day"* or *"Pain was present during some parts of the day but not during others,"* estimating daily variability is difficult when asked to recall over a substantial period of time. Nevertheless, within-day variability may be an important aspect of experience or physiological function that is often overlooked.

Variability may be associated with basic physiological processes of interest to researchers, it may be correlated with personal or environmental conditions that are modifiable (with potential treatment implications), and it may have predictive ability in its own right (e.g., pain variability predicting later dysfunction).

A specific type of variability is produced by diurnal patterns; variability created by rhythms may have special importance given what they may indicate about underlying physiological processes or about environmental conditions. To use an example from the psychoneuroendocrinology field, there is growing evidence that some individuals have less pronounced (flatter) diurnal patterns of cortisol (a very active hypothalamic-pituitary-adrenal hormone) than others (Stone, Schwartz, Smyth, et al., 2001) and that this variability may be related to survival duration in patients who are severely ill with cancer (Sephton, Sapolsky, Kraemer, & Spiegel, 2000). My guess is that many important insights will emerge from the study of diurnal rhythms with EMA.

Momentary variability is also part and parcel of a state-trait evaluation. When we think of a depressed individual, we probably imagine that their depressed affect is experienced constantly, or when we think of pain in a chronic pain condition, we imagine that pain is fairly constant. Yet, when studied with EMA, we learn that both momentary depressed affect and pain are highly, perhaps surprisingly, variable (Barge-Schaapveld, Nicolson, Berkhof, & deVries, 1999; Williams, Gendreau, Hufford, et al., 2004). More generally, many variables that are considered to be traits may actually have highly fluctuating levels over the course of a day. This is not to say that depressed or chronically ill people do not have higher average levels of depressed affect or pain—they do—but it is also the case that there is substantial moment-to-moment variation about those averages. Thus, many variables may have components of both traits and states, and real-time data collection is well suited to reveal these qualities.

A particularly interesting possibility is that the variability of momentary phenomena may have a special role when it comes to the cognitive heuristics that affect the accuracy of recall. An example of this idea is that the variability of the momentary pain is associated with how pain is recalled. Specifically, we found that more pain is remembered for those individuals with greater variability than those with less variability, even when these individuals' average pain throughout the week was equivalent (Stone, Schwartz, Broderick, & Shiffman, 2005). This leads to the speculation that intervening on particular aspects of real-time experience could strongly influence the recall of the experience. We know that beliefs about the past are predictive of later behavior (Redelmeier, Katz, & Kahneman, 2003), so it is important that we understand how remembrances are constructed, as this could lead to new interventions.

Status of EMA with Regard to Self-Report Bias

Several of this book's authors have made strong cases that real-time data avoid many problems associated with recall assessments, and this is certainly one of the major strengths of the methodology. The point I make here is that we should not be misled into thinking that eliminating recall bias is tantamount to eliminating **all** bias associated with self-report. In fact, Schwarz's chapter (Chapter 2) mentions some of the remaining issues that are associated with self-reports more generally, and I add to his concerns below.

Even if immediate experience is tapped by momentary assessment and recall is avoided (i.e., experiential memory, rather than episodic or semantic memories, is assessed; Robinson & Clore, 2002), how the information is translated into a response has the potential to influence ratings in ways that are unintended and unwanted. One way that can happen depends on a respondent's interpretation of the rating scale. For example, when vaguely worded scale labels are used, such as "not at all," "somewhat," "moderately," and "quite a lot," respondents make tacit assumptions about how to interpret these response options that depend upon their implicit comparison standard (Schwarz, 1999). If a respondent answers a question using a *"compared to how I usually am"* standard, for example, the response may be quite different than if he or she uses a comparison standard of *"compared to all other people."* Just as this issue presents a problem for interpreting retrospective self-report data, with the distinct possibility that different participants employ different standards, it may present problems for momentary data as well.

A similar problem may occur when researchers ask for more information than respondents know or can access from memory. Authors in this volume have argued that biasing occurs when long periods of recall are requested and memories are simply not available for accurately answering the question. However, the same phenomenon may occur during an immediate assessment if the respondent does not have access to the relevant information. When asked to report about their mood at the moment, for example, individuals may not always know how to answer the question. When their mood is particularly distinctive (very sad, very happy, very angry), answering the question may be easy. However, when not in a distinctive mood, how are such ratings made? In such cases, I expect that the same processes that have been identified for operating with global recall will be activated—namely, irrelevant information from the immediate situation or general beliefs the respondent holds may be used to address the question (Menon & Yorkston, 2000).

These are examples of issues that have not been adequately investigated in EMA assessments and that are, frankly, quite vexing. As the field matures, I hope that difficult issues like these will be tackled and resolved.

The Meaning of Momentary Versus Recalled Information

Findings from the well-known colonoscopy studies of Redelmeier and Kahneman (Redelmeier & Kahneman, 1996; Redelmeier, et al., 2003) help to illustrate this point. In these studies, patients reported on their real-time pain levels every minute during the procedure, and these levels were compared with recall of the pain immediately and 1 hour later. Analyses showed that memories of the procedure favored the peaks of pain and the level of pain at the end of the procedure, or what has become known as the peak-end effect. The average of the momentary reports of pain was less well associated with recall.

So, there are at least two different ways of representing the pain experience—the average of the momentary and recall—and it is my observation that scientists have strong opinions about which measure they prefer. Proponents of a real-time point of view believe that the momentary assessments were clearly what patients had experienced and the recall was clearly biased by memory processes. Proponents of a recall point of view believe that no matter how patients processed the information about the procedure, all that matters is the remembrance.

It is probably best to think of the momentary and recall variables simply as different ways of representing the pain of the procedure and that the decision to use one or the other depends upon the reason for wanting the information in the first place. The logic behind this position is demonstrated by example. If one were interested in predicting subsequent behavior that could be influenced by the degree of pain experienced during the procedure—for example, in trying to predict return for regularly scheduled colonoscopies—then the impression left in memory should be most predictive of future behavior. In fact, Redelmeier and colleagues (Redelmeier et al., 2003) demonstrated this in a recent study: repeat colonoscopies were predicted by recalled pain. On the other hand, if a researcher was interested in the effect of pain during a medical procedure on physiological activity, then the pain experience as presented by EMA (e.g., an area-under-the-curve measure) would logically be the most appropriate variable for analysis.

The point is that researchers and clinicians should carefully consider what they are trying to capture in an assessment. I believe that knowledge of the distinction just presented may usefully inform this kind of decision-making.

Respondent Compliance with Study Protocols and Its Effect on Data

EMA protocols are by their nature demanding. Participants in EMA studies are often interrupted during daily activities and are asked to complete brief diaries and/or take physiological readings or samples. As such, researchers have expressed concern about possibly poor compliance with EMA protocols. The issue of reported compliance, which is based on the time and dates participants record in their diaries, versus actual compliance, which is based on electronic verification of diary completion, was covered in Chapter 4. The conclusion of the few studies that have explicitly examined compliance associated with EMA protocols is that standard paper diaries, both with or without auditory reminders, yield relatively high levels of reported compliance and relatively low levels of actual compliance.

I will discuss two issues pertaining to compliance. The first concerns the generalizability of the compliance research mentioned above. The studies in question were conducted with particular sample schemes, patient samples, training materials, diary components, and so forth, and one can ask whether other sampling schemes, patient samples, and so forth, would yield the same compliance levels. Until the new studies have been conducted, any estimation of generalizability is limited to that based on logical analysis. In this regard, scientists have questioned aspects of the design that they believe may have resulted in relatively low levels of compliance for paper diaries. One of these questions is about the fixed-time schedule (the same three times were assessed every day) used in the studies. Perhaps randomly timed assessments and their associated unpredictability would induce better compliance.

Alternatively, perhaps patients who were being treated by their own physicians and felt that the monitoring task would be of benefit to them would be more motivated and have better compliance. And perhaps less demanding end-of-day protocols would yield higher compliance. I agree that these possibilities cannot be ruled out. A recent paper (Green, Rafaeli, Bolger, et al., 2006) and several commentaries on the paper (Bolger, Shrout, Green, et al., 2006; Broderick & Stone, 2006; Takarangi, Garry & Loftus, 2006; Tennen, Affleck, Coyne, et al, 2006) provide the interested reader with a detailed discussion of the complexities of this topic. Nevertheless, at this time I advise researchers to be skeptical about participants' reported compliance in EMA studies. When at all possible, data collection schemes that allow for verification of the compliance (electronic diaries, IVR, Web-based, for instance) should be considered.

The second issue concerning compliance and EMA is the possible effect that poor compliance has on the data. This is a complex issue, and the answer to the question depends upon many factors. It is probably foolhardy to simply assume that data with poor compliance rates are equivalent to those from studies with high levels of verified compliance. I say this because it is unlikely that the times when people do not make scheduled data entries (contributing to noncompliance) are representative of all possible samples. In other words, noncompliance does not occur in a random manner. It is more likely that participants are not compliant when they are particularly busy or stressed, are in highly sensitive situations (e.g., meeting with the boss, intimate relations), or simply do not wished to be disturbed (e.g., at the theater). If the outcome being measured is affected by the circumstances associated with the non-randomness, then the data from those with poor compliance will be different than the data from those with high compliance. Generally speaking, it is likely that many psychological and symptom variables will be associated with the circumstances mentioned above (e.g., more stress when with the boss or more pleasure when at the theater), although other classes of variables may not be affected. Thus, the impact of noncompliance is dependent on the reasons underlying the noncompliance and on the nature of the phenomenon being investigated. The field of real-time data collection needs considerably more information about both of these factors so that researchers can make informed decisions about EMA study designs and the proper interpretation of data.

An extension of the previous argument is that the effect of level of compliance may be related to the degree of variability in the phenomenon being studied. An extreme example makes the point: if an individual had a constant level of a variable being examined, then one randomly chosen momentary assessment would be sufficient for accurate assessment. But if the phenomenon had considerable variability from one measurement to the next (and this includes variability associated with trends in the level of the data over time), then a single assessment would not be adequate to accurately characterize an individual. The point is that the variability of momentary variables is another factor that can moderate the effects of noncompliance. My hunch is that certain of the factors mentioned above regarding generalizability will turn out to be important, yet others will not.

The Design and Reporting of EMA Studies

As the chapters in this book have shown, studies employing EMA have the potential to break new ground and add to our understanding of complex phenomena in the real world. For the field of real-time data capture to advance, the procedures employed in studies and the results must be clearly communicated to readers so they can evaluate the findings and, if they desire, replicate the study. For this reason, Saul Shiffman and I described the basic characteristics of an EMA that should be included in a study's write-up (Stone & Shiffman, 2002), and the paper is included as an appendix to this volume. It lays out basic design features that need to be described, as well as information about how the diaries performed in the study. I strongly recommend that readers who are considering running a diary study read this paper before designing the study. It will help in identifying some of the critical issues that need to be considered in the design and will ensure that the researcher is aware of information that needs to be collected during the execution of the study.

Does Using Real-Time Data Collection Alter the Phenomena Studied?

Most EMA applications require participants to make many diary entries, and this raises the possibility that the repeated assessments may themselves alter the data (known as reactivity). There certainly is a possibility that this happens, and several diary studies have looked for evidence of reactivity (e.g., Cruise, Porter, Broderick, et al., 1996; Stone, Broderick, Schwartz, et al., 2003). As Chapter 4 shows, to date the evidence is surprisingly negative: none of the studies detected signs of reactivity. There is little doubt that more evidence needs to be accumulated before we can be entirely confident about this, but the early indications are reassuring. Nevertheless, it is still difficult to believe that the apparent effects of self-monitoring that have been observed in the behavioral literature are illusory. One question that may be pertinent to this puzzle is, *"Are there differences between simple momentary assessment and self-monitoring in the context of a therapeutic intervention?"* My guess is that there may be something to this idea, and I hope that this is examined one day. Perhaps the cognitive set (namely, *"I am monitoring this behavior so that I can change it"*) induced by self-monitoring in a therapy context does create reactive arrangements, whereas the absence of this viewpoint does not.

Issues in the Analysis of EMA Studies

Studies using real-time data capture are capable of producing massive amounts of data that may prove, at least at times, overwhelming to all but the most capable data managers and statisticians. Imagine an example from the clinical trials world where 200 patients participate in a 12-week study. A six-times-per-day random sampling schedule is employed in the study and each diary entry is composed of 20 items (not unusual, considering the inclusion of context items, potential mediating variables, and the outcome measures). This yields 200 (patients) × 20 (items per diary) × 6 (entries per day) × 84 (number of days), yielding a total of 2,016,000 data points. Considerable planning for this large amount of data is necessary for a successful study, including careful specification of a priori hypotheses to be tested.

There are also many statistical challenges in the analysis of EMA data. Schwartz and Walls (chapters 5 and 17) address current thinking about approaches to EMA data and emerging techniques that may provide new insights into the structure of EMA data. Given the multilevel structure of EMA data, where observations are nested within people who themselves may be nested within groups, it is likely that researchers will have to modify their thinking about analyses, because some of the "old" rules associated with simpler designs may not apply. An optimistic viewpoint concerning this situation is that the structure of the data may highlight new, dynamic associations that have not been previously explored. A pessimistic viewpoint is that the complexity of the data and the analyses may obscure the underlying associations or lead to erroneous conclusions. Again, let me repeat that careful planning of analyses will reduce the possibility of a negative outcome.

Additional Challenges for the Field

As a researcher in the field and a colleague of many of the chapters' authors, I understand and have experienced several challenges conducting EMA studies. Here I mention a few of them. A practical issue concerns the resources necessary to conduct an EMA study, and among the considerations are the costs for the participants, the researchers, and the organizations funding the research. There are numerous details that are associated with real-time data collection, including the technical issues inherent in the complex programming of palmtop computers, the management of complex and large data sets, and the careful monitoring of participant compliance, to name a few. Real-time data capture research is also expensive, not just because the technology is inherently costly (though not prohibitively so), but also because of the intensive use of personnel in these studies. Researchers need to carefully plan and appropriately budget for EMA studies, and the best advice is to discuss this with someone who has experience running these studies. There is a strong tendency for those moving into the EMA field to underestimate these costs.

A second issue concerns the skills needed to analyze EMA data, a subject mentioned earlier. Although there are a number of statistical experts working on multilevel analyses, my concern is that non-statisticians working on EMA data will misapply the techniques. In particular, issues surrounding the autocorrelation structure of repeated observations, the appearance of "local minima" (which can paralyze a statistical program), the appropriate designation of variables as random versus fixed effects, issues surrounding the need to "center" data, and, in general, the difficulty in specifying models that test the appropriate effects are all potential pitfalls. The situation is further compounded by inadequate reporting of the statistical methods employed, making it difficult for readers to know exactly how data were analyzed. Chapters such as those in this volume and other publications will help with this problem, but extensive and comprehensive "how to" documents describing the details of handling EMA data would be very welcome.

Information about many basic properties of EMA data is also not available, so researchers designing real-time data capture studies are, to a degree, operating in the dark. Information about what is required to generate reliable person-level information from momentary variables is just beginning to be examined. More specifically, only sparse information is available to guide researchers' decisions about how many days should be sampled, over what period of time (is it better to sample 6 consecutive days or 3 days in each of 2 different weeks?), and with what density of within-day sampling. Parametric studies of several basic types of phenomena and their associated reliabilities are necessary for intelligently designing EMA studies.

Finally, considerably more information on the validity of momentary assessment of constructs versus recall methods is needed to inform the field. Development of the conceptual basis of studies investigating this question is itself challenging; studies will need to invoke creative approaches to evaluate construct validity. As mentioned earlier, the meaning of momentary versus recalled or global measurements may be very different, yet there has been little empirical work on this important topic. Similarly, we need robust estimates of the degree of bias associated with recall of particular variables. Without this information, researchers will have great difficulty determining whether real-time data capture is necessary for a particular study.

Conclusions

I have reviewed many aspects of the development, definition, and application of EMA in this chapter. There is no doubt for me that EMA and other forms of real-time data capture will continue to enhance our ability to tease apart the complexities of everyday life.

ACKNOWLEDGMENTS

I would like to thank the National Cancer Institute for supporting the conference on which this book is based and for supporting the production of the book. My thoughts about EMA have been developed and enhanced in conversations with many valued colleagues, including Joseph Schwartz, Saul Shiffman, Joan Broderick, Norbert Schwarz, Daniel Kahneman, and Leighann Litcher-Kelly.

References

Barge-Schaapveld, D. Q., Nicolson, N. A., Berkhof, J., & deVries, M. W. (1999). Quality of life in depression: Daily life determinants and variability. *Psychiatry Research, 88*, 173–189.

Broderick, J., & Stone, A. (2006). Paper and Electronic Diaries: Too Early for Conclusions on Compliance Rates and Their Effects—Comment on. *Psychological Methods, 11*(1), 106–111.

Bolger, N., Davis, A., & Rafaeli, E. (2003). Diary methods: Capturing life as it is lived. *Annual Review of Psychology, 54*, 579–616.

Bolger, N., Shrout, P., Green, A., Rafaeli, E., & Reis, H. (2006). Paper or Plastic Revisited: Let's Keep Them Both. *Psychological Methods, 11*(1), 123–125.

Cruise, C. E., Porter, L., Broderick, J. B., Kaell, A. T., & Stone, A. A. (1996). Reactive effects of diary self-assessment in chronic pain patients. *Pain, 67*, 253–258.

Green, A., Rafaeli, E., Bolger, N., Shrout, P., & Reis, H. (2006). Paper or Plastic? Data Equivalence in Paper and Electronic Diaries. *Psychological Methods, 11*(1), 87–105.

Menon, G., & Yorkston, E. A. (2000). The use of memory and contextual cues in the formation of behavioral frequency judgments. In A. A. Stone, J. S. Turkkan, C. A. Bachrach, J. B. Jobe, H. S. Kurtzman, & V. S. Cain (Eds.), *The science of self-report: Implications for research and practice* (pp. 63–79). Mahwah, NJ: Lawrence Erlbaum Associates.

Redelmeier, D. A., & Kahneman, D. (1996). Patients' memories of pain medical treatments: Real-time and retrospective evaluations of two minimally invasive procedures. *Pain, 66*, 3–8.

Redelmeier, D. A., Katz, J., & Kahneman, D. (2003). Memories of colonoscopy: A randomized trial. *Pain, 104*, 187–194.

Robinson, M. D., & Clore, G. L. (2002). Belief and feeling: Evidence for an accessibility model of emotional self-report. *Psychological Bulletin, 128*, 934–960.

Schwarz, N. (1999). Self-reports. How the questions shape the answers. *American Psychologist, 54*, 93–105.

Sephton, S. E., Sapolsky, R. M., Kraemer, H. C., & Spiegel, D. (2000). Diurnal cortisol rhythm as a predictor of breast cancer survival. *Journal of the National Cancer Institute, 92*, 994–1000.

Stone, A. A., Broderick, J. E., Schwartz, J. E., Shiffman, S. S., Litcher-Kelly, L., & Calvanese, P. (2003). Intensive momentary reporting of pain with an electronic diary: Reactivity, compliance, and patient satisfaction. *Pain, 104*, 343–351.

Stone, A. A., Schwartz, J. E., Broderick, J. E., & Shiffman, S. S. (2005). Variability of momentary pain predicts recall of weekly pain: A consequence of the peak (or salience) memory heuristic. *Personality and Social Psychology Bulletin, 31*, 1340–1346.

Stone, A. A., Schwartz, J. E., Smyth, J., Kirschbaum, C., Cohen, S., Hellhammer, D., & Grossman, S. (2001). Individual differences in the diurnal cycle of salivary cortisol: A replication of flattened cycles for some individuals. *Psychoneuroendocrinology, 26*, 295–306.

Stone, A. A., & Shiffman, S. (2002). Capturing momentary, self-report data: A proposal for reporting guidelines. *Annals of Behavioral Medicine, 24*, 236–243.

Takarangi, M., Garry, M., & Loftus, E. (2006). Dear Diary, Is Plastic Better Than Paper? I Can't Remember: Comment on. *Psychological Methods, 11*(1), 119–122.

Tennen, H., Affleck, G., Coyne, J., Larsen, R., & DeLongis, A. (2006). Paper and Plastic in Daily Diary Research: Comment on. *Psychological Methods, 11*(1), 112–118.

Williams, D. A., Gendreau, M., Hufford, M. R., Groner, K., Gracely, R. H., & Clauw, D. J. (2004). Pain assessment in patients with fibromyalgia syndrome: A consideration of methods for clinical trials. *Clinical Journal of Pain, 20*, 348–356.

Appendix

Capturing Momentary, Self-Report Data: A Proposal for Reporting Guidelines

Arthur A. Stone and Saul Shiffman

The following article was published in *Annals of Behavioral Medicine* in 2002.

Abstract

Self-report data are ubiquitous in behavioral and medical research. Retrospective assessment strategies are prone to recall bias and distortion. New techniques for assessing immediate experiences in respondents' natural environments (e.g., Ecological Momentary Assessment [1]; Experience Sampling [2]) are being used by many researchers to reduce reporting bias. This paper discusses seven aspects of momentary research that are often overlooked or minimized in the presentation of momentary research reports, yet which are critical to the success of the research: (1) the rationale for the momentary sampling design; (2) the details of momentary sampling procedures; (3) the data acquisition interface; (4) rates of compliance with the sampling plan; (5) the procedures used to train and monitor participants; (6) data management procedures; and, (7) the data analytic approach. Attention to these areas in both the design and reporting of momentary research studies will not only improve momentary research protocols, but will allow for the successful replication of research findings by other investigators.

Capturing Momentary, Self-Report Data: A Proposal for Reporting Guidelines

Self-reports of one's own behaviors, circumstances, and subjective experiences are commonly used in clinical practice and research (3). Some of the more salient examples of self-reported concepts are: quality of life (QOL) and subjective well-being, both which have been adopted as general endpoints for the evaluation of a wide variety of important societal concerns. Subjective health-related symptoms such as pain, fatigue, malaise, and energy levels are often employed as endpoints in medical research. Reports of behaviors, ranging from food or drug consumption through sexual activities, have been used as both predictors and outcomes in research. While self-report is often used to assess subjective states, self-report methodologies are also used to collect data about objective events that are most easily or conveniently observed by respondents. It may be safely concluded that self-report data play a significant role in activities that are central to clinical practice and research. In this report, we provide a brief overview of the rationale for momentary studies and then review issues in the reporting of momentary data and suggest guidelines for reporting.

A Brief Rationale for Momentary Studies

Much has been written about the challenge of collecting accurate and detailed self-reports of experiences with our most current assessment methodologies—retrospective questionnaire and interview methods. Of the various difficulties, the most vexing is the extensive memory distortion that pervades retrospective self-reports. Cognitive science has shown that the details of past experiences are neither fully encoded into memory nor fully decoded at the time of recall in unbiased ways (4). Autobiographical memory research has shown numerous ways in which recalled information is distorted and transformed by memory and summarization processes (5). In particular, this research suggests that retrieval and interpretation of past experience is heavily influenced by respondents' *current* state: for example, current pain influences recall of past pain (6, 7). More broadly, some experts consider recall more akin to reconstruction than retrieval, and it is thus subject to numerous biases at the time of recall (8). Many research and clinical inquiries require the respondent to not only recall past experience, but also to summarize it (e.g., How many times did that happen? How severe was it, on average?). The cognitive processes involved in summarizing can introduce further biases (e.g., giving undue weight to more salient or more recent experiences). These influences result not only in random error, but also in systematic bias, particularly when the context of recall is influenced by the research design (e.g., when recall occurs in a particular environment such as a research unit). Several articles and books are available that discuss these memory processes and their effects on recalled information (3, 5, 9).

A set of techniques has been developed to acquire self-report information with less distortion than is found in traditional recall methodologies. These new methods reduce distortion due to recall bias by assessing phenomena by means of instantaneous reports of immediate experience. Momentary assessments—that is, asking a person to report about how they feel or what they are doing *at the moment*—minimize recall bias, because the cognitive processes responsible for distortion should be reduced. These methods also circumvent the need for summary processing, since none is being requested of respondents—just a report of their immediate state. In lieu of summaries made by participants, these methods use aggregations of multiple momentary reports to characterize experience over a given period of time. For example, instead of asking patients to recall how much pain they experienced over the last week, as is common in research practice and clinical care, momentary techniques might instead average randomly selected momentary reports of pain taken several times a day for the entire week (see 10, 11). The reports are collected in peoples' natural environments, so as to sample real-world experience and to avoid the bias potentially introduced by artificial reporting contexts. The family of techniques that utilize these strategies is often referred to as the Experience Sampling Method (ESM [2]) or as Ecological Momentary Assessment (EMA [1]). EMA is a more broadly defined construct than ESM. ESM has traditionally focused on random time-sampling of experience, one important way of characterizing experience. EMA also includes other approaches, such as the recording of events. While ESM has traditionally been focused on private subjective experience, EMA also explicitly includes self-reports of one's own behaviors and physiological measures.

EMA methods rely on *sampling* patients' experiences. While it might be preferable to have continuous on-line measures of self-reports and to summarize these, no methodology exists for obtaining such reports without extreme burden and intrusiveness for study participants or patients. The emphasis on sampling is an essential element of EMA. Momentary experience is expected to vary over time being influenced by a number of factors, some that may be relevant to a given study (e.g., medication regimen) and others that may not be (e.g., weather). Thus, the characterization of a person depends on representative sampling of momentary states to estimate the whole, much in the way that representative sampling of subjects is seen as essential for valid inferences from a sample to a population of people.

Momentary data collection methods are increasingly appearing in the literature as a method to capture peoples' experiences in the real world as they go about their everyday activities. The scope of these methods ranges from complex sampling schemes assessing subjects several times a day to daily diaries, completed once a day, that are also intended to avoid or reduce the problems of retrospection. To date, several special issues of scientific journals have been devoted to the topic, and several books, many book chapters, and dozens of articles have used the methodology (for overviews, see 3, 12).

Guidelines for Reporting Momentary Studies

Unlike other well-established methodologies, few standards or guidelines are available to counsel those contemplating using momentary methods and to inform the consumer of momentary research to determine whether or not techniques were properly implemented. In this, as in any other area of methodology, understanding the details of the method is key to interpreting the resulting data; this requires that research reports include the relevant information. Research reports must meet two important criteria that go to the function of publication: first, to allow the reader to interpret the findings in light of the particular research methods, including making comparisons across studies. Second, they must allow the reader, at least in principle, to replicate the study procedures. Meeting these objectives requires detailed reporting of methods and methodological findings. It is our goal to propose a set of criteria that might serve as a starting point for informing users and consumers about momentary data collection methods. In doing so, we discuss many technical and conceptual aspects of conducting momentary research in order to show the importance of considering these topics and ensuring that descriptions of momentary protocols provide a level of detail that enables replication of the protocol. We hope these guidelines enable more effective communication among investigators conducting momentary research and more informed design and evaluation of momentary studies.

While our primary focus is on standards for *reporting* EMA studies, this is inextricably tied up with standards for *performing* EMA studies. In the course of proposing reporting standards, we describe why we believe certain aspects of the design and methods are crucial to the validity and interpretation of EMA research. Taking on this task, we understand that the guidelines presented will undoubtedly reflect our own emphases and concerns about conducting momentary studies. We fully expect readers of this paper to form their own opinions about what is most important in the conduct and reporting of momentary research, and we believe that this will help the field advance. To aid readers of this report, we have summarized the major points discussed in Table 1.

PROVIDE THE RATIONALE FOR THE MOMENTARY SAMPLING DESIGN

One of the first and most basic questions an EMA researcher faces in constructing their study design is the plan for sampling moments. It is essential to begin this task with a well-thought-out set of research questions and then to fashion the sampling scheme to match those questions. An example is presented to show how specific hypotheses inform the development of the sampling scheme. More detail about sampling strategies can be found in Delespaul (13) and Reis (12).

For purposes of discussion, we posit a hypothetical study examining daily level pain in two groups, where one group receives a new treatment for pain reduction and the other group receives placebo treatment. The key to this study hinges upon the idea that "daily level of pain" is the desired outcome measure. An EMA approach aims to assess daily experience by sampling a representative sample of moments throughout the day. The reason for this approach involves two key factors. The first is based on our preferring a momentary approach to reduce recall bias, which means that we will be asking about pain experienced at the moment as opposed to the recall of pain over several hours. Since we expect that pain will vary considerably from moment to moment (due to a host of psychological, biological, and environmental factors), we believe we should sample multiple moments so that our summary measure adequately represents the pain experienced throughout the day. Representatively sampling moments, the second factor, is necessary so that our samples are not entrained to particular situations or conditions that might be systematically related to pain level. For example, daily sampling at noon

Table A-1

Design issue	Reporting guidelines
1. Sampling	a. Rationale for sampling design b. Sampling density and schedule c. Implications for bias and validity
2. Momentary procedures	a. Description of prompting and recording methods b. Description and definition of subject-initiated event entries c. How non-responses are handled d. Whether response-delaying procedures were available e. Definition of an *immediate* and *timely* response
3. Data acquisition interface	a. Description of physical characteristics of diary or palmtop computer b. Mode of item presentation c. Discussion of important algorithm features d. Text of items and response options, and how they were derived or modified
4. Compliance	a. Rationale for compliance decisions b. Presentation of systematic compliance rates (% of required assessment episodes completed) c. Demonstration that compliance was accurately and objectively assessed
5. Participant training and monitoring	a. Description of training procedures b. Use of run-in or training periods c. Procedures to enhance compliance
6. Data management procedures	a. Discuss data management decisions that affect data analyses b. Define missing data criteria and actions
7. Data analysis	a. Rationale for aggregated or disaggregated approach b. Clearly specified model used in analyses c. Note details of procedures, such autocorrelation approach, random effect levels

could bias reports given the high probability that situational factors associated with lunch would influence the reports.

The best way to obtain a representative sampling is to ask participants to record their pain at random moments throughout the day. A stratified random sampling plan, a variant of pure random sampling of times and one of the more common EMA schemes, can work nicely to accomplish this aim. Briefly, a stratified sampling protocol randomly samples moments within blocks of times (e.g., 2-hour blocks) running throughout the day (13). A preprogrammed device such as a palmtop computer can provide an auditory signal alerting the participant to make a recording. This scheme ensures that the entire waking day is covered and that the moments sampled within blocks are random (although some small restrictions could be added to enhance the plan). Again, the rationale underlying these decisions should be clearly presented in the write-up.

There is an important implication of saying that the *entire* day should be sampled to adequately address this question: random sampling should begin from the point an individual awakens and should end upon their going to bed. This design feature was very difficult to implement with the early devices for signaling diary entries, such as pagers and preprogrammed wristwatches, because there was no practical way to make the signals conform to participants' schedules. Even individualizing prompt schedules to participants' typical daily schedules is not adequate, because participants' schedules are prone to natural variation. These variations are not random in nature (e.g., an individual is stressed and awakes earlier than usual or a weekend party lasts into the early morning) and omitting them threatens the validity of the resulting summary measure. Study reports should state what degree of time coverage was afforded by the sampling scheme, the rationale for that coverage, and the implications of any limitations on coverage.

The decision about how many samples or recordings per day are needed should also be guided by the nature of the phenomenon to be recorded. Referring to our example, knowledge about the behavior of pain intensity over the course of the day—for instance, whether or not the pain is constant or episodic, the duration of an episode, etc.—will inform the sampling density. Brief and infrequent episodes indicate that a high density of sampling is probably required, whereas longer episodes can be adequately assessed with a low density. It should also be noted that *very* brief episodes might never be captured by immediate momentary sampling, even when fairly dense sampling frequencies are employed. A variation of momentary reports that allow some retrospection might be necessary to capture such brief experiences.

Similarly, a daily sampling scheme should also be influenced by theoretical considerations. This is especially true when an investigator is interested in associations between two or more *within-subject* factors. In this case, a theoretical position about temporal relations among the variables is critical for specifying the sampling scheme that provides an adequate test of the hypothesized associations. In our example, knowing the time lag from medication administration to pain assessment may be paramount for interpreting the pain data, because pain relief is thought to decrease with increasing time from medication. In some instances, theory may justify a sampling scheme that oversamples certain times, based either on time of day or time since some event (e.g., 14). In any case, investigators should carefully consider how experience is sampled, taking into account the principles of representative sampling, their conception of the underlying phenomena, and the hypotheses being evaluated.

Having considered issues related to sampling, we next consider one of the most commonly used approaches to diary data: daily end-of-day (EOD) diaries. This approach has participants complete a diary at the end of the day, usually about the experiences and feelings of the entire day (e.g., assessing the day's mood, pain, or stressful events). Many researchers, including us, have used EOD study designs and have described the attractive features of EOD sampling designs (15). EOD studies generally do not impose excessive burden on participants and are thus very useful for studying people over long time periods (e.g., many weeks or several months). However, it is notable that EOD approaches do not adopt a sampling approach. The data are collected at end of day as a matter of convenience and rely on recall rather than momentary report. This is problematic when the constructs to be measured are prone to recall bias even within a day. For example, many EOD designs ask participants to rate their mood for the entire day. This may be a problem because we know that mood fluctuates considerably over the course of a day. The EOD mood summaries, which rely on recall and summary processes, may be subject to recency, peak, and summary biases.

On the other hand, if a researcher was interested in salient and relatively discrete occurrences, such as a simple count of migraine headaches or significant arguments with spouses, then EOD recall methods may adequately capture the desired information. Investigators considering EOD methods should also consider that the end of the day is not a representative time-point for many subjective states (e.g., subjects are likely to be tired, at home, not engaged in work, etc.). This adds to the potential for recall bias in EOD reports. In summary, careful thought must always go into the decision about the degree of retrospection that is acceptable taking into consideration whatever is known about the construct in question and about the rationale for selecting the timing of recording. The rationale for the decision should be reported in the introduction to the article.

Careful thought is also needed to decide the number of days to be sampled and the arrangement of those days over time (e.g., consecutive days or separated by some interval over a longer period of time). One consideration in our example is the degree of stability of pain over days (16). Generally, there is no simple answer to the question, How many samples per day should be taken and for how many days? Increasing the number of samples each day clearly provides increased temporal resolution and statistical reliability, but also increases the burden to participants. On the other hand, studying people over longer intervals (more days) may increase generalizability in terms of days, and allow one to observe a greater range of response. Statistical power is also affected by the number of samples per day and the number of days in the protocol. However, how power is affected depends upon the nature of the hypothesis being testing (e.g., between-persons versus within-persons) and the sources of variability in the outcome variables. Interested readers should refer to the work of Raudenbusch and colleagues (17) on this topic. In summary, considerations of sampling design do not lend themselves to formulaic answers, but require careful weighing of theoretical and statistical as well as practical considerations.

SPECIFY THE DETAILS OF SAMPLING PROCEDURES

Once the type of sampling scheme has been determined, there are a number of decisions that must be made concerning the implementation of the scheme. While this may at first glance appear to be a minor detail deserving only passing attention, many of the decisions have important implications for evaluating the validity of the assessment methodology.

SUBJECT DISCRETION IN RESPONDING. A research report should describe any provision that allows subjects to select when they record their data. When subjects can select the timing of recording, bias may inadvertently be introduced (e.g., subjects may remember to make reports of pain when they are feeling especially sharp pain or may find it more convenient to make reports when they are free of pain). If momentary assessments are to be made at particular times of day, the report should provide data about subjects' reported or documented compliance with the prescribed times.

MISSING AND DELAYED DATA. For many reasons, participants will on occasion not respond to the signal to make a momentary recording. The signaling device (pager, watch, palmtop) may fail, or subjects may not perceive the signal, because the signaling device has been left at some distance from them or they may be in an environment where the signal is drowned out by other noises (e.g., a sporting event). There isn't much to be done in this case and resulting data should be recorded as missing. A description of how signaling was implemented may be essential to understanding any biases that may have been introduced by the particulars of the signaling method.

In circumstances when the participant is unable to respond immediately to the prompt, the investigator has alternatives regarding the protocol. One alternative is to instruct the participant to simply ignore the prompt and resume data entry at the next signal. A second option is to allow the participant to complete the assessment some time later, but this raises a question about what the target of the reporting should be: recollection of the experience at the time of the missed signal or the experience at the (delayed) moment of recording? If the former, then we must ask ourselves how much elapsed time from the original signal is acceptable to consider the recollection valid? For example, some researchers are sanguine about recollections that are made within five to ten minutes of the prompt (generally, we are), but would be uncomfortable with delays of 30 minutes or more, fearing systematic bias akin to those associated with longer recall periods. These decisions need to be made thoughtfully and should be clearly presented in research reports. It is desirable to present an analysis contrasting immediate and delayed responses to assess potential bias.

Programs for computerized EMA have been developed that allow participants to delay making an entry if they are unable to respond when signaled.[1] Some programs allow repeated delays that can result in an entry being made many minutes after the original signal. While these entries may be viewed as valid by the investigators, it is incumbent upon investigators to inform the reader regarding definitions of an acceptable response. Importantly, early signaling methods (pagers and wristwatches) did not allow for this flexibility and did not provide information about when a response was actually recorded, a point we return to later.

SUSPENSION OF PROMPTING. Another feature of sophisticated computer EMA solutions is the option to suspend signaling for a period of time when auditory signals would be embarrassing or inconvenient. The duration of this period may range from a few minutes through several hours, although participants may also have the capability to discontinue the suspension if their circumstances change. Applied judiciously, such provisions may help subjects adapt a demanding protocol to their daily lives. If over-used, such provisions can undermine a well-conceived momentary sampling plan, and the frequency and duration of such suspensions of sampling should be reported so that readers can make their own appraisal of the data.

DESCRIBE THE DATA ACQUISITION INTERFACE

Successful EMA applications are based on many factors including user-friendliness, simplicity of design, and thoughtful uses of response interfaces. By the latter, we mean the various ways that participants can indicate their responses on either paper diaries or on the LCD screens of palmtop devices. Of course, the concerns we discuss apply to the design of any questionnaire, but EMA applications present two additional issues. The first is that participants will be assessed frequently, usually many times a day. This means that each sampling occasion must be relatively brief (e.g., 1 to 3 minutes). Otherwise, participants may quickly become annoyed with the task, resulting in poor compliance (assessments either not completed or completed sloppily) and dissatisfaction with the study. Care in the design of questions and response formats can greatly reduce the burden by enabling minimal response time and by making the task more pleasant. To date, this important practical issue has not received much attention in the momentary assessment literature. Research reports should communicate how questions were presented and how responses were gathered.

The second set of concerns is based on the unique formatting demands that EMA diaries have. So that they may be easily carried throughout the day, EMA diaries use very small formats, ranging from pocket-size booklets (for written diaries) to small palmtop computer screens (such as Palm Pilots). This small format means that compared to typical questionnaires, relatively little real estate is available for questions and response keys. Because questions are often presented in a telegraphic format in order to conserve space, care must be taken to ensure that the original meaning of the full question (and responses) are preserved in the momentary application. Additionally, because EMA items are presented multiple times, brevity and clarity are important virtues: subjects simply stop 'seeing' items that are long or verbose. We recommend that investigators consider the optimal display of items for an EMA application, and routinely report the text of their primary EMA questions and any procedures undertaken to 'translate' items from their original versions and to validate the translation.

A corollary of this issue arises from the flexibility that is possible with palmtop computers. Many palmtop applications run real-time algorithms that alter their behavior according to predefined parameters set by the programmer. For example, in one of our own studies, the sampling rate increased when participants indicated that they were experiencing moderate or high levels of psychological stress (18). Other investigators have used similar branching schemes to change the question content presented to participants based upon responses to earlier questions (e.g., skip-out routines). While this plasticity is welcome and empowering to creative research protocols, it creates a level of complexity hitherto unknown to the field.[2] For this reason, we believe it is necessary for investigators to report on the algorithm employed for computer-based EMA applications in the methods section of the resulting paper. Only the essential principles need be reported in order to allow other investigators to replicate the study.

REPORT COMPLIANCE WITH THE SAMPLING PLAN

Success of an EMA study depends upon a high degree of participant compliance with the sampling scheme protocol; the validity of the assessment scheme is threatened by noncompliance. Using the pain example presented above, if participants did not respond to a high proportion of prompts, say 20% or more, the investigator might question the representativeness of the sampling[3] and, thus, the validity and generalizability of the findings. Random noncompliance is certainly more acceptable than systematic noncompliance, but we believe that most noncompliance is systematic rather than random. Using pain as an example, it is easy to imagine ways that pain intensity could systematically influence responding. When in considerable pain, participants might choose to ignore a prompt because it is too overwhelming given their current condition; in doing so, the resulting average level of pain for the period studied would be falsely underestimated (the variability of momentary pain scores would be reduced as well). Alternatively, participants may not complete a signaled assessment when free of pain, mistakenly believing that the researchers are only interested in reports when the patient is in pain. The effect of this response behavior would be to increase overall pain summary scores, because pain-free intervals would be systematically under-represented. Effective training in the momentary protocol, discussed below, may largely eliminate this type of response bias. Our point, though, is that missing data is likely to be systematic and may be a threat to a study's validity.

A related issue involves the possibility that participants are not completing momentary reports according to the protocol, but are completing reports at a later time. An extreme example of this problem occurs when an entire day's reports are hoarded and completed at the end of the day or, even worse, days later. Furthermore, participants may indicate that they have completed the reports according to the protocol schedule when in truth they were completed at another time. This deception may at first glance appear unlikely, but recent studies of patient compliance with medication regimens suggest this occurs frequently (19). For instance, studies using aerosol inhalers that were outfitted with electronics to monitor when a patient used the device have shown quite dramatic instances of hoarding wherein many doses of medication were logged by patients immediately before a scheduled appointment with their physician (20).

Measurement of compliance is difficult when responses are recorded on paper. The investigator knows when the recordings were *to be made* and what date and time *were entered* on the record form, but there is no way of knowing when responses were actually recorded. Some investigators have developed procedures wherein diaries are returned to the investigator on the day following completion, allowing the checking of postmarks. At best, this procedure only ensures that responses have not been delayed longer than 24 hours. However, participants could still complete diaries the day after they should have been completed, while still meeting the study postmark criteria. Other investigators have developed ingenious schemes wherein a programmed wristwatch provides a unique numerical code at the time of the signal and the code is to be recorded on the diary. This procedure probably improves compliance given the message it explicitly imparts to participants about compliance, but participants may defeat the plan by jotting down the codes and entering them later when the entire diary is completed. Of concern is that there have been some informal reports of this happening based on participant debriefing at the close of studies.

We recently completed a study that confirmed our concerns about compliance with paper-and-pencil diaries. Using a specially instrumented paper diary binder that enabled us to covertly monitor the openings and closings of the diary (with a computer embedded in the diary), we were able to document actual timely completion of diaries and compare it to the time and date subjects entered on the written diary cards. Across a three-week reporting period, subjects submitted cards corresponding to 89% of the assessment occasions. However, only 11% of entries were actually compliant (based upon the diary binder being open and having a completed diary card for the corresponding time). Moreover, there were indications of frequent hoarding of diaries across days. This result suggests that poor compliance is a major issue in research using paper diaries.

A solution to accurate recording of compliance is to have a mechanism wherein each diary completion is time- and date-stamped in real time in a manner that is not accessible to participants. This has been implemented in several palmtop EMA solutions and we strongly recommend this approach. Without such procedures, the investigator simply will not know the true degree of compliance. However, if faced with the absolute necessity of having to run a protocol without objective time and date stamping, we recommend that a thorough debriefing of participants be included in the protocol, as some studies have shown that a portion of noncompliant individuals readily admit to their noncompliance and, somewhat surprisingly, to their faking of timely reports (19). It is essential that methods for ascertaining compliance be included in scientific reports, along with the resulting data.

Beyond assessing and recording compliance, investigators should do what they can to achieve high compliance. This often requires a combination of subject training, monitoring and feedback, incentives, and other procedures (21). For example, the study reported above with paper diaries also examined compliance rates with a similar protocol using an electronic diary and compliance-enhancing procedures. The electronic diary system achieved 93% compliance.

We have four recommendations concerning reporting of compliance. First, investigators should always report the missing data rates in some detail. We have seen momentary studies where no mention is made of missing data, implying the improbable situation where the completion rate was 100%. In addition to reporting the average number of missed assessments, the report should also characterize the range. Analyses should consider whether subjects' missing data rates are associated with the time of day. Second, the "rules" an investigator uses for designating a diary or a subject as valid or invalid should be explicitly stated and justified. The number of subjects excluded on these grounds should be reported, and attention paid to the potential for group differences and attendant bias. Again, this will provide consumers of the research with adequate information to replicate the data management scheme employed in a particular study, and to assess the validity of the reported findings. Third, compliance should be assessed against the original subject protocol. Specifically, investigators should report the percentage of study assessments that were missed. The definition of compliance should correspond exactly to the original protocol specification, rather than defining some new (more liberal) standard for compliance (e.g., 22). Fourth, we believe that it is now incumbent upon researchers to demonstrate that their compliance rates are accurate, given the data we presented from the instrumented diary study. It is important to remember that the compliance rate in that study as reported by patients was 90%, but the actual compliance rate indicated by objective measures was only about 11%.

Report on the Procedures Used to Train and Monitor Participants

EMA studies usually place considerable demands on participants. They must be willing to complete repeated assessments in a timely way. In sampling protocols, they must be willing to be signaled throughout their waking days, must carry materials with them at all times, and must be willing to devote considerable time and effort to a project. Therefore, participants in momentary studies require thorough knowledge of what is expected of them and thorough training in the materials they will be using. Effective training increases the likelihood that procedures are followed correctly and improves compliance, especially when participants are viewed as partners in the research endeavor.

Some investigators have opted for extensive training on procedures, including training on the meaning of items and the available alternative responses. The return on investment in training is likely to be favorable, since participants complete the assessment many times. Documentation may also be provided in the assessment itself, whether on paper or on computer. Such training should be documented in the research report.

To date, we have seen only sparse descriptions of training methods in the procedure sections of papers employing momentary methods. Nevertheless, we know that the range of training experiences offered by EMA investigators is broad. Some investigators employ rather casual, individualized training whereas others employ systematic, comprehensive training involving demonstrations of momentary data collection and participant practice with feedback during the training. Some investigators extend training into the field by having participants use the diary for several days and then return for feedback about their data. In some cases, feedback continues periodically throughout the study. We strongly suspect that the thoroughness of the training and feedback given to participants affects compliance and the validity of the data. It is difficult to interpret the missing data rates (if reported) without knowledge of the training methods. Just as importantly, the field will not advance unless investigators are able to replicate each other's findings; this is impossible to do accurately without the provision of training details. Training may be especially important for protocols using palmtop computers since some participants may not be familiar with these devices. In any case, procedures for training and for providing technical support and feedback (if any) to subjects should be reported.

Report on the Data Management Procedures

One of the surprising discoveries that confronts a first-time momentary investigator is the mountain of data these techniques generate. A relatively simple protocol with 50 participants reporting on their pain, affect, and environmental settings (activity, place, etc.) 8 times a day for one week will generate over 50,000 data points (assuming 20 data items per momentary assessment). If the protocol is implemented on a palmtop computer running a sophisticated EMA program, then the number of data points may increase dramatically, because there are many additional records generated each day concerning other transactions and compliance-related data. More complex protocols generate much more data.

The investigator must design a plan for checking the data to ensure that they are valid and describe data-handling methods well enough that other investigators know exactly what was done. Data management procedures are needed in all empirical investigations, but data from EMA studies require many decisions that are not faced by studies that yield less complex data sets. A couple of examples provide the reader with a sense of these decisions. In the pain study described above, let us imagine that a participant went to a party and did not go to sleep until 2 a.m. Should the pain reports that occurred after midnight be included as part of the first or second day? This decision may have important implications for day-of-the-week analyses, for instance. Another example concerns how a partially completed diary should be handled. What proportion of data is required to count a set of entries as missing? There are a host of decisions along these lines that experienced EMA investigators are all too familiar with. In the spirit of full disclosure, we suggest that investigators carefully consider which of their decisions have implications for the analyses and report those in their papers.

The volume of data referred to above must not only be managed, but analyzed. As with all large, complex data sets, an *a priori* plan of attack that sets the course for analyses is incredibly important, lest the researcher become caught up in pursuing incidental analyses. Because analysis of EMA data is not a settled area, descriptions of the precise methods and statistical procedures that were used for analyzing the data and testing hypotheses should be reported. Many standard statistical techniques (e.g., repeated measures ANOVA, ordinary least squares regression, etc.) are usually appropriate methods of analysis if the momentary data have been aggregated to the subject level. Even so, aggregate momentary data presents unusual, though manageable, issues that must be addressed in the report (e.g., whether the number of observations in the aggregate varies across subjects and leads to differential reliability). As we and others have previously discussed (23–26), different methods are needed when the momentary data are not aggregated. Investigators should discuss the rationale for selection of aggregate or disaggregate analysis and report them in enough detail so that other investigators are able to reproduce their analytic methods. Because different modes of analysis are available, care must be taken that the analytic approach matches the hypothesis being pursued. Again, experienced EMA investigators are familiar with the vagaries of these complex analytic procedures, which not only demand technical expertise, but experience with complex statistics and unusual data structures (e.g., such as when a maximum likelihood procedure converges to a local minimum or choosing the particular autocorrelation structure that best fits the observations).

Conclusion

We recognize that there are no hard and fast rules about conducting studies and publishing their results in any area of research. Nevertheless, given the burgeoning interest in EMA approaches to self-reported phenomena and our own experience with these methods, as well as the fact that EMA studies require particularly careful thought in conception, design, implementation, analysis and reporting, we think it reasonable to propose these general guidelines. We also wish to acknowledge that there are issues that we have not discussed that are nonetheless important for this research area. As a starting point, however, we believe it is essential that EMA studies adopt and convey a systematic approach to sampling and assessment, and that papers reporting EMA studies contain standard and detailed accounts of the methods and methodological results. This will allow readers to better interpret EMA findings and, over time, allow the field to assess the suitability of diverse methodological approaches. It is our hope that consideration of the factors discussed here will better enable researchers to make informed decisions about their momentary study designs and will result in more complete and useful published reports about their efforts.

ACKNOWLEDGMENTS

The authors thank Dr. Joseph Schwartz and Dr. Michael Hufford for comments on an early draft of the paper. This article originally appeared in *Annals of Behavioral Medicine,* 2002 (issue 24, p. 236–243). Reprinted with permission.

Notes

1. Some of these programs also allow the participant to specify a reason for the delay in response, which can be useful for interpreting the data.

2. This complexity also increases the probability of errors in programming that may be especially hard to detect in field applications. Extensive pretesting and validation of EMA computer programs is essential.

3. This criterion level of response is arbitrary and an argument could be made that it should be considerably more stringent depending upon the reasons for the missing data.

References

1. Stone A, Neale J, Cox D, Napoli A, Valdimarsdottir H, Kennedy-Moore E. Daily events are associated with a secretory response to an oral antigen in humans. Health Psychology 1994;13:440–6.

2. DeVries M. The Experience of Psychopathology. Cambridge, England: Cambridge University Press, 1992.

3. Stone A, Turkkan J, Jobe J, Bachrach C, Kurtzman H, Cain V. The science of self report. NJ: Erlbaum, 2000.

4. Bradburn N, Rips L, Shevell S. Answering autobiographical questions: The impact of memory and inference on surveys. Science 1987;236:151–67.

5. Gorin AA, Stone AA. Recall biases and cognitive errors in retrospective self-reports: A call for momentary assessments. In: Baum A, Revenson T, Singer J, editors. Handbook of Health Psychology. NJ: Erlbaum, In press. p 405–13.

6. Erskine A, Morley S, Pearce S. Memory for pain: A review. Pain 1990;41:255–65.

7. Salovey P, Sieber W, Jobe J, Willis G. The recall of physical pain. In: Schwarz N, Sudman S, editors. Autobiographical memory and the validity of retrospective reports. New York: Springer-Verlag, 1993. p 89–106.

8. Schwarz N. Self-reports. How the questions shape the answers. American Psychologist 1999;54:93–105.

9. Schwarz N, Sudman S. Autobiographical memory and the validity of retrospective reports. New York: Springer-Verlag, 1994.

10. Salovey P, Smith A, Turk D, Jobe J, Willis G. The accuracy of memory for pain: Not so bad most of the time. American Pain Society Journal 1993;2:181–91.

11. Stone A, Broderick J, Porter L, Kaell A. The experience of rheumatoid arthritis pain and fatigue: Examining momentary reports and correlates over one week. Arthritis Care and Research 1997;10:185–93.

12. Reis H, Gable S. Event-sampling and other methods for studying everyday experience. In: Reis H, Judd C, editors. Handbook of research methods in social and personality psychology. Cambridge: Cambridge University Press, 2000. p 190–223.

13. Delespaul P. Assessing schizophrenia in daily life — The Experience Sampling Method. Maastricht: Maastricht University Press, 1995.

14. Shiffman S. Real-time self-report of momentary states in the natural environment: Computerized Ecological Momentary Assessment. In: Stone A, Turkkan J, Jobe J,

Bachrach C, Kurtzman H, Cain V, editors. The science of self-report: Implications for research and practice. Mahwah, NJ: Lawrence Erlbaum Associates, 2000. p 277–96.

15. Stone A, Valdimarsdottir H, Katkin E, Burns J, Cox D, Neale J, et al. Stressed-induced autonomic reactions are associated with altered mitogen responses. Psychosomatic Medicine 1991;2:211–2.

16. Stone A, Neale J. Development of a methodology for assessing daily experiences. In: Advances in Environmental Psychology: Environment and Health (Volume 4). Hillsdale, New Jersey: Erlbaum, 1982.

17. Raudenbush S. Statistical analysis and optimal design for cluster randomized trials. Psychological Methods 1997;2:173–85.

18. Marco C, Schwartz J, Neale J, Shiffman S, Stone A. Do appraisals of daily problems and how they are coped with moderate mood in everyday life? Journal of Consulting and Clinical Psychology 1999;67:755–64.

19. Litt M, Cooney N, Morse P. Ecological Momentary Assessment (EMA) with treated alcoholics: Methodological problems and potential solutions. Health Psychology 1998;17:48–52.

20. Rand C, Nides M, Cowles M, Wise R, Connett J. Long-term metered-dose inhaler adherence in a clinical trial. American Journal of Respiratory & Critical Care Medicine 1995;152:580–8.

21. Shiffman S, Hufford M, Paty J. Subject Experience Diaries in Clinical Research. Part 1: The Patient Experience Movement. Applied Clinical Trials 2001;10:46–56.

22. Raymond S, Ross R Electronic Subject Diaries in Clinical Trials. Applied Clinical Trials 2000;9:48–58.

23. Affleck G, Tennen H, Keefe F, Lefebvre J, Kashikar-Zuck S, Wright K, et al. Everyday life with osteoarthritis or rheumatoid arthritis: Independent effects of disease and gender on daily pain, mood, and coping. Pain. 1999 Dec;83(3):601–9.

24. Michela J. Within-person correlational design. In: Hendrick C, Clark M, editors. Review of Personality and Social Psychology Series, 1990. p 279–311.

25. Schwartz J, Stone A. Data analysis for EMA studies. Health Psychology 1998;17:6–16.

26. West S, Hepworth J. Statistical issues in the study of temporal data: Daily experiences. Journal of Personality 1991 September;59(3):609–62.

Index